Teratology of the Limbs

Teratology of the Limbs

Fourth Symposium on Prenatal Development
September 1980, Berlin

Edited by H.-J. Merker, H. Nau, D. Neubert
With the assistance of B. Steyn, J. Klein-Friedrich, R. Kreft

Walter de Gruyter · Berlin · New York 1980

Editors:
Professor Dr. H.-J. Merker
Professor Dr. H. Nau
Professor Dr. D. Neubert
Institut für Toxikologie und Embryonal-Pharmakologie,
Freie Universität Berlin, Garystraße 9, D-1000 Berlin 33,
West-Germany

247 Figures (13 in color)

CIP-Kurztitelaufnahme der Deutschen Bibliothek

Teratology of the limbs / 4. Symposium on Prenatal Development,
September 1980, Berlin. Ed. by. H.-J. Merker . . .
With the assistance of B. Steyn . . . –
Berlin, New York: de Gruyter, 1980
ISBN 3-11-008462-7
NE: Merker, Hans-Joachim [Hrsg.]; Symposium on Prenatal
Development (04, 1980, Berlin, West)

Library of Congress Cataloging in Publication Data

Main entry under title:

Symposium on Prenatal Development (4th: 1980: Berlin, Germany)
Teratology of the limbs.
Includes index.
1. Extremities (Anatomy) – Abnormalities – Congresses.
2. Extremities (Anatomy – Abnormalities – Animal models –
Congresses.
3. Teratogenic agents – Congresses.
I. Merker, Hans-Joachim, 1929 – II. Nau, Heinz, 1943 –.
III. Neubert, Diether. iv. Title.
DNLM: 1. Extremities – Abnormalities – Congresses. W3 SY542N
4th 1980 / WE 800 S989 1980t

QM695.E95S95 1980 616'.043 81-4985
ISBN 3-11-008462-7 AACR2

 Printing: Karl Gerike, Berlin. – Binding: Lüderitz & Bauer, Buchgewerbe GmbH, Berlin. – Cover design: Rudolf Hübler, Berlin. – Printed in Germany.

Preface

The 4th Symposium on Prenatal Development - "Teratology of the Limbs" was held in Berlin from September 25 to 27, 1980. It was organized by the Institut für Toxikologie und Embryonal-Pharmakologie, Freie Universität Berlin (Sonderforschungsbereich 29 - Embryonale Entwicklung und Differenzierung).

During the past few years, various groups of the Sfb 29 have concerned themselves with the problems of normal and impaired limb development. A number of the results obtained so far are included in this book. We have not included the extensive in vitro studies as these will be the subject of our next Symposium in 1981.

The Sfb 29 and the Institut für Toxikologie und Embryonal-Pharmakologie are indebted to the Deutsche Forschungsgemeinschaft and the Freie Universität Berlin for their generous financial support. The contributions of Messrs. Helopharm KG, Berlin, Luitpold-Werk, München, Schering AG, Berlin, Dr. Karl Thomae, Biberach an der Riss, and Dr. Ralf Krowke are gratefully acknowledged.

Our special thanks to Mrs. Ingrid Wolff, Mrs. Ulla Schwikowski, Mrs. Ulrike Krüger and Mrs. Erika Klein-Gabski for their excellent art work.

We also wish to thank the Administration Department of the Sfb 29, and especially Mrs. Anita Kath and Mr. Peter Abt for their help in the organization of the symposium.

Introduction

When planning our 4th Symposium on Prenatal Development, several reasons prompted us to select the topic "Teratology of the Limbs".

In addition to deformities of the head region, double monsters and dwarfs, limb defects are considered to be a classical example of malformations. The evaluation of a teratogenic risk in animal experiments focuses on the investigation of changes of the skeleton, including the limb region. For these reasons alone, it is important to create the basis for elucidation of limb abnormalities, the conditions of their induction and developmental mechanisms.

It was our intention to bring together scientists from four fields of research on normal and pathological limb development and teratology i.e.:

1) experimental research of normal development - where great progress has lately been made;

2) teratological investigations: Substances are applied during pregnancy and the resulting malformations investigated at birth. This procedure undoubtedly suffices for practical purposes, such as the administrative registration of drugs but causal and formal genesis, modes of action of a substance etc. are more intricate to disclose.

3) clinical research: Findings are collected, systemized and classified for epidemiological and therapeutic reasons. Surgical methods, prognosis and postoperative treatment are determined.

4) Genetic investigations.

There are certainly wide gaps in the understanding of these various areas, especially normal developmental biology, experimental teratology and human teratology. Closer co-operation, or even the creation of a common language, would yield greater progress. Without this co-operation a number of problems cannot be tackled or solved. This is especially evident when major problems concerning species specificity or drug specificity of teratogenic substances are to be investigated. Normal and impaired limb development may serve as examples for discussions of very important tasks of the future, such as the elucidation of basic mechanisms of the induction of abnormalities.

Approximately 1,000 substances are newly synthesized and introduced every year. However, the field of prenatal toxicology has expanded to such an extent in the last two decades that it is difficult to subject each of these substances to all teratological tests available today. This problem can only be solved by the selection of a limited number of efficient methods. Their establishment and responsible application can only be satisfactory, if basic models and mechanisms are known and may be attributed to certain chemical properties. On the basis of our present knowledge limb development is, in our opinion, well suited to investigate some of these problems.

The intention of our Symposium as well as its Proceedings is to stimulate colleagues working in related fields of research to join in their efforts in tackling the tasks of the future.

Table of Contents

I. BASIC PROBLEMS OF NORMAL LIMB DEVELOPMENT

I. Basic Problems of Normal Limb Development

Developmental Control of Spatial Sequences of Structures

Hans Meinhardt

Max-Planck-Institut für Virusforschung
Spemannstraße 35, D-7400 Tübingen

1. Pattern formation

Important clues about the control of normal development have been derived from abnormal developments occurring either spontaneously or after experimental interference. However, these observations do not allow a direct elucidation of the molecular mechanisms on which normal development is based. One has to make hypotheses and compare their consequences with experimental observations. To be sure that these hypotheses are free of internal contradictions and to allow a more quantitative comparison, it is very helpful to have the hypothesis in a precise mathematical form. We have developed a general theory for pattern formation in developing organisms (GIERER and MEINHARDT, 1972; GIERER, 1977; MEINHARDT, 1978 a; MEINHARDT and GIERER, 1980). Under the assumption that sequences of structures are generated by communication between neighbouring cells, two principally different mechanisms can be envisaged which are both probably realized during development:

(i) The sequence is formed by a mutual induction of structures. In this case, a relatively short-ranging communication is required. We have shown which conditions have to be satisfied so that a sequence of structures emerges which is more stable than just one (very large) element or the alternation of only two elements (MEINHARDT and GIERER, 1980). This mechanism controls correct neighbourhoods of structures and can lead to a self-regulatory intercalary regeneration of missing elements. An example in which this type of sequence formation appears to be realized is the internal organization of insect segments.

(ii) An alternative consists in the generation of positional information and its interpretation (WOLPERT, 1969, 1971), which in its simplest form would involve setting up a graded concentration of a substance - the morphogen - whose local concentration determines the fate of the individual cells.

We have shown that a graded concentration profile can be generated in two ways:

1. by a dynamic process in which an autocatalytic substance, the activator, interacts with its long-ranging antagonist, the inhibitor. A homogeneous distribution of both substances is unstable, since any small local deviation of the homogeneous distribution will, due to the autocatalysis, grow further leading through long-ranging inhibition to stable activator maxima (GIERER and MEINHARDT, 1972). This mechanism allows the generation of a pattern in an initially more or less homogeneous tissue, such as in very early embryonic development. An activator maximum has many properties of a classical organizer, e.g., it can be induced in a rather unspecific way, or removed parts can regenerate. Fig. 1 shows the generation of a graded and of a periodic pattern.

Teratology of the Limbs

2. For the formation of structures within a subfield, such as the leg, it is no longer necessary to generate a pattern in a more or less homogeneous tissue. On the contrary, a pattern can be formed by "cooperation of compartments" (MEINHARDT, 1980). For instance, if two patches of differently determined cells ("compartments") have to collaborate to produce a substance which acts as morphogen, collaboration and therefore production of the morphogen is possible only at the common boundary. If the morphogen spreads out by diffusion and decays everywhere, a ridge-like morphogen concentration is formed, centered over the common boundary (see Fig. 3 d).

If only the cells of one "compartment" can respond, they are exposed to an expotential morphogen distribution. There are several lines of evidence that the antero-posterior determination of the vertebrate limb is controlled by a morphogen gradient (TICKLE, SUMMERBELL and WOLPERT, 1975). SLACK (1977 a, b) demonstrated that a collaboration between a competent and a polarizing region is necessary to generate the antero-posterior positional information in the axolotl.

Interpretation of positional information

Can the local concentration of a substance be measured with sufficient precision so that a selection of one out of, for instance, ten alternative pathways becomes possible? The analysis of the early insect development indicates that the cells do not measure the local concentration at once but that they are shifted step by step under the influence of the morphogen into more posterior determination states (MEINHARDT, 1977). The local morphogen concentration defines how far this stepping-through will go. The experimental observation in the chick limb (TICKLE, SUMMERBELL and WOLPERT, 1975) indicates a completely analogous behavior. The promotion-like change in the cell determination argues against a series of binary decisions (KAUFFMAN, 1975), but indicates a ladder-like sequence of decisions.

A mechanism which is able to select a particular gene out of a set of alternative genes has been proposed (MEINHARDT, 1978 b). A possible realization on the gene level is shown in Fig. 2 a. A set of genes is assumed. Each gene has a feedback on its own via a gene activator gi. This allows that a gene, once activated, remains active. Every gene of the set produces and responds to a common repressor which assures that only one gene can be active within one cell. The morphogen enables a transition: activity passes from one particular gene to the next. The stepping-through comes to a rest if the determination achieved corresponds to the local morphogen concentration. This mechanism enables a precise and unequivocal interpretation of the local morphogen concentration (Fig. 2 b). Each step is essentially irreversible. After the stepping-through has been completed, a removal of a morphogen source is without effect. This could be the reason why the pattern formation in the chicken wing bud proceeds normally even after removal of the organizer for the antero-posterior dimension, the ZPA (FALLON and CROSSBY, 1975).

The proximo-distal axis

In the experiments of TICKLE et al. (1975) and SLACK (1976, 1977 a, b) a duplication of the antero-posterior (A - P) axis is connected with the establishment of a second proximo-distal (PR - DI) axis. Two almost complete limbs have been observed. This indicates that the formation of both axes is intimately coupled. A straightforward extension of the "collaboration of compartments" hypothesis can account for this feature.

Let us assume (Fig. 3) that the primary subdivision of an embryo is made by an antero-posterior gradient formed as shown in Fig. 1 and converted into a stable pattern of gene activities as shown in Fig. 2. Among the areas specified is the competent (C) and the polarizing (P) area (see SLACK, 1976, 1977 a, b). A second dorso-ventral gradient (Fig. 3 c) specifies the bilateral symmetrical areas D and V (Fig. 3 b). As described above, the boundary region can become the source region of a morphogen which then obtains a ridge-like distribution (Fig. 3 d, e). The positional information for the proximo-distal (PR - DI) dimension could be produced by the cooperation of the two coordinate systems (Fig. 3 f). A high distal point would be produced if, and only if, an intersection of both the AP and the DV borders is given.

What is explicable under this assumption? Let us first consider the amphibian leg with its high ability for regeneration.

(i) The condition of CP and DV intersection is of course satisfied during early embryonic development, leading to the formation of the coordinate system for the normal limb development.

(ii) After removal of the tip of the limb bud and closing the wound, a new intersection of the P, C, D and V region is formed, leading to a new high distal point and regeneration.

(iii) An experimentally produced limb consisting of two posterior halves regenerates a symmetrical limb after amputation (SLACK and SAVAGE, 1978). According to the model, two points of intersection are given and therefore two PR - DI axis are formed.

(iv) In contrast, an experimentally produced limb consisting of two anterior halves does not regenerate distally (STOCKUM, 1978), since in such a case no posterior (polarizing) tissue is present and therefore no intersection of both borders is given.

(v) Amputation, 180° rotation and reimplantation or grafting of a limb to the contralateral side generally lead to the outgrowth of one or two supernumerary legs (BRYANT and ITEN, 1976). In such operations new intersections of borderlines are created at the tip-stump connection, leading to new PR - DI axes in that region.

This model has some similarities with the polar coordinate model of FRENCH, BRYANT and BRYANT (1976), but avoids its problems and is easier to interpret in molecular terms. In the model proposed, it is only of importance that the two borderlines intersect, whereas, in the polar coordinate model the presence of all elements of the antero-posterior (or circumferential) structures has no influence.

In the chicken wing bud neither the apical ectodermal ridge (AER) nor the zone of polarizing activity (ZPA), which is responsible for the antero-posterior organization, can be regenerated after removal. However, a similar cooperation of both systems is presumably required, since a new axis is formed only if an additional ZPA is grafted close to the AER (WOLPERT et al., 1975).

The structures of the proximo-distal sequence are formed, one after the other, during outgrowth of the limb bud. This seems to contradict a positional information scheme. If a constant morphogen source is assumed at the tip, newly added cells would be exposed to the same positional information as existing cells and new structures could not be added during outgrowth. SUMMERBELL, LEWIS and WOLPERT (1973), therefore, proposed a very different mechanism, the progress-zone model in which the number of cell divisions are used as a measure for the PR - DI position. We have shown (MEINHARDT and GIERER, 1980) that this problem vanishes if a feedback between the achieved determination and the strength of the morphogen source is assumed. With such a mechanism, the antero-posterior and the proximo-distal determination would be very similar. It also allows a correct regeneration of removed parts and carries with it the danger of an instability that the most distal structure, the digits, can be formed in a premature proximal position, which has been observed in children whose mothers had taken the drug thaladomide during pregnancy.

In summary, pattern formation can be explained by autocatalysis and lateral inhibition. The pattern can be converted into stable differentiated states by a stepwise activation of mutually exclusive genes. In this way ordered sequences of structures in space can be generated. The "cooperation of compartments" allows the formation of positional information for the third, the proximo-distal axis of appendices.

REFERENCES

Bryant, S.V., Iten, L.E., 1976, Supernumerary limbs in amphibians: experimental production in Notophthalmus viridescens and a new interpretation of their formation, Develop. Biol., 50, 212 - 234.

Fallon, J.F., Crossby, G.M., 1975, Normal development of the chick wing following removal of the polarizing zone, J. exp. Zool., 143, 449 - 455.

French, V., Bryant, P.J., Bryant, S.V., 1976, Pattern regulation in epimorphic fields, Science, 193, 969 - 981.

Gierer, A., 1977, Biological features and physical concepts of pattern formation exemplified by hydra, Curr. Top. Develop. Biol., 11, 17 - 59.

Gierer, A., Meinhardt, H., 1972, A theory of biological pattern formation, Kybernetic, 12, 30 - 39.

Kauffman, S., 1975, Control circuits for determination and transdetermination: interpreting positional information in a binary epigenetic code, in: "Cell patterning" (Ciba Found. Symp. 29), pp. 201 - 214, Associated Scientific Publ., Amsterdam.

Meinhardt, H., 1977, A model for pattern formation in insect embryogenesis, J. Cell Sci., 23, 117 - 139.

Meinhardt, H., 1978 a, Models for the ontogenetic development of higher organisms, Rev. Physiol. Biochem. Pharmacol., 80, 48 - 104.

Meinhardt, H., 1978 b, Space-dependent cell determination under the control of a morphogen gradient, J. theor. Biol., 74, 307 - 321.

Meinhardt, H., 1980, Cooperation of compartments for the generation of positional information, Zeitschr. f. Naturforsch., (in press).

Meinhardt, H., Gierer, A., 1980, Generation and regeneration of sequences of structures during morphogenesis, J. theor. Biol., 85, 429 - 450.

Slack, J.M.W., 1976, Determination of polarity in the amphibian limb, Nature, 261, 44 - 46.

Slack, J.M.W., 1977 a, Determination of antero-posterior polarity in the axolotl forelimb by an interaction between limb and flank rudiments, J. Embryol. exp. Morph., 39, 151 - 168.

Slack, J.M.W., 1977 b, Control of antero-posterior pattern in the axolotl forelimb by a smoothly graded signal, J. Embryol. exp. Morph., 39, 169 - 182.

Slack, J.M.W., Savage, S., 1978, Regeneration of reduplicated limbs in contravention of the complete circle rule, Nature, 271, 760 - 761.

Stocum, D.L., 1978, Regeneration of symmetrical hindlimbs in larval salamanders, Science, 200, 790 - 793.

Summerbell, D., Lewis, J.H., Wolpert, L., 1973, Positional information in chick limb morphogenesis, Nature, London, 244, 492 - 496.

Tickle, C., Summerbell, D., Wolpert, L., 1975, Positional signalling and specification of digits in the chick limb morphogenesis, Nature, 254, 199 - 202.

Wolpert, L., 1969, Positional information and the spatial pattern of cellular differentiation, J. theor. Biol., 25, 1 - 47.

Wolpert, L., 1971, Positional information and pattern formation, Curr. Top. develop. Biol., 6, 183 - 224.

Wolpert, L., Lewis, J., Summerbell, D., 1975, Morphogenesis of the vertebrate limb, in: "Cell patterning" (Ciba Found. Symp. 29), pp. 95 - 118, Associated Scientific Publ., Amsterdam.

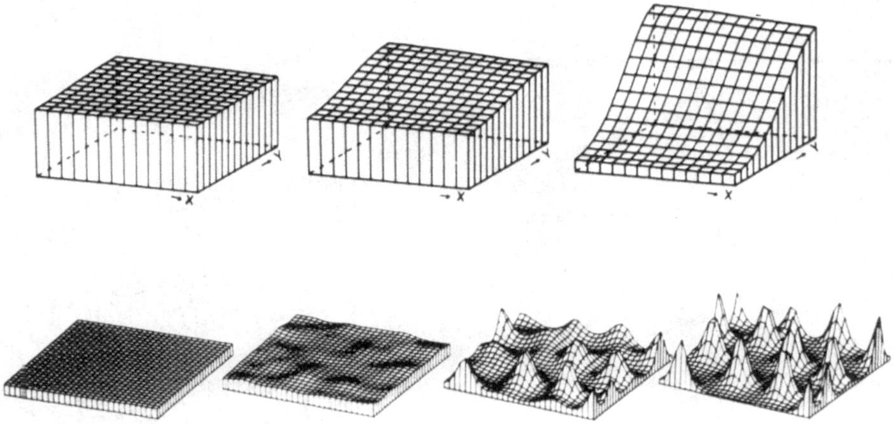

Fig. 1: Generation of a pattern from an initially homogeneous situation by autocatalysis and lateral inhibition (GIERER and MEINHARDT, 1972; MEINHARDT, 1978 a). The activator distribution is shown at different times.
Top row: if the diffusion range of the autocatalytic substance is of the order of the field size, a graded concentration profile e-merges.
Bottom row: if the range is smaller, a quasi-periodic, bristle-like arrangement of isolated maxima appears.

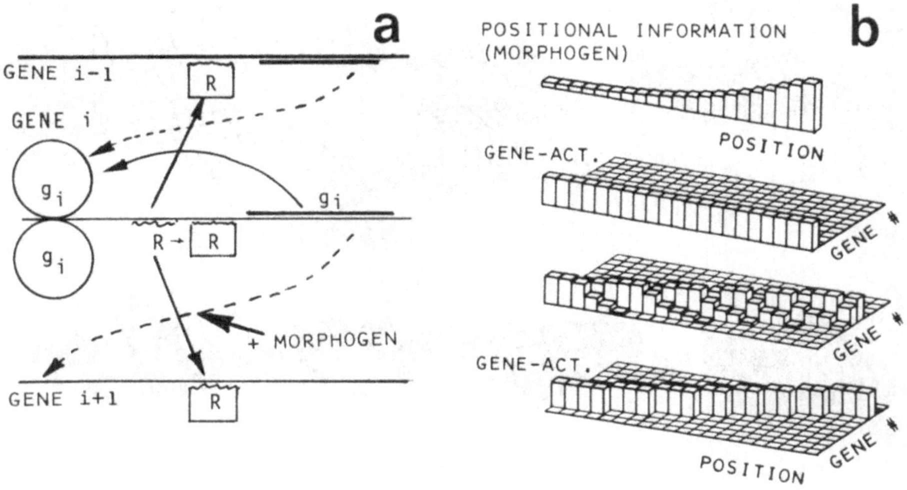

Fig. 2: Interpretation of positional information. The graded distribution of a morphogen can be converted into a stable activation of genes.
(a.) A set of autocatalytic genes which compete with each other via a common repressor. Only one gene of the set can be active within one cell. A transition from one gene to the next is possible under the influence of the morphogen.

(b.) Computer simulation: positional information (morphogen gradient) as well as the initial, intermediate and final state in the activation of a particular gene is shown. The ultimately activated gene corresponds to the local morphogen concentration. The cells respond in a discrete manner, although the positional information is smoothly distributed (MEINHARDT, 1978 b).

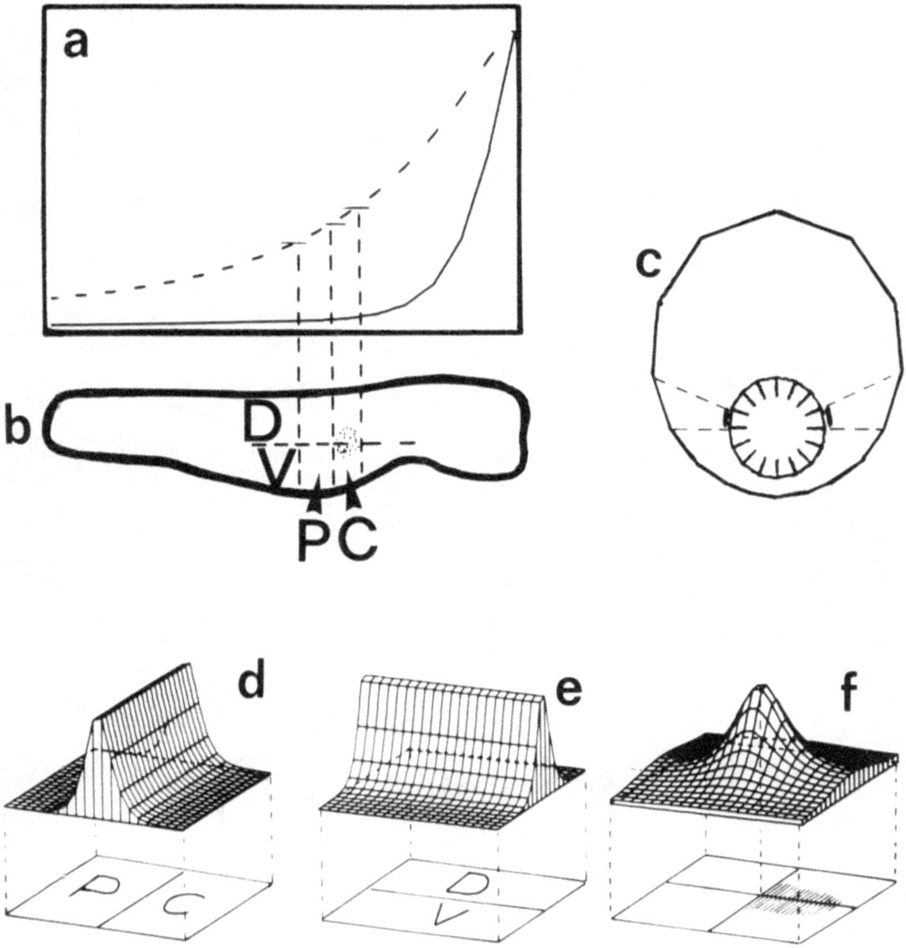

Fig. 3: Formation of positional information for the proximo-distal dimension (for details, see text).

Antero-Posterior Positional Signalling in the Developing Chick Limb

Lawrence S. Honig

Lab. of Developmental Biology, School of Dentistry, University of Southern California, University Park, GER-317, Los Angeles, Cal. 90007, U.S.A.

Pattern formation in primary embryonic fields such as whole embryo body patterns needs not involve growth, is essentially morphallactic, and entails global phenomena (COOKE, 1975). In secondary fields, such as the vertebrate limb, much growth occurs during the time of tissue determination, and two basic classes of communication mechanisms within the framework of positional information have been proposed, which either employ: (a) only local interactions between neighbouring or near-neighbouring cells of fixed positional values, or (b) long-range signalling by organizer regions, such as seems to occur in primary embryonic fields. In this latter process, cells may have their positional values changed. Work reported here pertains to the chick limb antero-posterior axis. In higher vertebrates, a region called the zone of polarizing activity has generally been accepted as being responsible for organization of the limb (MacCABE et al., 1973; TICKLE et.al., 1975). But recently, attention in some other systems has focused on models in which local interactions are responsible for pattern formation (FRENCH et al., 1976) and it has been suggested that in secondary fields the "organizers", such as polarizing regions, may simply be territories having densely clustered positional values, and differ only quantitatively from other parts of the field. Results here suggest that the limb polarizing region has qualitatively different properties from anterior limb tissue, and that the polarizing region appears to be able to signal information over long distances of about 20 - 30 cell diameters in direct contradiction to models based on local interaction.

The Specialness of the Polarizing Region

A central question in limb development is whether or not there is a special organizing region, either at the limb margin or outside the limb field. The polarizing region was originally identified as tissue with unique properties: grafted into different locations it induced the formation of extra limb structures. Tissue grafts from other, more anterior or interior positions, when emplaced as substitute pieces of tissue did not generate any extra limb structures but rather were integrated into normal-looking limbs (MacCABE et al., 1973); this regulation in which tissue with an original anterior presumptive fate was apparently respecified might be effected under the influence of the limb polarizing region, by adjustment to its new environment. However, when extra tissue is added to a host limb (Fig. 1), regulation does not always occur and the definitive limb developing from a bud with extra tissue inserted at its apex may show additional cartilage elements (AMPRINO and CAMOSSO, 1965; ITEN and MURPHY, 1980). These results may be interpreted as evidence for local signalling by grafts which do not consist of polarizing region tissue (ITEN and MURPHY, 1980). Alternatively they may represent self-differentiation, owing to inability to regulate the excess, under the influence of the host polarizing region. In an effort to discriminate between these two possibilities, the remarkable resistance of the quail polarizing region to X-irradiation (SMITH et al., 1978) was used to advantage. Doses of up to 150 Gy (1 Gy = 100 rad) do not appreciably affect quail polarizing activity, although comparatively lower

Teratology of the Limbs

doses eliminate contribution of the cells to the final limb by arresting cell division (SMITH, 1979). For example, percentage polarizing activity (HONIG et al., 1980) following wedge grafts of irradiated (75 Gy) polarizing regions was 67%, with 2.2 extra digits average per limb, (compared with unirradiated wedges: 100% activity, and 2.8 extra digits average). Since much higher doses of radiation are required to abolish signalling than to abolish cell proliferation, quail anterior wedges were irradiated to examine whether they could 'signal' without contributing to supernumerary outgrowths, in the way posterior wedges from the polarizing region can.

Control quail anterior wedge grafts (Fig. 1) were performed with results similar to those of ITEN and MURPHY (1980) using chicks,except that fewer of the operations resulted in extra digit structures (irrespective of whether chick or quail were used). Following 30 quail grafts opposite somites 18/19 or 19/20, a full 87% gave extra limb structures although only 60% gave extra digits such as in Fig. 2 A (overall average: 1.0 extra digit per limb). But among 43 operated limbs which received quail wedges irradiated with 75 Gy (27 cases), 38 Gy (10 cases) or 12 Gy (6 cases), there were no examples in which any extra limb structures were produced (Fig. 1, 2 B), regardless of whether the anterior wedge was placed opposite somites 18/19 (13 cases) or opposite somites 19/20 (20 cases). The irradiated grafts opposite somites 19/20 resulted in normal limbs, but those opposite somites 18/19 frequently (83%) resulted in abnormal limbs having either reduced, missing, or fused host digits rather than possessing any extra structures.

These results show that even slight doses of irradiation which impair cell proliferation (12 Gy), completely abolished extra digit formation by anterior tissue, while much larger doses of 75 Gy were required to have even partial effect on the ability of polarizing region tissue to induce reduplicated digits using the same grafting procedure.

The same general conclusions hold when using chick wings as donors. Control wedge grafts opposite somites 19/20 caused extra cartilage structures in 88% of cases and extra digits in 63% of the operated limbs (overall average: 1.0 extra digit per limb). Wedges irradiated with 19 Gy gave no extra structures while wedges irradiated with 12 Gy yielded in 2 out of 6 cases only small unidentifiable extra cartilage nodules. With chicks, the contrast between results of anterior wedge and polarizing region wedge grafts was less striking since chick polarizing activity by this assay was sizeably reduced (33% activity, 1 digit extra per limb) after doses of 19 Gy. Nonetheless, the dose required to completely eliminate polarizing region graft activity was more than an order of magnitude higher than that required to abolish the ability of anterior tissue wedge graft operations to result in extra limb structures.

The distance over which the polarizing region acts

The action of the polarizing region has frequently been explained by models in which a gradient of diffusible morphogen occurs across the limb (TICKLE et al., 1975; SUMMERBELL, 1979). Such a gradient plausibly could be produced if, for example, the polarizing region was, exclusively a source or sink. The positional value of each cell could than depend on morphogen concentration, solely a function of the distance from the polarizing region. However, direct evidence for a long-range signal in the chick limb has been lacking. The experiments discussed here show such an action.

Double grafts were performed in which leg anterior tissue was interposed as a living 'barrier' between a grafted wing polarizing region and the distal host wing tissue posterior to it (Fig. 3). Leg tissue was used because when grafted in this manner it produces recognizable toes (SAUNDERS et al., 1959); in many cases quail tissue which has a histological marker was also used. Following 66 grafts, 61 contained, as expected, recognizable toes. What was of interest, was that the polarizing region graft was able to influence host wing tissue on the distant side of the leg barrier. In 27 cases reduplicated wing digits were present posterior to toes (Fig. 4 A). In the other 34 cases, mostly containing leg barrier grafts of greater width, only host wing digits were found posterior to the leg tissue 'barrier' (Fig. 4 B).

Control operations in which leg anterior tissue alone was grafted usually yielded the normal complement of digits, and never resulted in limbs with reduplicated wing elements. Hence it was the long-range influence of the grafted polarizing region, not the interaction of host and leg anterior tissue which gave rise to the extra wing digits in the 'barrier' experiment. Also, if proximal anterior tissue from older (st. $\geq$ 22) leg or wing buds was used as a 'barrier', there was never any long-range influence by the polarizing region.

The results show that the polarizing region can influence cells at distances of 150 - 300 µm.

Antero-posterior pattern formation

Results of many grafting experiments in the avian limb are consistent with either local intercalation type models (FRENCH et al., 1976) or long-range signalling models, such as the diffusable morphogen model of TICKLE et al. (1975). The results of a grafting experiment predicted by the two types of models may frequently coincide. Especially if the effective range of a diffusible morphogen is very small and if a local interaction model encompasses a slightly extended notion of neighbourliness, the two models may experimentally be nearly indistinguishable. Nevertheless, mechanistically there is a real discrepancy. Local models assume fixed positional values among cells, which values must still have arisen at some earlier time. Interaction would most likely involve surface-surface recognition. Long-range models need not invoke a strict positional memory, and interaction might be via freely diffusible molecules, molecules transferred between cells, electric potentials, or even cell-to-cell propogated signals in which no actual substance might be interchanged.

Results presented here strongly support the idea of long-range signalling in the chick limb. The polarizing region is a unique region, whose signalling properties do not depend on the manner of grafting (i.e. whether host tissue is removed or not) or cellular contribution of the graft to resulting supernumerary outgrowths. The influence of the polarizing region does not extend to cells in the chick limb that are over 300 µm away, but it does extend to cells over distances of 20 - 30 cell diameters, in contradistinction to models in which only local neighbour-neighbour interactions prevail. The long-range communication by the polarizing region may be by means of a freely diffusing morphogen or might be through some equivalent cell-mediated signal which diminishes with distance.

ACKNOWLEDGEMENT

Work described here was supported by the Anna Fuller Fund (Fellowship No. 487) and the Medical Research Council of Great Britain.

REFERENCES

Amprino, R., Camosso, M.E., 1965, La régulation d'excédents de l'ébauche de membres du poulet, Arch. Anat. Microscop., 54, 781 - 810.

Cooke, J., 1975, The emergence and regulation of spatial organization in early animal development, Ann. Rev. Biophys. Bioeng., 4, 185 - 217.

French, V., Bryant, P.J., Bryant, S.V., 1976, Pattern regulation in epimorphic fields, Science, N.Y., 193, 969 - 981.

Honig, L.S., Smith, J.C., Hornbruch, A., Wolpert, L., 1980, Effects of biochemical inhibitors on positional signalling in the chick limb bud, J. Embryol. exp. Morph., (in press).

Iten, L.E., Murphy, D.J., 1980, Pattern regulation in the embryonic chick limb: supernumerary limb formation with anterior (non-ZPA) limb bud tissue, Develop. Biol., 75, 373 - 385.

MacCabe, A.B., Gasseling, M.T., Saunders, J.W., Jr., 1973, Spatiotemporal distribution of mechanisms that control outgrowth and antero-posterior polarization of the limb bud in the chick embryo, Mech. Age. Dev., 2, 1 - 12.

Saunders, J.W., Jr., Gasseling, M.T., Cairns, J.M., 1959, The differentiation of prospective thigh mesoderm grafted beneath the apical ectodermal ridge of the wing bud in the chick embryo, Develop. Biol., 1, 281 - 301.

Smith, J.C., 1979, Studies of positional signalling along the antero-posterior axis of the developing chick limb, PhD. thesis, University of London.

Smith, J.C., Tickle, C., Wolpert, L., 1978, Attenuation of positional signalling in the chick limb by high doses of X-radiation, Nature, 272, 612 - 613.

Summerbell, D., 1979, The zone of polarizing activity: evidence for a role in normal chick limb morphogenesis, J. Embryol. exp. Morph., 50, 217 - 233.

Tickle, C., Summerbell, D., Wolpert, L., 1975, Positional signalling and specification of digits in chick limb morphogenesis, Nature, 254, 199 - 202.

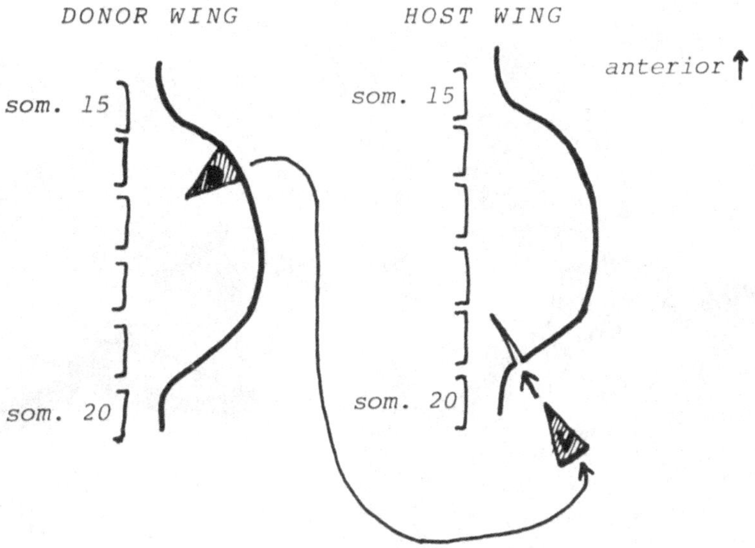

Fig. 1: Diagram showing anterior wedge graft. Chick or quail donor embryos were, when required, irradiated *in ovo* through use of a Vickers-Armstrong Mark IV#^{60}Co irradiation unit (dose rate of 12 Gy/min) and used within 1 hour of irradiation. Wedges of anterior margin tissue opposite somites 16/17 were excised from donor wings and grafted, dorsoventrally reversed, into a slit (AMPRINO and CAMOSSO, 1965; ITEN and MURPHY, 1980) in the posterior margin of a host chick wing opposite somites 18/19 or 19/20. In some cases, a pin made from platinum wire of 25 µm diameter was used to hold in the graft. Donors and hosts were stages 19 - 22. The windowed host embryos were resealed with cellotape and reincubated at 38° for 6 to 8 days.

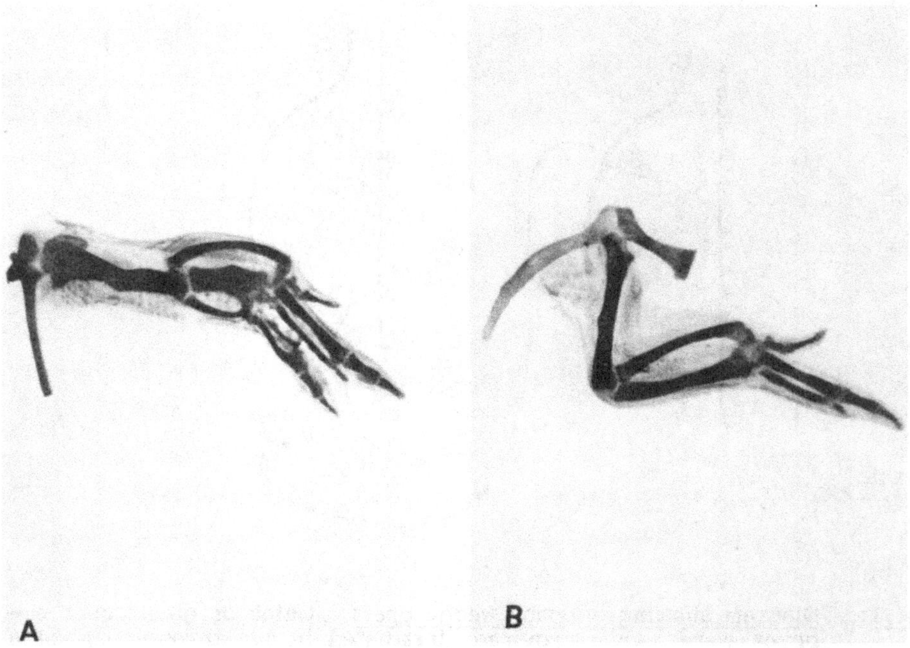

Fig. 2: Chick limbs following grafts of anterior wedge tissue to a slit in the posterior margin. See Fig. 1 for details of operation. Resulting 10-day limbs are shown as whole mounts following fixation, staining with Alcian Green 2GX, dehydration, and clearing with methyl salicylate (SUMMERBELL, 1979). Magnifications are about 6X.

(A) Extra limb structures following anterior wedge graft of unirradiated quail tissue into position opposite host somites 19/20; the digit pattern is 2 3 4 3 4 listed in anterior to posterior order.

(B) Essentially normal limb with digit pattern 2 3 4, resulting from graft of irradiated (12 Gy) quail anterior tissue wedge opposite host somites 19/20.

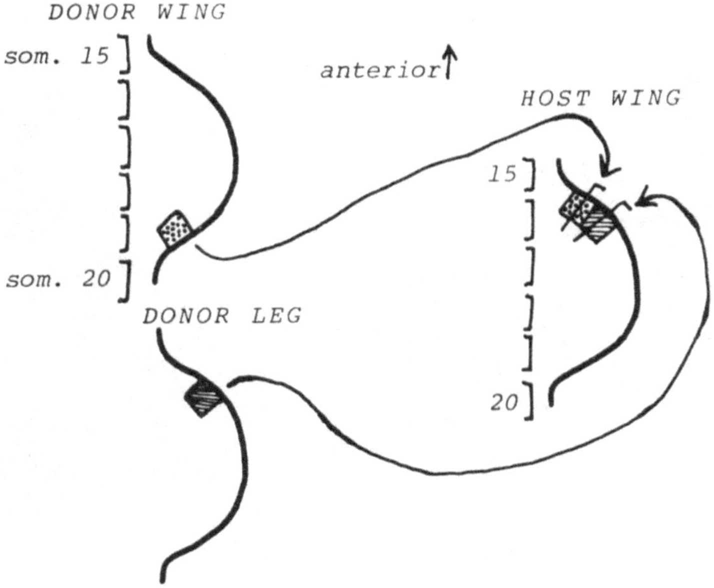

Fig. 3: Diagram of double graft: polarizing region plus leg responding anterior tissue. Wing polarizing region tissue (dotted) and leg anterior tissue (cross-hatched) were grafted into a hole prepared by removing tissue from a host chick wing bud, as shown. Platinum pins were used to hold in the grafts.

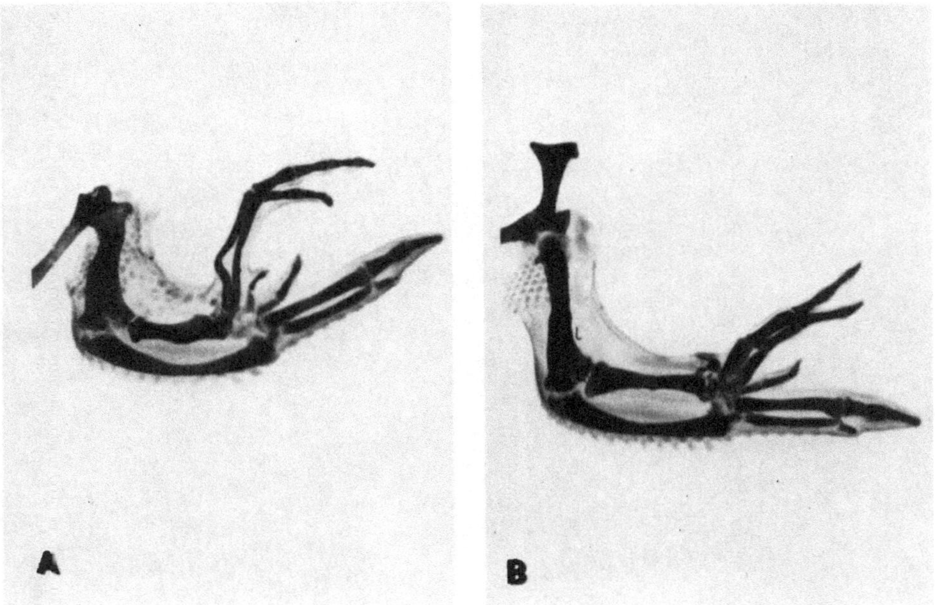

Fig. 4: Chick limbs following double grafts of polarizing region and leg responding tissue 'barrier'. See Fig. 3 for details of operation. Toes are listed as Roman numerals.

(A) Limb in which posterior host tissue was influenced through the leg 'barrier'; the digit pattern is III II 2 2 3 4.

(B) Limb in which host tissue was not affected, with digit pattern III II 2 3 4.

Morphological and Histochemical Aspects of the Subridge Mesoderm in Avian and Mammalian Limb Buds

Jean Milaire

Laboratoire d'Anatomie et d'Embryologie humaines de la Faculté de Médecine, Université Libre de Bruxelles, 97, rue aus Laines, B-1000 Brussels, Belgium

Modern theories about the mechanisms of limb morphogenesis have focused on the undifferentiated "subridge" mesoderm, which, under the influence of the apical ectodermal ridge (a.e.r.) is thought to be maintained in a state of complete lability with respect to its further regional specification. According to different experimental investigations performed in the chick embryo, the ridge's influence would extend over a distance varying from 150 to 300 µm (SUMMERBELL et al., 1973; STARCK and SEARLS, 1973; SUMMERBELL and LEWIS, 1975; CAIRNS, 1975). As a result of active and continuous cell proliferation inside this so-called "progress zone", the deeper cells are gradually pushed to more proximal levels until they escape the ectodermal influence.

Whatever the precise mechanisms may be which trigger the regional specification in the distal mesoderm of growing limb buds, and without underestimating their major importance in further efforts to increase our knowledge of limb morphogenesis, it appears that more detailed information is required on the structural and histochemical properties of the subridge mesoderm. Although in some respects they are still incomplete, the comparative results presented here have been obtained in different descriptive studies performed in the developing limb buds of chick (MILAIRE, 1967; MILAIRE and DUCHESNES, 1979), mouse (MILAIRE, 1965), rat (MILAIRE, 1971) and monkey (unpublished data) embryos. I am greatly indebted to Professor W. SCOTT (Cincinatti) who kindly provided the *Macacus rhesus* material.

1. Tissular organization and cell morphology:

As soon as the limb bud starts its lengthwise outgrowth, two areas of different cell densities can be distinguished in its mesodermal field: a central core of loose mesoderm and a thick subectodermal layer of dense mesoderm which, according to the limb bud shape, can be divided into ventral and dorsal layers joining together into a thick marginal layer. At early stages when the a.e.r. still extends along the entire cephalo-caudal margin of the bud, the subridge mesoderm and the marginal mesoderm are indistinguishable. At later stages, when the growing limb bud acquires pre- and postaxial edges and the a.e.r. is gradually shifted in a distal direction, the structural organization of the marginal mesoderm is maintained in the only subridge area. A loosening occurs simultaneously in the mesoderm of the pre- and postaxial marginal zones which, in the chick embryo, become the seat of selective necrotic changes described as the ANZ (wing and leg buds) and the PNZ (wing buds). They are probably related to the local regression of the corresponding proximal portion of the a.e.r.; however, no such necrotic areas have ever been observed at corresponding stages in mammalian limb buds.

The same histological and cytological features characterize the subridge mesoderm during the whole morphogenetic period, i.e. until the presumptive mesoderm of all limb segments has been laid down according to a continuous proximo-distal progression. They may be summarized as follows:

Teratology of the Limbs

Histologically, the most striking feature is the genesis of a cephalocaudal venous network in the deeper cell layers of the subridge mesoderm. In most mammalian embryos this network develops into a large marginal venous sinus. Initially, this vessel is only a limited part of a large vascular network which, at more proximal levels, lies parallel to the ectoderm between the outer premuscular mesoderm and the central core of preskeletal mesoderm (SEICHERT and RYCHTER, 1978; CAPLAN and KOUTROUPAS, 1973). Later on, the terminal branches of the central artery open into the marginal vein which then functions as the main venous channel of the limb bud. For unknown, though most probably important morphogenetic reasons, the marginal vein exhibits close chronological and topographical relationships with the a.e.r.: not only are its genesis and later involution strictly simultaneous with those of the ectodermal thickening, but during the whole morphogenetic period the vessel runs parallel to the ridge, remaining at a constant distance of it, which in the chick embryo does not exceed 150 µm. This results from a continuous rebuilding of the vessel by numerous vascular buds (SEICHERT and RYCHTER, 1978). In rat and mouse embryos, the venous sinus lies closer to the ectoderm than in the chick embryo. This is especially true of the preaxial half. As shown by the histochemical demonstration of a non-specific ATP-phosphohydrolase, which in most species selectively characterizes the endothelium of embryonic vessels, the mesoderm lying distal to the marginal vein is completely free of any blood vessel.

In most species, the subridge mesoderm itself consists of a thick homogeneous layer of densely packed and actively proliferating undifferentiated cells. In chick limb buds, however, a transitory change in cell density occurs in the subridge mesoderm during the period extending from stage 20 to stage 26 (Fig. 1). As soon as the marginal venous network begins to assemble in the deeper cell layers, a decrease in cell density takes place in the more distal cell layers which lie under the apical ectoderm. As it concerns a larger subectodermal area pre- than postaxially, the proximodistal thickness of the loose outer mesoderm increases in a caudo-cephalic direction. At stage 26, a late increase in cell density occurs in the distal layer of subridge mesoderm which from that time on recovers a uniform distribution up to the end of the morphogenetic period. Mitotic indices measured inside the subridge area of stage 22 hind limb buds did not reveal any significant difference in proliferative activity, neither between the dense and loose cell layers, nor between their pre- and postaxial constituents, respectively. Until a better explanation can be found, I suggest that the transitory heterogeneity taking place in the subridge mesoderm of chick limb buds might be a consequence of a sudden acceleration of the ectodermal growth occurring in relation with the genesis of the limb bud footplate. According to the maps of presumptive limb segments established by STARK and SEARLS (1973), the material laid down during the corresponding period is that of the proximal part of the autopod, that is the basipod and the proximal metapod. The phenomenon would thus have no particular morphogenetic significance as far as the behaviour and specific properties of the subridge mesoderm are concerned. In mammalian limb buds, however, in which an increase in the rate of growth similarly characterizes the genesis of the autopod rudiment, no particular change occurs in the pattern of cell density of the subridge mesoderm.

Generally assembled in clusters of 5 to 10 units, the mesodermal cells of the subridge area display ultrastructural features similar to those of other undifferentiated cells of the mesodermal field (JURAND, 1965). Bordered by numerous outer projections making contact with neighbouring cells or with the subectodermal basement membrane, or lying free in the exocellular spaces, the cytoplasm has a rather limited volume with respect to that of the nucleus. It contains numerous free polyribosomes, elongated mitochondria, a limited number of rough-surfaced endoplasmic reticulum profiles, and usually one small group of Golgi membranes of various size and shape. Interphase nuclei generally contain two or more large nucleoli.

2. Histochemical properties:

Like all actively proliferating cell populations, the subridge mesoderm exhibits large amounts of cytoplasmic and nucleolar RNA, which accounts for its affinity for pyronine and other basic dyes. No selective histochemical property was found in this particular area of mouse and mole limb buds. Selective glycogen deposits were demonstrated in limited pre- and postaxial areas of rat limb buds; this is most probably an early metabolic change related to degenerative phenomena occurring at later stages in the corresponding areas. Together with a differential pattern of mesodermal growth, they contribute to the relative involution of digit I and V (MILAIRE, 1976).

In both fore- and hind limb buds of chick and monkey embryos, the outer subridge mesoderm located between the marginal vein and the a.e.r. exhibits a similar pattern of dephosphorylating activity towards monophosphate mononucleotides, among which AMP was the most frequently used as substrate (Fig. 2 a, d, e). The reaction is distinctly stronger in the postaxial half of the area, whence it spreads over the whole marginal mesoderm up to its junction with the body wall; it is particularly strong in the postaxial one third of the subridge area, but suddenly decreases preaxially according to an obvious caudo-cephalic gradient. As development proceeds, the reaction gradually disappears in the marginal area of the postaxial border, being thus selectively maintained in the subridge area, where it exhibits the same gradient of intensity. It suddenly decreases at stage 24 in the limb buds of chick embryos, but remains present longer in monkey embryos, where it still characterizes the apical mesoderm of the postaxial digital outgrowths in the limb buds of 36-day embryos (Fig. 2 f). In chick limb buds, the same mesodermal areas containing AMP-phosphohydrolase activity also exhibit a non-specific ATP-phosphohydrolase reaction, with the same pattern of intensity (Fig. 2 b, c). This latter reaction, however, is still very strong at stage 26 in the older limb buds examined. At early stages which have not yet been investigated in monkey embryos, both reactions characterize the whole mesodermal field of chick limb buds. The ATP-phosphohydrolase is present in the entire lateral mesoderm as soon as gastrulation stages; the AMP-phosphohydrolase, on the other hand, selectively appears in the limb bud mesoderm as it starts outgrowing at late stage 17. The histochemical reactions in question here were performed in non-deparaffinized sections of cold-ethanol fixed limb buds. A methodological comparative study of the same reactions performed in paraffin and cryostat sections of chick limb buds at stages 17 to 20 (GOFF and MILAIRE, 1974) has shown that they effectively reveal the products of two different and relatively unspecific enzymes. The pattern of enzymatic reactions is the same in both technical conditions. At the ultrastructural level, the sites of activity of the AMP-phosphohydrolase have been recently investigated in longitudinal sections of glutaraldehyde fixed chick limb buds at stage 22. For still unknown reasons, no difference was found in the pattern or in the intensity of the mesodermal reactions demonstrated in the subridge area and in other territories of the mesodermal field. Two sites of activity are present in each mesodermal cell, one in the nucleus and the other in the cytoplasm. A fine granular reaction is found uniformly scattered in the nucleoplasm; it is more concentrated along the inner nuclear membrane and becomes very densely packed in the nucleoli of resting cells (Fig. 3 a, c) as well as in the chromatin masses of dividing cells (Fig. 3 d).

The cytoplasmic reaction is represented by groups of multiple heavy deposits of variable sizes and shapes; one single group is usually present in each cell (Fig. 3 b, c). Unfortunately, the poor preservation of cytoplasmic infrastructure in incubated tissues did not permit more precise correlations between the reaction sites and their ultrastructural support. According to the shape of the lead phosphate deposits, they might be associated either with endoplasmic reticulum profiles, or with Golgi membranes, or both. Until more information can be obtained on the biochemical and morphogenetic significance of the dephosphorylating activities demonstrated in the subridge mesoderm of chick and monkey limb buds, the two following hypotheses of equal probability may be suggested. According to their caudo-cephalic gradient of activity, the enzymatic reactions might first be a metabolic expression of the polarizing properties which were shown to be exerted in vivo by the postaxial marginal mesoderm (SUMMERBELL, 1979; MacCABE and PARKER, 1979; MacCABE et al., 1979); for similar reasons they might, however, be related with the a.e.r. maintenance factor which shares some unsettled similarities with the polarizing influence (SUMMERBELL, 1974). According to the second hypothesis, the enzymatic reactions might somehow reflect the state of lability into which this material is supposed to be maintained under the influence of the a.e.r. If this is true, the effective thickness of the progress zone would obviously be established around 150 µm, as it was concluded by CAIRNS (1975) on the basis of experimental results. In spite of the fact that the observed enzymatic reactions were found ineffective towards cyclic AMP, they suggest, however, a correlation with recent results obtained by KOSHER et al. (1979), who found that cyclic AMP derivatives can stimulate chondrogenic differentiation of the subridge mesoderm in the chick embryo.

REFERENCES

Cairns, J.M., 1975, The function of the ectodermal apical ridge and distinctive characteristics of adjacent distal mesoderm in the avian wing bud, J. Embryol. exp. Morph., 34, 155 - 169.

Caplan, A.I., Koutroupas, S., 1973, The control of muscle and cartilage development in the chick limb: the role of differential vascularization, J. Embryol. exp. Morph., 29, 571 - 583.

Goff, R.A., Milaire, J., 1974, A comparative analysis of the histochemical dephosphorylation of ATP and AMP in cryostat and paraffin sections of early chick embryos, Acta histochem., 51, 220 - 254.

Jurand, A., 1965, Ultrastructural aspects of early development of the forelimb buds in the chick and the mouse, Proc. Roy. Soc. B, 162, 387 - 405.

Kosher, R.A., Savage, M.P., Chan, S.C., 1979, Cyclic AMP derivatives stimulate the chondrogenic differentiation of the mesoderm subjacent to the apical ectodermal ridge of the chick limb bud, J. exp. Zool., 209, 221 - 228.

MacCabe, J.A., Parker, B.W., 1979, The target tissue of limb bud polarizing activity in the induction of supernumerary structures, J. Embryol. exp. Morph., 53, 67 - 73.

MacCabe, J.A., Lyle, P.S., Lence, J.A., 1979, The control of polarity along the anteroposterior axis in experimental chick limbs, J. exp. Zool., 207, 113 - 120.

Milaire, J., 1965, Etude morphogénétique de trois malformations congénitales de l'autopode chez la souris (syndactylisme-brachypodisme-hémimélie dominante) par des méthodes cytochimiques, Mémoires in 4° de l'Acad. roy. Belg., classe des Sciences, 16, 1 - 120.

Milaire, J., 1967, Etude histochimique des premiers stades de la genèse des membres chez le poulet (stades 13 à 19), Arch. Biol., (Liège), 78, 289 - 346.

Milaire, J., 1971, Etude morphogénétique de la syndactylie postaxiale provoquie chez le rat par l'hadacidine. II. Les bourgeons de membres chez les embryons de 12 à 14 jours, Arch. Biol., (Liège), 82, 253 - 322.

Milaire, J., 1976, Rudimentation digitale au cours du développement normal de l'autopode chez les Mammifères, Coll. intern du C.N.R.S., Mécanismes de la rudimentation des organes chez les embryons de Vertébrés, 266, 221 - 233.

Milaire, J., Duchesnes, Ch., 1979, Etude de quelques propriétés structurales et histochimiques du mésoblaste marginal des bourgeons de membres de l'embryon de poulet (stades 20 à 26), Arch. anat. microscop., 68, 169 - 193.

Seichert, V., Rychter, Z., 1978, Development of the vascularization of the anterior limb in chick embryo, XIXth Morph. Congress Symp.,Charles Univ. Prague, (E. Klika, ed.), pp. 59 - 63.

Stark, R.J., Searls, R.L., 1973, A description of chick wing bud development and a model of limb morphogenesis, Develop. Biol., 33, 138 - 153.

Summerbell, D., 1974, Interaction between the proximo-distal and antero-posterior co-ordinates of positional value during the specification of positional information in the early development of the chick limb bud, J. Embryol. exp. Morph., 32, 227 - 237.

Summerbell, D., 1979, The zone of polarizing activity: evidence for a role in normal chick limb morphogenesis, J. Embryol. exp. Morph., 50, 217 - 233.

Summerbell, D., Lewis, J.H., Wolpert, L., 1973, Positional information in chick limb morphogenesis, Nature, (Lond.), 244, 492 - 496.

Summerbell, D., Lewis, J.H., 1975, Time, place and positional value in the chick limb bud, J. Embryol. exp. Morph., 33, 621 - 643.

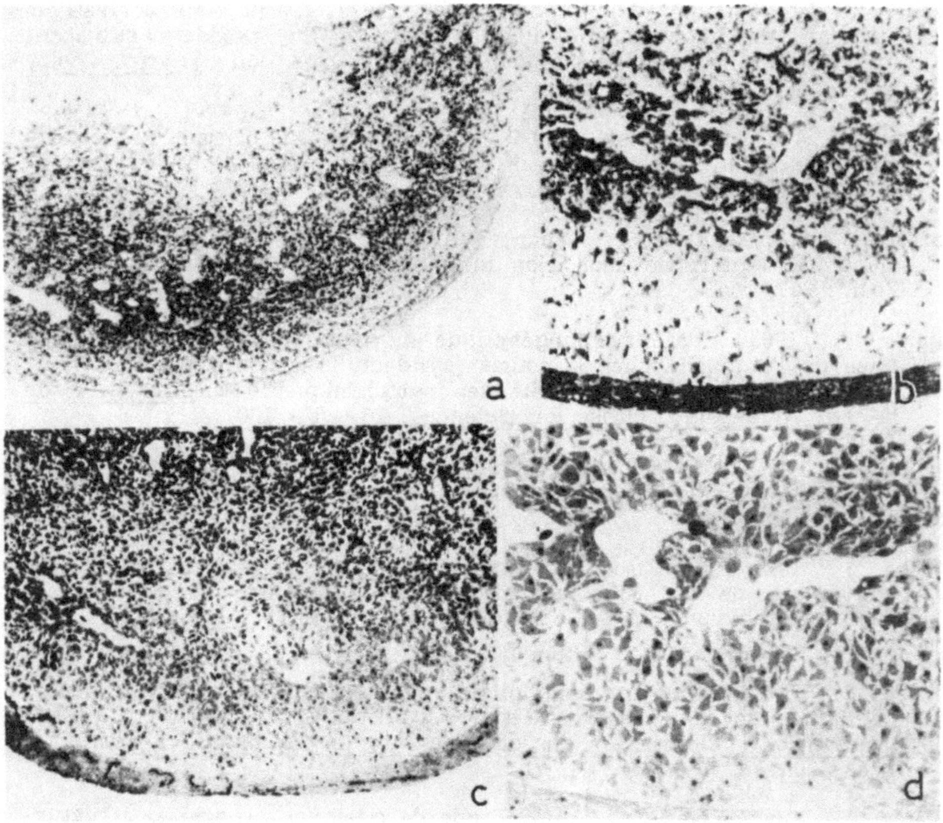

Fig. 1: Pattern of differential cell density in the subridge mesoderm of chick limb buds as demonstrated in paraffin (a, b) and thick Epon sections oriented longitudinal through the ectodermal ridge,
a) wing bud, stage 20, pyronine-methyl green;
b) wing bud, stage 24, pyronine-methyl green;
c) and d) leg bud, stage 22, toluidine blue.

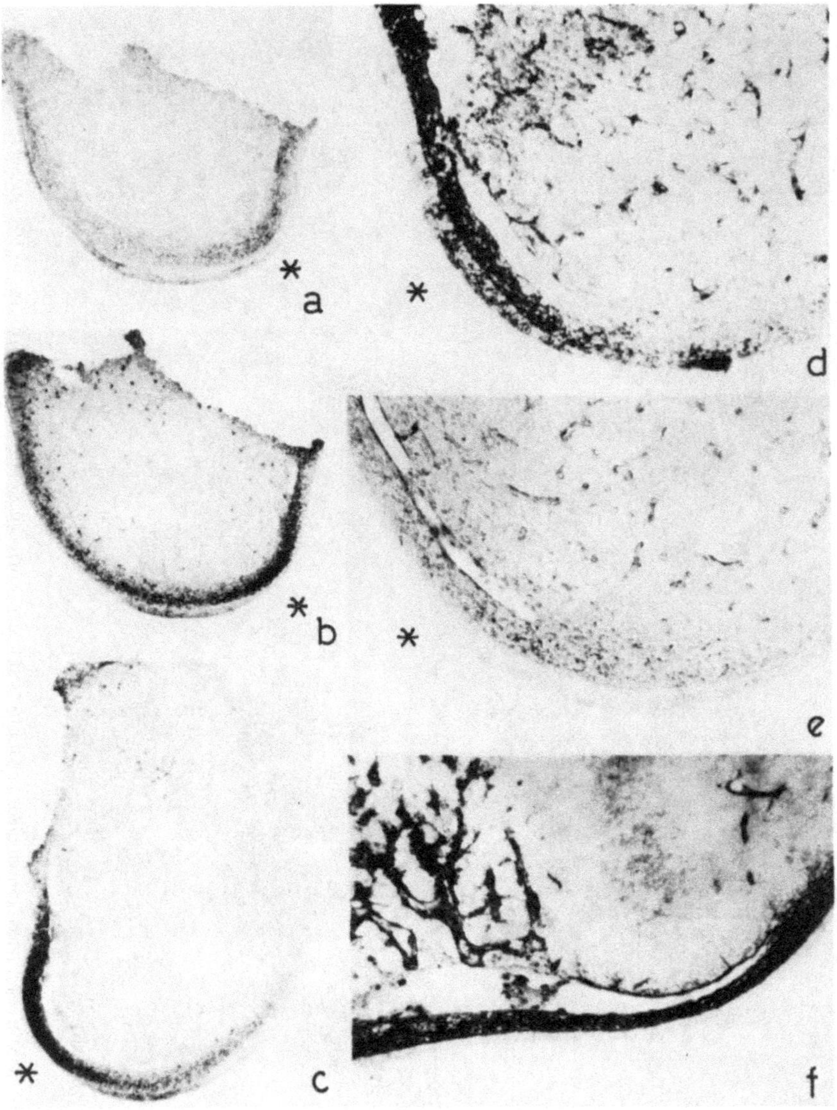

Fig. 2: Sites of AMP- and ATP-phosphohydrolase (PH) activities demonstrated in longitudinal sections of developing limb buds. The asterisk indicates the postaxial side of the section.

a) AMP-PH, chick leg bud, stage 22;
b) ATP-PH, chick leg bud, stage 22;
c) ATP-PH, chick leg bud, stage 24;
d) AMP-PH, 32-day stage Macacus hindlimb bud,
e) AMP-PH, 32-day stage Macacus forelimb bud,
f) AMP-PH, 36-day stage Macacus hindlimb bud.

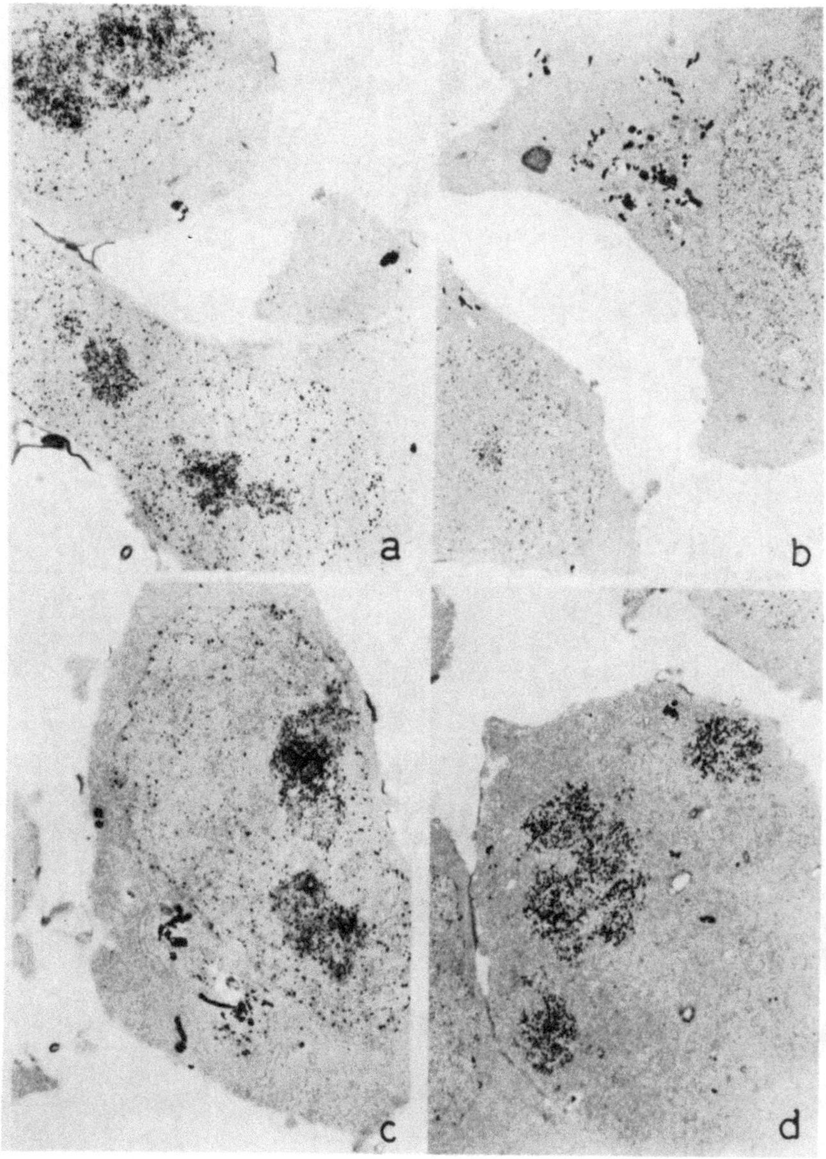

Fig. 3: Ultrastructural sites of AMP-phosphohydrolase activity demonstrated in the subridge mesoderm of chick hind limb buds at stage 22 (100 μ -thick cryostat sections incubated 6 hours at 37°C after glutaraldehyde fixation).

a) nuclear reaction;
b) cytoplasmic reactions;
c) nuclear and cytoplasmic reaction;
d) reaction in the chromatin masses of a dividing cell (x 10 000).

Control by the Posterior Border of Cell Death Patterns in Limb Bud Development of Amniotes: Evidence from Experimental Amputations and from Mutants

J. R. Hinchliffe

The University College of Wales, Department of Zoology
Penglais, Aberystwyth SY23 3DA, U.K.

Amniote limb development is characterised by large scale mesenchymal cell death (Review in SAUNDERS and FALLON, 1967; HINCHLIFFE and JOHNSON, 1980; HINCHLIFFE, 1981). This paper will briefly review the areas of cell death, their morphogenetic significance, and cellular control mechanisms. Variations in the normal cell death pattern are clearly related to certain limb abnormalities, and this paper proposes a hypothesis to explain the changed patterns in cell death found in certain mutants and following experimental amputations of limb bud parts.

In two classical papers on the chick limb morphogenesis, SAUNDERS (SAUNDERS et al., 1962; SAUNDERS and FALLON, 1967) directed attention to significant cell death at stages 23 - 26 in the anterior and posterior necrotic zones (ANZ, PNZ) and later in the interdigital mesenchyme (INZ) of the leg at stage 32. Mapping these areas with such vital dyes as Neutral Red has proved a useful technique. Analysis of control of the cell death has been at several levels. At the cellular level, the following sequence of events has been found: (i) mesenchyme cells develop autophagic vacuoles rich in acid phosphatase (AP), an enzyme which is a useful lysosomal marker, (ii) autolysis begins with the autophagic vacuoles releasing their contents into the cell cytoplasm which becomes damaged, while simultaneously the cell fragments, (iii) the cell debris is phagocytosed by viable neighbouring mesenchymal cells which become transformed into large macrophages containing up to 20 dead cells in process of digestion in AP-rich vacuoles (HURLE and HINCHLIFFE, 1978; HINCHLIFFE, 1981). While cell death is characterised by early lysosomal activation, there is little evidence that this is the primary cause. Protein and nucleic acid synthesis falls off before any cytochemical deterioration can be detected, and it may well be that a certain level of deterioration triggers an auto-destruct mechanism through loss of control of the intracellular digestion system. In a different approach, SAUNDERS (1966) has analysed the progressive determination of the prospective PNZ cells, by in vitro and grafting experiments which emphasise the importance of the position of the prospective area in relation to other parts of the wing bud.

Only in the case of the INZ is a morphogenetic role unequivocally indicated. Throughout amniotes the INZ clearly separates and shapes the digits by removing the interdigital soft tissue (SAUNDERS and FALLON, 1967). This is confirmed by studies on web-footed species (e.g. the duck, PAUTOU, 1974) and by mutant embryos showing soft-tissue syndactyly such as talpid in the chick (HINCHLIFFE and THOROGOOD, 1974) and polysyndactyly in the mouse (JOHNSON, 1969) where the interdigital cell death is inhibited. In web-footed species, INZ inhibition is a matter of degree, since the INZs are still substantial, but they are of shorter duration and less extensive in area than in the chick. In the chick the injection of Janus Green also greatly reduces the INZ, resulting in soft tissue syndactyly in the foot (SAUNDERS and FALLON, 1967).

Teratology of the Limbs

The role of ANZ and PNZ in early limb buds is much more puzzling. Tempting though it is to suggest a shaping role, in fact SAUNDERS (1966) found he could experimentally suppress the PNZ and still obtain a normally shaped wing. One possibility is that the zones are a device by which a correctly-sized limb bud is formed by regulating mesodermal cell number, in the same way as spinal ganglia regulate their cell number in relation to 'peripheral loading'. But if the quantity of stage 18 - 21 wing bud mesoderm is reduced experimentally, although the limb buds soon regulate for the deficiency (WOLFF, 1958), they do not do so at the expense of either ANZ or PNZ (HINCHLIFFE, 1981).

Phylogenetic considerations indicate another possibility. ANZ and PNZ, unlike INZ, seem to be confined to birds (Fig. 3, A - C), while in such mammals as the rat and mouse, there is only a minor anterior zone (MILAIRE, 1967) and this is associated with a limb bud very wide distally which forms the full number of digits (5) of the pentadactyl limb. In the very specialized limbs of birds, however, the digit number is reduced, and in much narrower bird limb buds ANZ and PNZ may control skeletal pattern by limiting the amount of available mesenchyme.

In a number of mutants, increases or decreases in ANZ and PNZ are correlated with decreases or increases in digital number. In the talpid mutant, whose mesenchyme is resistant to mal-treatment, ANZ and PNZ are both absent, and the limb buds become very broad and form up to 8 digits (HINCHLIFFE and EDE, 1967). In the wingless mutant, the ANZ is precocious and enlarged (Fig. 3 D) and accounts for the wingless condition (HINCHLIFFE and EDE, 1973).

So far ANZ and PNZ have been considered together, though in fact in both wing and leg buds, the ANZ may be more important since it is larger and persists for a longer period. The remainder of the paper will set out evidence for the hypothesis that the ANZ is ultimately under ZPA control, and that variation in its size may reflect variation in the control system.

Experimental support is provided by a series of controlled wing bud amputations carried out by HINCHLIFFE and GUMPEL-PINOT (1981). If the posterior half of the chick wing bud (stage 17 - 22) is excised, the anterior half subsequently forms only a single skeletal element, either humerus or humerus fused with radius (Fig 1 B). Independent experiments with chimeric chick-quail wing buds show that the anterior half normally contributes to the skeleton radius and digit 2, the posterior half forming ulna and digits 3 - 5 (GUMPEL-PINOT and HINCHLIFFE, 1981). Thus the isolated anterior half forms less than its prospective fate, and in fact vital staining reveals that beginning at 18 hours after operation the AER regresses and increased cell death first enlarges the ANZ (Fig. 3 E) and then spreads into the distal mesenchyme (Fig. 3 F). By contrast, if the anterior half of the chick wing bud (stages 17 - 22) is excised, the posterior half develops as in the normal bud, and forms humerus (part), ulna and digits 3,4 and 5. Such posterior halves develop no more mesenchymal necrosis than the normal contro-lateral wing buds and the AER remains healthy (Fig. 3 G). Further, if the excision of the posterior part is made in such a way as to leave in place a part of the zone of polarizing activity (ZPA), a normal wing with complete skeleton is formed (Fig. 2).

Recent studies on the ZPA have aroused great interest following the discovery by SAUNDERS (1972) that the ZPA has the capacity to cause limb duplication when grafted pre-axially in the wing bud. Moreover, it appears to control the antero-posterior axis of the duplicated limb. But because a normal wing bud with ZPA removed still develops normally (FALLON and CROSBY, 1975), there has been disagreement between those who believe the ZPA controls antero-posterior differentiation in the normal limb (WOLPERT, 1978; SUMMERBELL and TICKLE, 1977) and those who deny such a role (SAUNDERS, 1977). Our amputation experiments suggest that in order to survive and differentiate, the anterior part of the wing bud needs a factor supplied by the posterior part containing the ZPA. FALLON'S results may be explained by the fact that sufficient mesenchyme of intermediate ZPA activity (an area removed in our amputation experiments) was left to polarize the limb.

There appears to be a close parallel between our amputation results, and the development of genetic winglessness. In sex linked winglessness (ws), the ANZ shows the same enlargement, and movement in a postero-distal direction, accompanied by AER regression, which follows posterior amputations which remove the ZPA (Fig. 3 D, compare 3 E, F). In the American wingless mutant (ZWILLING, 1956; wg, an autosomal recessive), there is also increased cell death though its pattern is less specific (SAUNDERS, quoted in HINCHLIFFE and EDE, 1973) while the AER regresses or never forms. Significantly, MacCABE (quoted in SAUNDERS, 1972) has shown that the posterior mesenchyme of wingless (wg) wing buds lacks ZPA properties. In ws, the wing bud has not been tested for ZPA properties, but this possibility is currently being examined.

The nature of the factor supplied by the ZPA is still unknown (MacCABE et al., 1977), but SUMMERBELL (1979) argues on the basis of barrier experiments that the ZPA acts as the source of a diffusible morphogen which declines along the A-p axis and specifies differentiation according to its concentration along this axis. A modification of this model would explain both the amputation and mutant findings. If limb mesenchyme dies below a certain low threshold of morphogen, then normally only the extreme anterior mesenchyme (the ANZ) falls below this threshold. When a posterior part of the limb including ZPA is amputated, thus removing the morphogen source, the level falls with the consequence that more of the anterior mesenchyme is below the critical level and thus it dies (Fig 2 B).

While only two mutants have been discussed, a number of others are known which are rather similar. Thus, in the mouse mutant, oligosyndactylism (GRÜNEBERG, 1963) the 11 day limb bud is narrowed preaxially and according to MILAIRE (1967) this is due to an extension of the small area of anterior necrosis found in normal fore limb buds. As a consequence the digits are close together, or one is lost. In dominant hemimelia the limb bud develops a preaxial mesenchymal excess attributed by MILAIRE (1970) to absence of this normal area of anterior necrosis. In fact both in mutants generally and following X-irradiation, skeletal anomalies of the limb are more common pre-axially than post-axially (GRÜNEBERG, 1963; HINCHLIFFE and EDE, 1973; WOLFF, 1958). While there is no direct experimental evidence from mammalian limbs, these observations are consistent with the view that such anomalies result from interference with the normal signal (ZPA factor) -response (anterior and distal mesenchyme) system. Possible variations include attenuation of, or increase in, the ZPA signal, or gene effects via the cell surface on diffusion from cell to cell, or cell to environment modifying signal propagation. Finally, one should perhaps emphasise that such a hypothesis remains essentially speculative, and that many major issues (such as whether the mode of action of ZPA is via mesoderm or ectoderm, the relationship of ZPA factor to ZWILLING'S maintenance factor, or the identity of the factor itself) remain to be resolved.

REFERENCES

Fallon, J.F., Crosby, G.M., 1975, Normal development of the chick wing following removal of the polarizing zone. J. exp. Zool., 193, 449 - 455.

Grüneberg, H., 1963, "The pathology of development". Blackwell, Oxford.

Gumpel-Pinot, M., Hinchliffe, J.R., 1981, The fate map of the skeletal areas of the chick wing bud along the antero-posterior axis: a study by chimeric grafting, J. Embryol. exp. Morph., (In preparation).

Hinchliffe, J.R., 1981, Cell death in embryogenesis. in: "Cell Death", (I.D. Bowen, R.A. Lockshin, eds.), Chapman and Hall, London.

Hinchliffe, J.R., Ede, D.A., 1967, Limb development in the polydactylous talpid3 mutant of the fowl, J. Embryol. exp. Morph., 17, 385 - 404.

Hinchliffe, J.R., Ede, D.A., 1973, Cell death and the development of limb form and skeletal pattern in normal and wingless (ws) chick embryos, J. Embryol. exp. Morph., 30, 753 - 772.

Hinchliffe, J.R., Gumpel-Pinot, M., 1981, Control of maintenance and antero-posterior differentiation of the anterior mesenchyme of the chick wing bud by its posterior margin (the ZPA), J. Embryol. exp. Morph. (In press).

Hinchliffe, J.R., Johnson, D.R., 1980, "The Development of the Vertebrate Limb", Oxford Univ. Press.

Hinchliffe, J.R., Thorogood, P.B., 1974, Genetic inhibition of mesenchymal cell death and the development of form and skeletal pattern in the limbs of talpid3 mutant chick embryos, J. Embryol. exp. Morph., 31, 747 - 760.

Hurle, J., Hinchliffe, J.R., 1978, Cell death in the posterior necrotic zone (PNZ) of the chick wing bud: a stereoscan and ultrastructural survey of autolysis and cell fragmentation, J. Embryol. exp. Morph., 43, 123 - 236.

Johnson, D.R., 1969, Polysyndactyly, a new mutant gene in the mouse, J. Embryol. exp. Morph., 21, 285 - 294.

MacCabe, A.B., Gasseling, M.T., Saunders, J.W., Jr., 1973, Spatiotemporal distribution of mechanisms that control outgrowth and antero-posterior polarization of the limb bud in the chick embryo, Mechanisms of Ageing and Development, 2, 1 - 12.

MacCabe, J.A., Calandra, A.J., Parker, B.W., 1977, In vitro analysis of the distribution and nature of a morphogenetic factor in the developing chick wing, in: "Vertebrate Limb and Somite Morphogenesis", (D.A. Ede, J.R. Hinchliffe, M. Balls, eds.) pp. 25 - 39, Cambridge Univ. Press.

Milaire, J., 1967, Histochemical observations on the developing foot of normal, oligosyndactylous (Os/+) and syndactylous (sm/sm) mouse embryos, Archs. Biol., Liège, 78, 223 - 288.

Milaire, J., 1970, Evolution et déterminisme des dégénerescences cellulaires au cours de la morphogenèse des membres et leurs modifications dans diverses situations tératologiques, in: "Malformations congénitales des mammifères", (H. Tuchmann-Duplessis, ed.) pp. 131 - 149, Colloque Pfizer : Amboise.

Pautou, M.P., 1974, Evolution comparée de la nécrose morphogène interdigitale dans le pied de l'embryon de poulet et de canard, C.r. hebd. Séanc. Acad. Sci., Paris, 278D, 2209 - 2212.

Saunders, J.W., Jr., 1966, Death in embryonic systems. Science N.Y., 154, 604 - 612.

Saunders, J.W., Jr., 1972, Developmental control of three-dimensional polarity in the avian limb, Ann. N.Y. Acad. Sci., 193, 29 - 42.

Saunders, J.W., Jr., 1977, The experimental analysis of chick limb bud development, in: "Vertebrate Limb and Somite Morphogenesis", (D.A. Ede, J.R. Hinchliffe, M. Balls, eds.), pp. 1 - 24, Cambridge Univ. Press.

Saunders, J.W., Jr., Fallon, J.F., 1967, Cell death in embryonic morphogenesis, in: "Major Problems in Developmental Biology", (M. Locke, ed.), pp. 289 - 314, Academic Press, New York, London.

Saunders, J.W., Jr., Gasseling, M.T., Saunders, L.C., 1962, Cellular death in morphogenesis of the avian wing, Devl. Biol., 5, 147 - 178.

Summerbell, D., 1979, The zone of polarizing activity: evidence for a role in normal chick morphogenesis, J. Embryol. exp. Morph., 50, 217 - 233.

Summerbell, D., Tickle, C., 1977, Pattern formation along the anteroposterior axis of the chick limb bud, in: "Vertebrate Limb and Somite Morphogenesis", (D.A. Ede, J.R. Hinchliffe, M. Balls, eds.), pp. 41 - 57, Cambridge Univ. Press.

Wolff, E., 1958, Le principe de compétition, Bull. de la Soc. Zool. de France, 83, 13 - 25.

Wolpert, L., 1978, Pattern formation in biological development, Scient. Am., 239, 124 - 137.

Zwilling, E., 1956, Interaction between limb bud ectoderm and mesoderm in the chick embryo. IV. Experiments with a wingless mutant, J. exp. Zool., 132, 241 - 253.

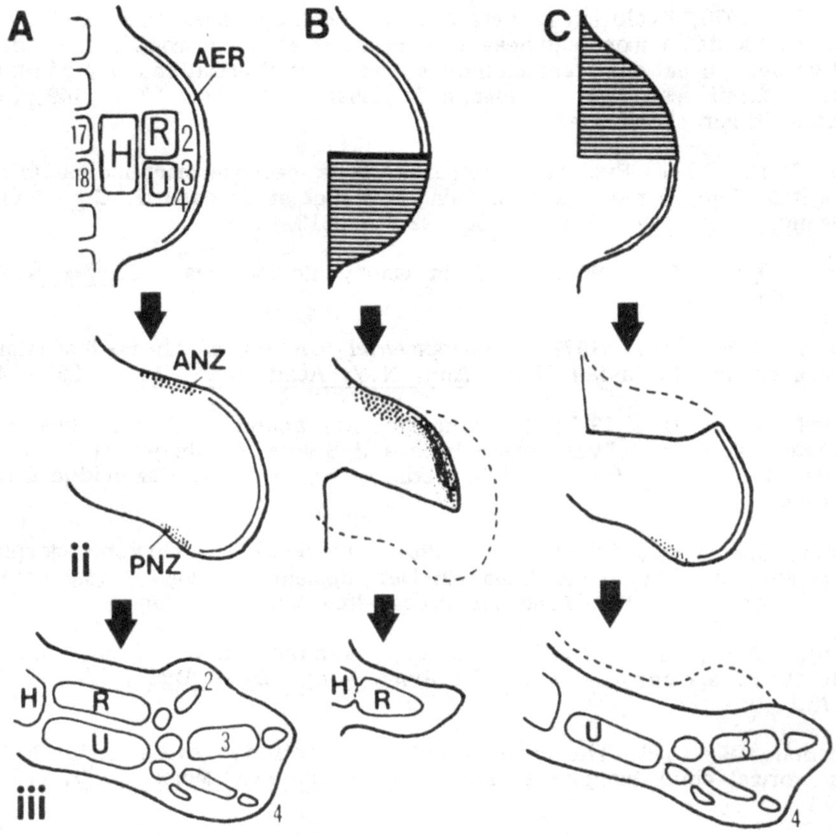

Fig. 1: (A), the normal chick wing bud at stage 21 with prospective areas and somites, (ii) at stage 26 with ANZ and PNZ, and (iii) the definitive skeleton at 7 days. In (B), the posterior half of the wing bud has been amputated, resulting after 24 hrs. in increased anterior cell death, (ii). Note increased ANZ (in macrophages; large dots), early stages of cell death in the distal mesenchyme (small dots) and AER regression. Only a fused humerus-radius (reduced) forms (iii). In (C) the anterior half of the wing bud has been amputated. Subsequently, after 24 hrs. there is no increase in mesenchymal cell death, and the AER remains healthy (ii). At 7 days, a wing skeleton lacking only radius and digit 2 has formed, (iii). Abbreviations: H, humerus; R, radius; U, ulna; 2,3,4, digits.).

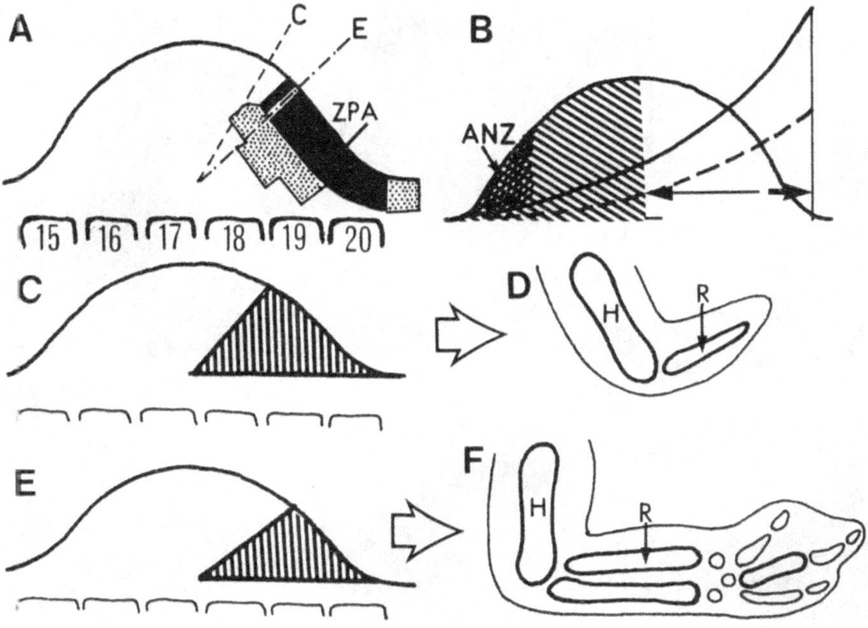

Fig. 2: (A), diagram of areas of high (black) and intermediate ZPA (dots) activity, as mapped by MacCABE et al. (1973). The dotted lines represent the amputations made in C and E. (B), interpretation of ZPA amputation experiments, based on the idea that the ZPA is the source of a morphogen which declines along the antero-posterior axis (see text). The solid line represents the normal morphogen profile: only the extreme anterior mesenchyme (ANZ) falls below the critical level (large arrow) and dies (dots). If a posterior part including ZPA is amputated (e. g. C) the morphogen profile declines (dotted line), so that all the shaded anterior mesenchyme now falls below the critical level (small arrow) and dies. (C - F), posterior amputations and their results. In (C), the ZPA has been amputated, subsequently skeletal development is restricted to humerus and radius, (D). In (E), part of the ZPA is left, and a normal wing skeleton forms (F).

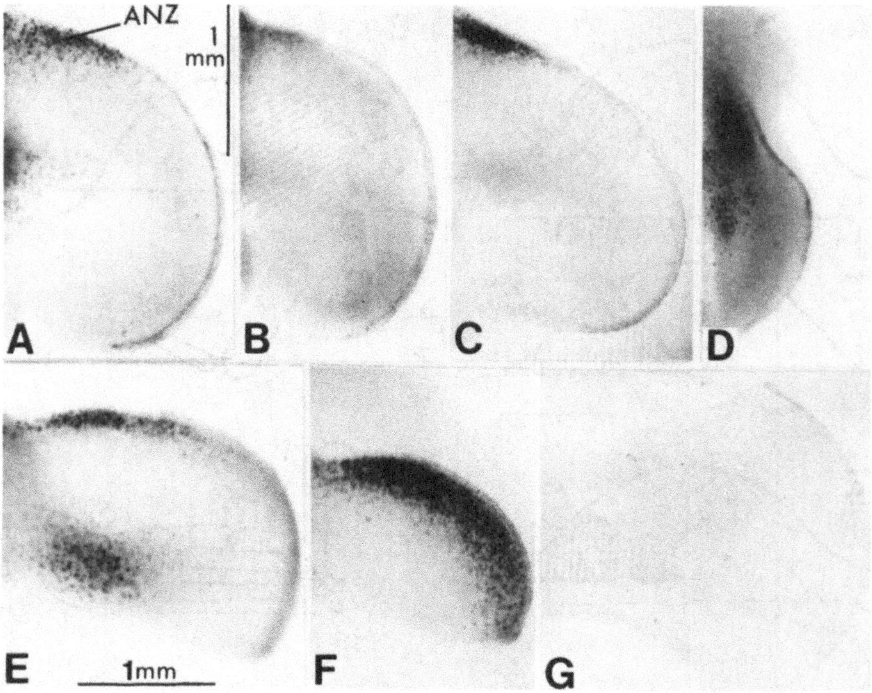

<u>Fig. 3</u>: Cell death in the anterior mesenchyme of various limb buds as revealed by vital staining. All except (B) from chick. (A), normal stage 23 wing bud (ANZ anterior necrotic zone), (B) Herring gull stage 23 wing bud, (C) normal stage 23 leg bud, (D) wingless mutant stage 21 wing bud with enlarged and precocious ANZ and regressing AER. (E) - (G), the pattern of cell death at 1 day following amputations. (E), posterior 1/3 amputation at stage 21: note enlarged ANZ. (F), posterior half amputations at stage 17/8: note cell death throughout distal mesenchyme. (G), anterior 1/2 amputation at stage 20/1. The AER is healthy and there is no mesenchymal cell death.

Characterization of Embryonic Cholinesterase in the Chondrogenic Core of the Chick Limb Bud and Demonstration of a Specific Acetylcholine Receptor

Ulrich Drews, Christoph Schröder, Heinrich Schmidt
Anatomisches Institut,
Österbergstraße 3, D-7400 Tübingen 1

Several years ago we described single cholinesterase-active cells in the chick blastoderm which migrated from the ectodermal into the mesodermal and endodermal layers (DREWS et al., 1966). Cholinesterase (ChE) activity in embryonic cells later turned out to be a general phenomenon. In all organs studied in various species, expression of cholinesterase was correlated to morphogenetic movements. The activity disappeared when the respective organ structure had formed (DREWS, 1975).

In the early limb bud, ChE activity is confined to the ectoderm and to the apical ectodermal ridge (Fig. 1 a) (DREWS and DREWS, 1972). At stage 20 ChE appears in the mesenchyme. At stage 24 and 25 it concentrates in the central chondrogenic core (Fig. 1 b). From stage 25 onwards, ChE active single myoblasts and invading nerve fibres also become visible. After fusion, activity in the myotubes is further enhanced so that formation of individual muscles can be followed. The ChE activity in the chondrogenic core disappears when the cartilaginous anlagen of the long bones have been formed (Fig. 1 c, d).

We were particularly interested in the ChE active chondrogenic core of the limb bud. Since chondroblasts do not express ChE activity in the differentiated state, they appear to be a suitable model for further studies on the functional meaning of embryonic ChE. In a tissue culture experiment we therefore analysed the correlation between ChE activity and morphogenetic movement (DREWS and DREWS, 1973). Chick limb bud mesenchyme of stage 20 to 24 was disaggregated by trypsination. The cell suspension was seeded out into tissue culture dishes. On the bottom of the dish ChE active cartilage nodules developed which were surrounded by myoblasts (Fig. 2). The movements of ChE active chondroblasts and ChE negative fibroblastic cells were recorded on time lapse film. It turned out that the ChE active chondrogenic cells adhered together performing only very slight aggregation movement, whereas the ChE negative fibroblastic cells randomly moved around on the surface of the culture dish guided only by contact inhibition.

Furthermore, we cultivated the cell suspension originating from limb bud mesenchyme in a roller culture system using small bags of Haereus Biofolie. In suspension culture small organoids formed. They contained a central cartilage nodule surrounded by connective tissue covered by a layer of myotubes. The myotubes successively degenerated and were lost in the culture medium. During development of the nodules, chondroblasts, myoblasts, and soft tissue cells segregated. The chondroblasts aggregating in the center and the myoblasts migrating outward showed ChE activity (Fig. 3).

Up to that stage, our results on embryonic cholinesterase had been entirely based on histochemical observations. We therefore characterized the enzyme from chick limb bud by colorimetry and disc gel electrophoresis. We used the colorimetric assay of ELLMANN, and for distinction of buty-

Teratology of the Limbs

ryl- and acetylcholinesterase, the blocker system according to FLUCK and STROHMAN (1973), which these authors used for the study of ChE activity in myoblast cultures. The development of butyryl- and acetylcholinesterase activity in the limb bud from stage 20 through 29 is shown in Figure 4. Between stage 20 and 25 both enzymes had about the same activity. At stage 25 a steep rise of AChE occured. Comparison with the histochemical results showed that the rise in AChE coincided with the appearance of myoblasts and development of myotubes. If at stage 29 only the tip of the anlage was assayed where myotubes had not yet formed, AChE activity was again in the range of BChE.

For disc gel electrophoresis limb buds of stage 24 were used. At this stage the ChE activity was mainly derived from chondroblasts and respresented typical embryonic ChE. The rationale of our experiment was to compare ChE from the chondrogenic core of stage 24 limb bud with ChE of myotomes of the same embryo. Figure 5 a shows five gels with a triton extract of limb bud homogenate, Figure 5 b, gels with the respective triton extract of myotome material, and Figure 5 c, gels with a mixture of both extracts. Limb bud and myotomes showed the same banding pattern. Three major bands appeared, the upper one with two subbands. The bands were blocked by eserine, inhibited by BW 284c51, not inhibited by iso-OMPA, and did not hydrolyse butyrylcholine. In the mixture of both extracts no additional bands appeared. The isoenzymes resolved from the limb bud and from the myotomes thus represented AChE. Since at stage 24 the ChE of the limb bud is located in the chondrogenic core, we conclude that the embryonic ChE of chondroblasts is AChE and is identical to the enzyme from striated muscle.

The pronounced BChE activity observed by colorimetry was only found in gels of crude homogenate and was represented by a faint band in both limb bud and myotomes. For further discussion see SCHRÖDER (1980).

After partial biochemical characterization of embryonic ChE as AChE, receptor binding studies were performed in order to demonstrate the presence of an acetylcholine receptor. Figure 7 shows the binding of ^{3}H-QNB (quinuclidinylbenzylate) to homogenate of chick limb bud of stage 25/26, measured by a filter assay. Specific binding was defined as the difference between total binding and unspecific binding measured after blocking the specific receptor sites by 1 µM atropine. The K_d in two experiments was 0.11 nM and 0.16 nM, the binding capacity was 15.7 fmol (^{3}H)QNB / mg protein and 12.0 fmol (^{3}H)QNB / mg protein, respectively.

QNB is a specific ligand for acetylcholine receptors of the muscarinic type. Data on displacement of the specifically bound (^{3}H)QNB by various nicotinic and muscarinic ligands confirmed the muscarinic nature of the receptor. Muscarinic ligands inhibited the (^{3}H)QNB binding, whereas nicotinic ligands caused no inhibition at pharmacological concentrations. A detailed description by SCHMIDT (1980) will be published soon.

Specific binding of QNB could also be demonstrated in the limb bud at stage 24. Myoblasts and myotubes did not express the muscarinic but the nicotinic acetylcholine receptor. We therefore assume that the embryonic cholinergic system demonstrated in the limb bud is of the muscarinic type.

REFERENCES

Drews, U., 1975, Cholinesterase in embryonic development, Progr. Histochem. Cytochem., 7, 3.

Drews, U., Drews, U., 1972, Cholinesterase in der Extremitäten-entwicklung des Hühnchens: I. Phasen der Cholinesterase-Aktivität in der jungen Knospe und bei der Abgrenzung von Knorpel- und Muskelanlagen, Wilhelm Roux' Arch., 169, 70 - 86.

Drews, U., Drews, U., 1973, Cholinesterase in der Extremitäten-entwicklung des Hühnchens: II. Fermentaktivität und Bewegungs-verhalten der präsumptiven Knorpelzellen in vitro, Wilhelm Roux' Arch., 173, 208 - 227.

Drews, U., Kussäther, E., Usadel, K.H., 1966, Cholinesterase bei Gestaltungsvorgängen in der Hühnerkeimscheibe, Naturewissenschaften, 53, 556.

Fluck, R.A., Strohman, R.C., 1973, Acetylcholinesterase activity in developing skeletal muscle cells in vitro, Develop. Biol., 33, 417 - 428.

Schmidt, H., 1980, Muscarinic acetylcholine receptor in chick limb bud during morphogenetic movement, Histochemistry, in press.

Schröder, C., 1980, Characterization of embryonic cholinesterase in chick limb bud by colorimetry and disk electrophoresis. Histochemistry, in press.

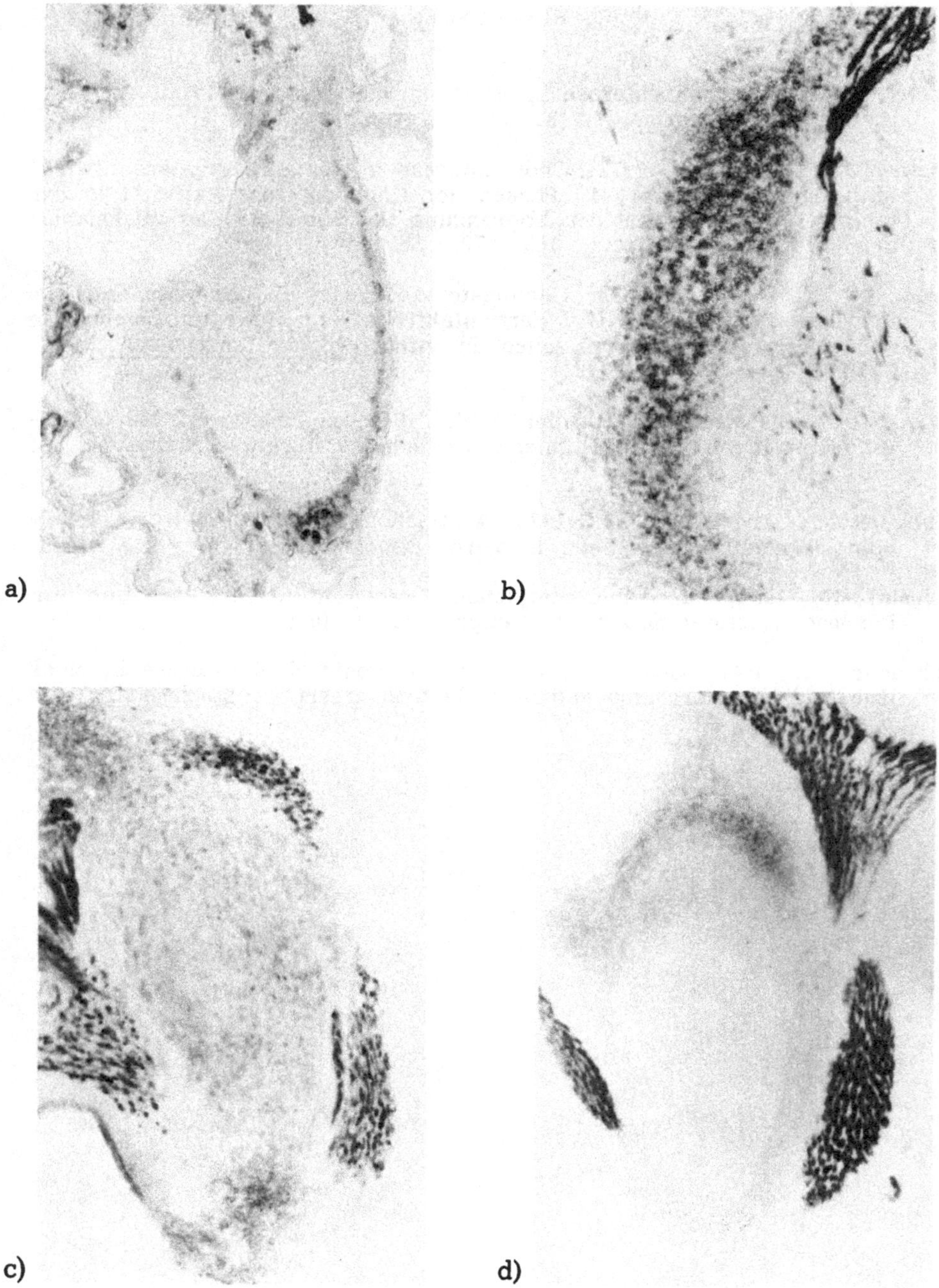

Fig. 1: ChE activity in the chick wing bud. Embedding in carbowax. ChE-reaction after KARNOVSKY and ROOTS,
a.) stage 19;
b.) stage 25;
c.) stage 27,
d.) stage 29.

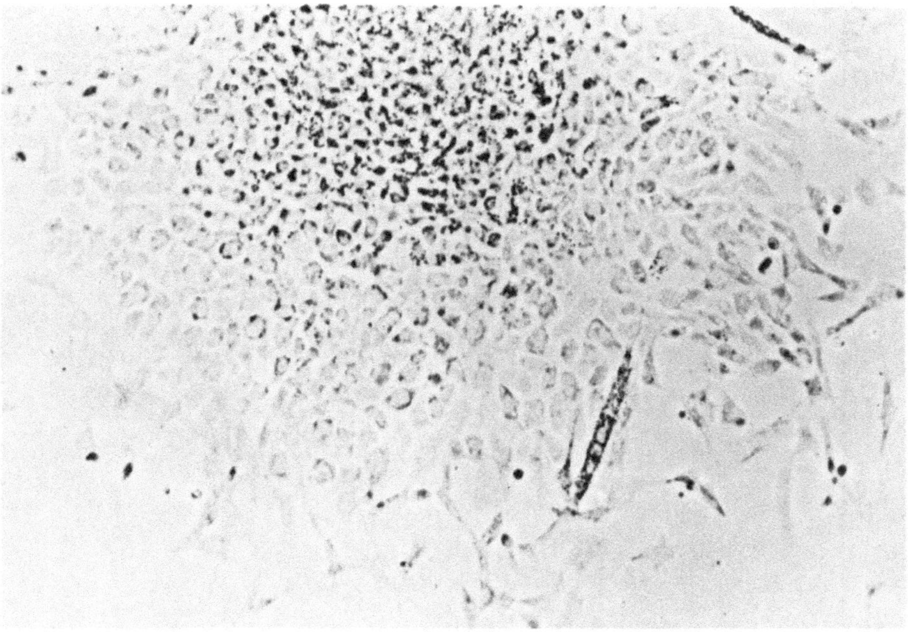

Fig. 2: ChE reaction in a monolayer culture of limb bud mesenchyme. ChE activity in aggregating chondroblasts.

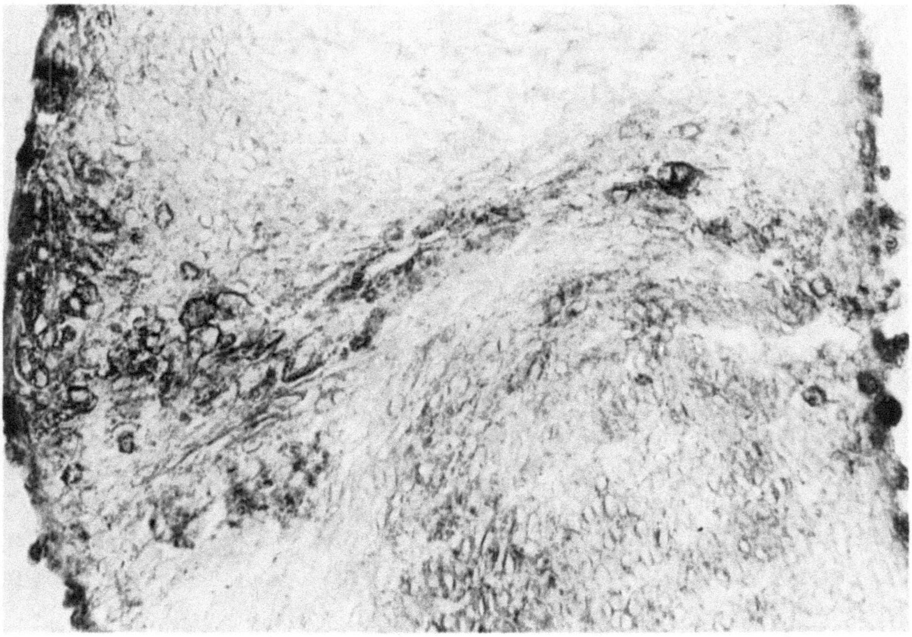

Fig. 3: ChE reaction in a suspension culture of limb bud mesenchyme. Activity in segregating myoblasts and chondroblasts.

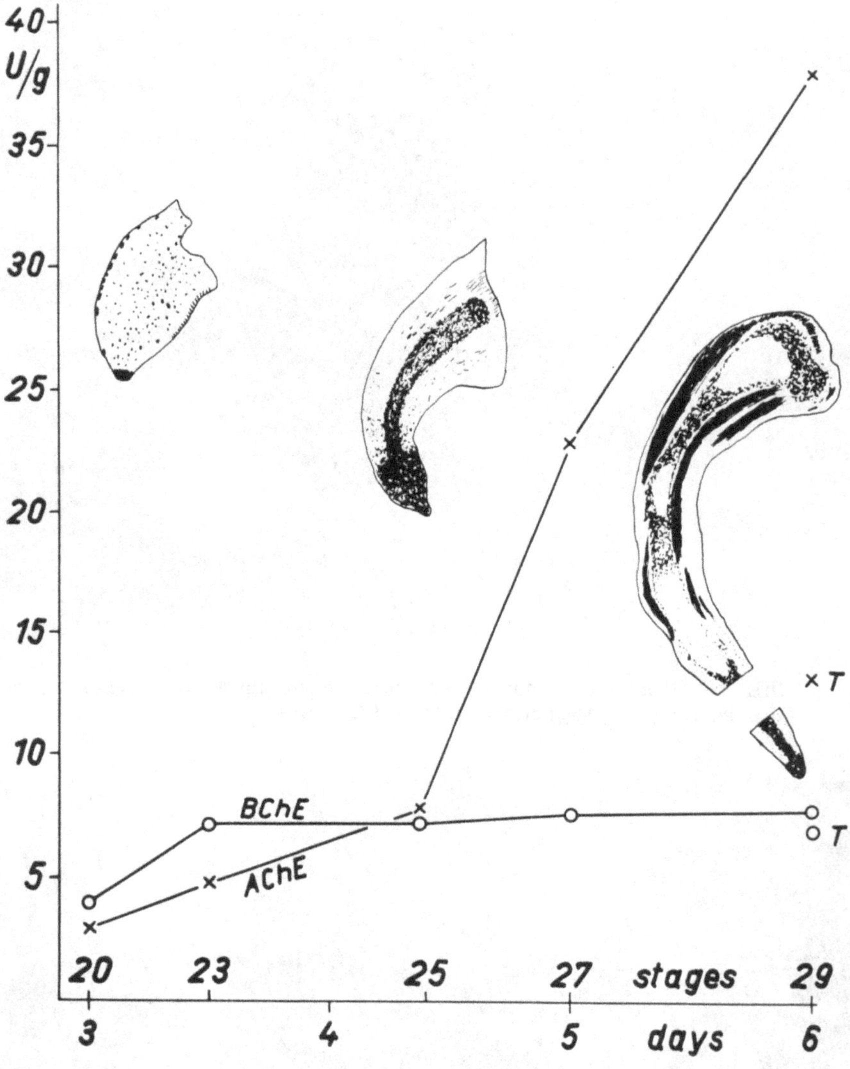

Fig. 4: Colorimetric determination of ChE activity in the chick limb anlage. Butyrylcholinesterase activity (BChE) is defined as rate of hydrolysis of butyrylthiocholine blocked by iso-OMPA, and acetylcholinesterase activity as rate of hydrolysis of acetylthiocholine blocked by BW 284c51.

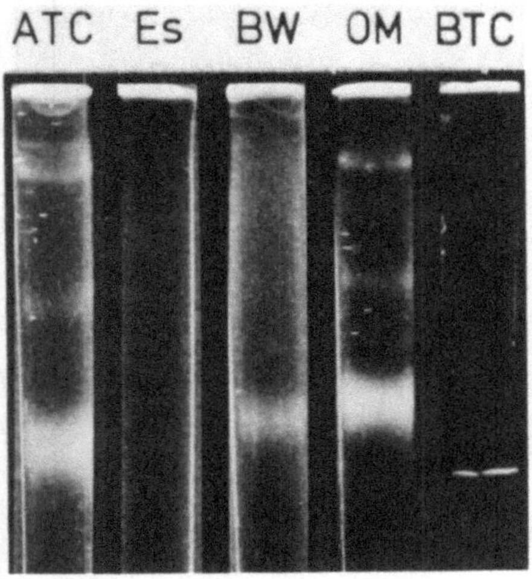

a)

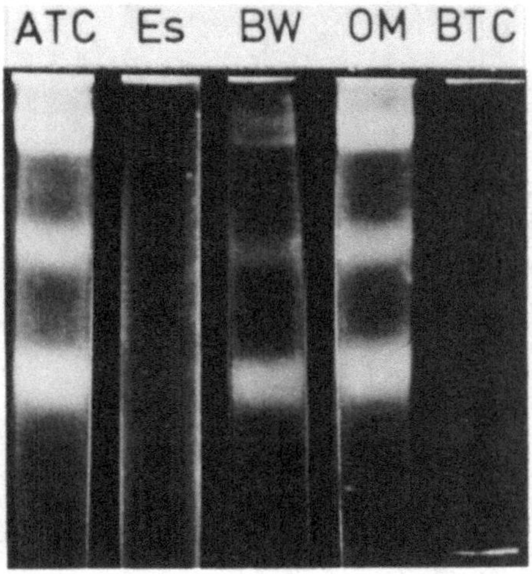

b)

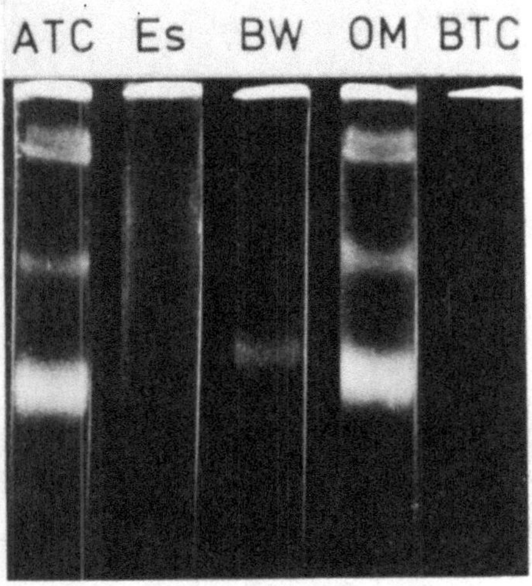

c)

Fig. 5: Cholinesterase from limb bud and myotomes. 7% polyacrylamide gels performed with 1% triton extracts.
a.) limb bud stage 24;
b.) myotomes stage 24;
c.) mixture of both extracts.
ATC: 7 mM acetylthiocholine; Es: eserine 10^{-5}M;
BW: BW 284c51 10^{-5}M; OM: iso-OMPA 10^{-5}M;
BTC: 7 mM butyrylthiocholine.

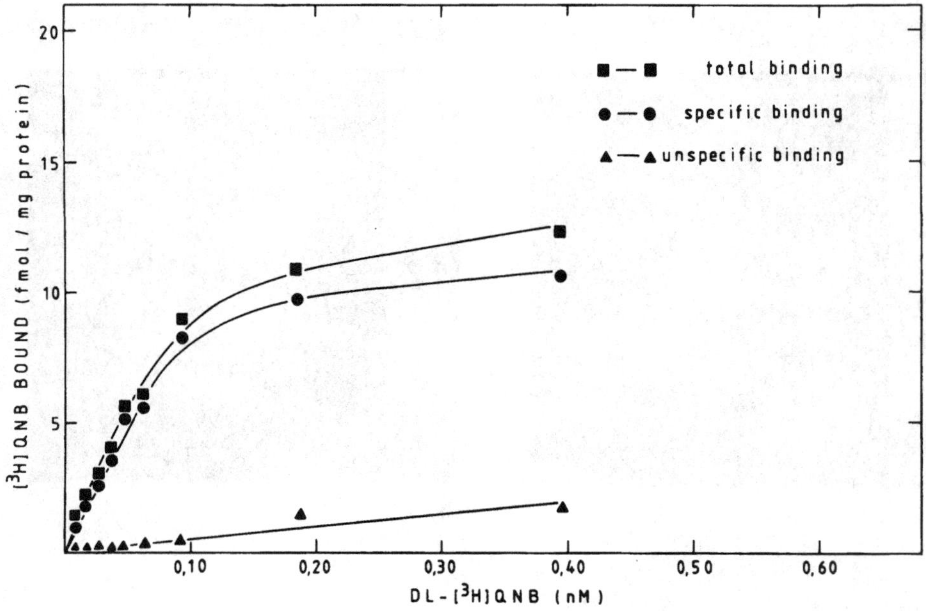

Fig. 6: Binding of ^{3}H-QNB in homogenate of chick limb buds at stage 25/26.

Limb Chondrogenesis: Interactions between Ectoderm and Mesoderm

Madeleine Gumpel-Pinot
Institut d'Embryologie 49 bis,
Avenue de la Belle-Gabrielle, F-94130 Nogent-sur-Marne, France

INTRODUCTION:

In the chick embryo, the wing primordium develops from the somatopleure. The limb rudiment is thus composed of mesoderm covered by ectoderm. It has been demonstrated during the last decades, that the limb develops through a series of interactions between ectoderm and mesoderm (for review, see ZWILLING, 1961).

More recent work (GUMPEL-PINOT, 1974; CHEVALIER et al., 1976, 1977, 1978; CHRIST et al., 1974, 1977) has shown that the limb-forming mesoderm is not exclusively of somatopleural origin; the striated muscles are derived from somitic mesoderm, while the somatopleural mesoderm gives rise to feather and vascular smooth muscle (KIENY et al., 1979), tendons (KIENY and CHEVALIER, 1979), connective tissue and skeleton.
In the present paper the differentiation of the cartilaginous skeleton will be discussed.

MATERIAL and TECHNIQUES:

White Leghorn chick embryos were used throughout. The exact stage reached at the time of wing primordium excision was specified by the number of somites and by HAMBURGER and HAMILTON (1951) stages.

CULTURE TECHNIQUES:

Two culture techniques were used. In the first series of experiments explants were cultured on WOLFF and HAFFEN (1952) semi-solid medium, wrapped in a fragment of vitelline membrane according to a procedure recommended by WOLFF (1961). In the last series, the technique of transfilter culture on liquid medium has been preferred.

Dissociation of the wing bud:
When necessary, ectoderm was separated from mesoderm by means of trypsin or collagenase digestion.

HISTOLOGICAL and CYTOLOGICAL TECHNIQUES:

Light microscopy:
The explants were fixed in BOUIN'S or CARNOY'S fluid. The sections were stained with hematoxylin-alcian blue.

Electron microscopy:
For scanning or transmission electron microscopy, the explants were fixed in glutaraldehyde and post-fixed in osmic acid. They were then dehydrated and embedded in Epon or critical point dried.

All these techniques, with special references for each experiment, have been described in detail in previous papers (GUMPEL-PINOT, 1972, 1973, 1980, 1981).

Teratology of the Limbs

RESULTS:

Culture of the entire wing primordium (Tab. 1):
The wing primordia were excised from embryos of 15 somites to 5 days of incubation. They were cultured on the semi-solid medium, wrapped in the vitelline membrane. In order to maintain the mass of explanted material at a constant level, several rudiments from the earliest stages were grouped. Table 1 shows that cartilage differentiated in the great majority of the explants regardless of their stage.

Effect of the ectoderm on chondrogenesis (Tab. 2):
As mentioned above, the wing bud is composed of ectoderm and mesoderm. What is the role played by the ectoderm in chondrogenesis? In order to answer this question, the wing bud was excised at stages 16 to 21 (HAMBURGER and HAMILTON, 1951). Ectoderm and mesoderm were dissociated by trypsin treatment. Control explants (M) consisted of mesoderm alone, experimental explant (M + E) of mesoderm reassociated with ectoderm. The proportion of reconstituted explants (M + E) which formed cartilage was very high at all stages studied. By contrast, in the absence of ectoderm stage 15 - 16 mesoderm appeared to be incapable of cartilage differentiation. Later on, chondrogenesis became progressively independent of the ectoderm. However, the ectoderm exerted a strong stimulation on cartilage formation at all stages; the proportion of explants which formed cartilage was higher in the presence of ectoderm, the quantity of cartilage produced was greater and the quality of differentiation was improved.

Thus, the ectoderm has a double effect:
1) It induces cartilage formation in a mesoderm incapable of autonomous chondrogenesis.
2) It stimulates cartilage differentiation.

Specificity of the ectodermal effects (Tab. 3):
The mesoderm of the wing from which the ectoderm had been previously removed was cultured in association with different tissues: ectoderm or epidermis from different sites, neural tube and notochord and various tissues or organs of different embryological origin. The control explant (M) consisted of mesoderm alone. When the wing mesoderm was associated with non-limb ectoderm (tail ectoderm or epidermis from the dorsal skin of 7- and 8-day embryos) the results were comparable to those obtained with limb ectoderm: non-limb ectoderm induced cartilage differentiation at stage 15 - 16 and stimulated chondrogenesis. When the wing mesoderm was associated with neural tube and notochord or with tissues such as mesonephros, lung, heart, allantois or Wolffian duct, the inductive effect was not observed. These tissues were only capable of exerting a stimulating effect on chondrogenesis.

Thus the inductive effect is specific of ectoderm or epidermis whatever their origin. By contrast, the stimulating effect is non-specific.

According to SAXEN (1977), the inductive systems can be classified into two main groups:

1) long-range transmission when the cells are separated by a gap of the order of 50.000 nm,

2) short-range transmission when the cells are in direct contact, i.e. their membranes are separated by a distance of the order of 5 - 10 nm.

Is contact necessary between ectoderm and mesoderm for the induction of cartilage?

Transfilter (Nuclepore) cultures (Tab. 4, 5):
In transfilter cultures of wing bud ectoderm and mesoderm, the mesodermal response as measured by chondrogenesis was directly related to the pore size (0.2 to 1 µm) of the filter. With filters of 0.2 µm pore size and 10 µm thickness, there was no increase in chondrogenesis over that of mesoderm cultured alone.

Scanning electron microscopy of the surface of the filters:
The lower face of filters on the upper face of which mesoderm or ectoderm had been cultured was studied by scanning electron microscopy. When ectoderm was cultured no processes crossed the filter. By contrast, cell processes from mesoderm crossed the filter and this was related to the pore size. The chondrogenic response was correlated to the mass and density of processes crossing the filter. No processes were observed with filters of 0.2 µm pore size.

Thus, induction of cartilage in limb mesoderm cannot be classified as a long-range transmission system. Ectoderm and mesoderm have to be separated by a narrow gap only and this condition can be brought about in vitro by extension of mesodermal processes through the filter close to the ectoderm (GUMPEL-PINOT, 1980).

A basement membrane is always present in vivo between ectoderm and mesoderm. What are the relations between ectoderm and mesoderm transfilter cultures?

Transmisson electron microscopy study of transfilter cultures:
The relations between ectoderm and mesoderm appeared to be similar in vivo and in transfilter cultures. In culture conditions, the filter was embedded in mesodermal cell outgrowths which formed a continuous mesodermal cover on the filter (Fig. 1). A basement membrane was present between the mat of mesodermal cell processes and the ectoderm (GUMPEL-PINOT, 1981).

CONCLUSIONS:

The ectoderm induced cartilage differentiation in the limb bud. The induction appears to be specific. The system requires conditions of "contact". However, a basement membrane is always present between ectoderm and mesoderm. This suggests that the basement membrane and the associated extracellular material plays an important role in the interaction.

Table 1: Culture of entire wing primordia.

Stage of donor embryos (H and H)	No. of explants	Differentiation of cartilage
19 and post.	31	30 (96%)
17 - 18 (29 - 36s)	47	39 (83%)
15 - 16 (24 - 28s)	25	18 (72%)
14 (21 - 23s)	37	31 (83%)
12 - 13 (15 - 20s)	68	52 (76%)

Table 2: Culture of mesoderm with or without ectoderm. Role of ectoderm in chondrogenesis.

Stage of donor embryos (H and H)	No. of pairs explants	M (mesoderm alone) CARTILAGE	M + E (mesoderm + ectoderm) CARTILAGE
19 - 21	43	34 (79%)	43 (100%)
18 (33 - 36s)	28	11 (39%)	23 (82%)
17 (29 - 32s)	31	4 (12%)	26 (83%)
15 - 16 (24 - 28s)	33	1 (3%)	27 (81%)

Table 3: Differentiation of cartilage from limb mesoderm cultured either isolated or associated with various tissues or organs.

	Control "M" mesoderm alone		M + limb ectoderm		M + non-limb ectoderm		M + neural tube and notochord		M + various tissues	
Stage of donor embryos	No. of explants	cartilage	No. of explants	cartilage	No. of explants	cartilage	No. of explants	cartilage	No. of explants	cartilage
17 (29 - 32s)	107	13 (12%)	31	26 (83%)	18	15 (83%)	36	11 (30%)	22	13 (59%)
15 - 16 (24 - 28s)	111	3 (2%)	33	27 (81%)	24	16 (66%)	32	1 (3%)	22	1 (4%)

Table 4: Results according to the stage of explantation. Pore size of the filter: 0.4 and 0.6 µm.

Stage of donor embryos (H and H)	Total no. of pairs of explants	Experiment. Differentiation of cartilage	Control. Differentiation of cartilage
14 (21 - 23s)	12	7 (60%)	0
15 - 16 (24 - 28s)	29	17 (58%)	2 (6%)
17 (29 - 32s)	33	27 (81%)	19 (57%)
18	4	4	4

Table 5: Stage 15 - 16. Results according to the pore size of the filter.

Pore size	Total no. of pairs of explants	Experiment. Differentiation of cartilage	Control. Differentiation of cartilage
0.2 µm	18	1 (5%)	0
0.4 µm	9	4 (44%)	0
0.6 µm	20	13 (65%)	2
0.8 to 1 µm	15	12 (80%)	0

REFERENCES

Chevallier, A., Kieny, M., Mauger, A., 1976, Sur l'origine de la musculature de l'aile chez les Oiseaux, C.R. Acad. Sci. (Paris), 282, 309 - 311.

Chevallier, A., Kieny, M., Mauger, A., 1977, Limb-somite relationship: origin of the limb musculature, J. Embryol. exp. Morph., 41, 245 - 258.

Chevallier, A., Kieny, M., Mauger, A., 1978, Limb-somite relationship: effect of removal of somitic mesoderm on the wing musculature, J. Embryol. exp. Morph., 43, 263 - 278.

Christ, B., Jacob, H.J., Jacob, M., 1974, Experimentelle Untersuchungen mit Wachtel- und Hühnerembryonen, Experientia, 30, 1446 - 1448.

Christ, B., Jacob, H.J., Jacob, M., 1977, Experimental analysis of the origin of the wing musculature in avian embryos, Anat. Embryol., 150, 171 - 186.

Gumpel-Pinot, M., 1972, Culture in vitro de l'ébauche de l'aile de l'embryon de Poulet. Role de l'ectoderme sur la chondrogenèse, C.R. Acad. Sci. (Paris), 274, 2786 - 2789.

Gumpel-Pinot, M., 1973, Culture in vitro du bourgeon de l'aile de l'embryon de Poulet. Differenciation du cartilage, Ann. Biol., 12, 417 - 428.

Gumpel-Pinot, M., 1974, Contribution du mésoderme somitique à la genèse du membre chez l'embryon d'Oiseau, C.R. Acad. Sci. (Paris), 279, 1305 - 1308.

Gumpel-Pinot, M., 1980, Ectoderm and mesoderm interactions in the limb bud of the chick embryo studied by transfilter cultures: cartilage differentiation and ultrastructural observations, J. Embryol. exp. Morph., 59, 157 - 173.

Gumpel-Pinot, M., 1981, Ectoderm-mesoderm interactions in relation to limb bud chondrogenesis in the chick embryo: transfilter cultures and ultrastructural studies, J. Embryol. exp. Morph., (submitted).

Hamburger, V., Hamilton, H.L., 1951, A series of normal stages in the development of the chick embryo, J. Morph., 88, 49 - 92.

Kieny, M., Chevallier, A., 1979, Autonomy of tendon development in the embryonic chick wing, J. Embryol. exp. Morph., 49, 153 - 165.

Kieny, M., Mauger, A., Chevallier, A., Sengel, Ph., 1979, Origine embryologique des muscles lisses cutanés chez les Oiseaux, Arch. Anat. micr., 68, 283 - 290.

Saxen, L., 1977, Morphogenetic tissue interactions: an introduction, in: "Cell interactions in differentiation", (M. Karkinen-Jaäskeläinen, L. Saxen, L. Weiss, eds.), pp. 145 - 151, Academic Press, New York.

Wolff, Et., 1961, Utilisation de la membrane vitelline de l'oeuf de Poule en culture organotypique. I. Technique et possibilités, Develop. Biol., 3, 767 - 786.

Wolff, Et., Haffen, K., 1952, Sur une méthode de culture d'organes embryonnaires in vitro, Texas Rep. Biol. Med., 10, 463 - 472.

Zwilling, E., 1961, Limb morphogenesis, in: "Advances in Morphogenesis", (M. Abercrombie, J. Brachet, eds.), pp. 301 - 330, Academic Press, New York.

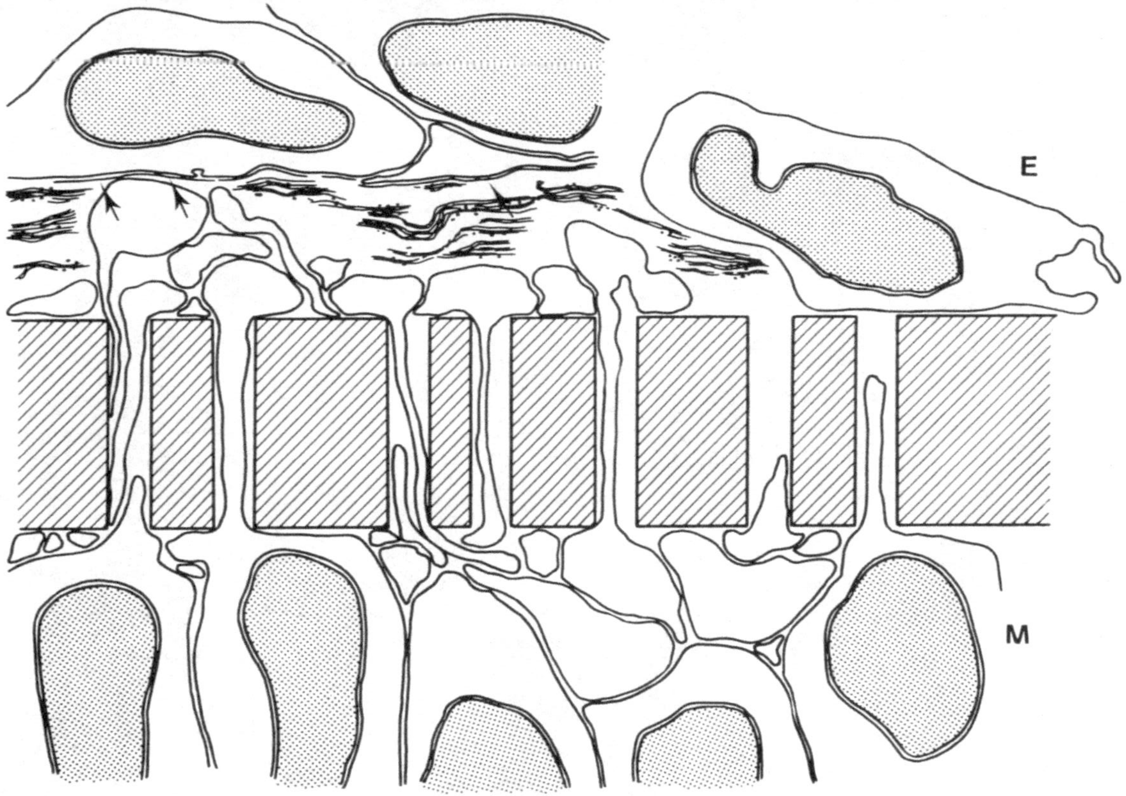

<u>Fig. 1</u>: Schematic representation of the relation between limb ectoderm and mesoderm through a Nuclepore filter (the thickness of the filter has been considerably reduced).
E = ectoderm; M = mesoderm; → = basement membrane

Role of the Ectoderm in Limb Development of Normal and Mutant Mouse (Disorganization, Pupoid Foetus) and Fowl (Talpid[3]) Embryos

D. A. Ede

Department of Zoology, University of Glasgow, Developmental Biology Building, 124 Observatory Road, Glasgow G12 9LU, U.K.

Disorganization (Ds)

This mouse mutant (Fig. 1, 2) has been described by HUMMEL (1958, 1959) and is probably the most complex ever to have been investigated, in respect of the variety of its pathological effects. It is a particularly difficult mutant to investigate and maintain since the effects of the gene are rarely the same in different individuals; futhermore, the penetrance of the gene is low; ranging, as HUMMEL found, from 9% in 129 hybrids to 89% in C3H hybrids. Three types of abnormality are commonly manifested in heterozygotes of this mutant.

(1) In about 1/3 there are abnormalities of the limbs, which often take the form of polydactyly, but of a particular sort (Fig. 3 - 6). Unlike most mutant polydactylies, any limb may be affected, usually not more than one, and the polydactyly is of no particular type, i.e. it may be preaxial, central or postaxial, and the number of individual digits may be greatly increased up to approximately twice the normal number. Also, there are sometimes additional limbs situated close to the normal limbs and smaller limb-like projections in other regions of the body, particularly on the belly.

(2) The second type of abnormality is represented by papillae of variable size and shape projecting from the surface of the body. These merge in type with the limb-like projections I have mentioned, when they contain cartilage and bone, but others resemble urogenital papillae and some are merely filled with loose connective tissue.

(3) The third type of abnormality, which occurs in about half of the embryos, is cranioschisis and exencephaly, i.e. failure of the neural tube to close in the brain region and exposure of this tissue as a large mass in the head region.

Clearly in this mutant both neural ectoderm and epidermis are affected and the series of stuctures ranging from virtually empty cyst-like projections to projections which have the basic form of limbs suggests that the polydactyly might also be of ectodermal origin, that is, abnormal outgrowth of ectoderm adjoining the limb bud may occur, which would become filled with the proliferating mesoderm of the limb bud which would then differentiate accordingly. If far away from the normal limb field, such projections would show only a parody of normal limb development, but within the field they might contribute to the limb itself and be subject to normal limb bud controls. This would be consistent with the view of AMPRINO (AMPRINO and AMBROSI, 1973; AMPRINO, 1977) that an important aspect of limb development is the biomechanical modelling role exerted by the ectoderm on the underlying mesoderm. On the other hand, besides the papillae arising from the surface of the embryo, other misplaced organoids and tissues occur within the body, as reported by HUMMEL, in the form of nodules embedded in musculature or suspended in body cavities. These appear to have no ectodermal component whatever.

Teratology of the Limbs

The Disorganization mouse represents at present an embryological mystery. Its effects in heterozygote are manifested at a relatively late stage since there is no indication, although there are many instances of later organizational duplications, of duplications of the primary organizer. Some basic cellular defect appears to occur throughout the body affecting control of transcription or possibly translation of the genetic message. However this cellular defect is controlled or regulated in most places, and in some or many individuals depending upon the strain, it is controlled in all places so that normal embryos are produced, but sometimes and in some places the genetic control is disrupted so that totally abnormal cell systems of proliferation and differentiation are produced in quite inappropriate positions in the body. It appears that one of the most common sites for this abnormal proliferation and differentiation, in which it is sometimes harmonized with the developing organ at that site, is in the limb fields.

Pupoid foetus

Pupoid foetus is an almost equally bizarre mouse mutant but one which is much easier to investigate since all homozygous mice are affected. In this case the mutant is distinctly an ectodermal one. Once again embryos complete their development to birth but are invariably eaten by the mothers since they are grossly abnormal. The mutant was originally described by MEREDITH (1965) who picked it out in a search for limb mutants. The limbs appear at first sight to be extremely short and undifferentiated but in fact the whole embryo is cocooned in an epidermis which shows evidence of unusually great cellular proliferation. Within this epidermal cocoon the remaining structures of the embryo, including all internal organs, are virtually normal, with some distortions of the skeleton which can probably be attributed to the mechanically constricting effect of the epidermis during growth (Fig. 7 , 8).

The abnormality is manifested comparatively late in development and appears first between 11 and 12 days of development as patches in which the boundary between the ectodermal and mesodermal layers of the skin is hard to define. These areas are related to regions which first become innervated by nerves growing out from the neural tube to form the peripheral sensory nerves. The relation between the termination of these nerves and the abnormal skin areas becomes increasingly obvious as development proceeds and in both regions, neural and epidermal, there appears to be an abnormal growth causing undue thickening of the epidermal region to form patches of abnormal skin which become larger and gradually merge with each other and beneath them peripheral nerve endings which themselves become excessively branched and actually in some cases penetrate into the epidermis and beyond it so that their terminations are free within the amniotic fluid. Furthermore, it appears that cells break through from the underlying mesenchyme onto the surface of the skin to form an additional layer of cells. It seems most likely (EDE and WATSON, in preparation) that these cells are in fact Schwann cells which are proliferated in excessive numbers and migrate along the peripheral nerves, burst through the epidermal mesodermal boundary and emerge onto the surface of the skin. Although MEREDITH believed that the limbs were affected, it appears that the effect is a purely mechanical one. They are indeed considerably shorter than the normal limbs and while all of the proximal elements are present the limb appears to stop short at the metacarpal and metatarsal bones, the phalanges being virtually undeveloped (Fig. 9 - 12). Histologically the limbs are perfectly normal and it appears that the failure of outgrowth is entirely the result of the mechanical restriction imposed by the abnormal epidermis.

Talpid^3

In this mutant of the fowl, studies by EDE and co-workers (reviewed EDE, 1976) have concentrated upon the effects which the gene has upon the limb and in particular upon abnormalities in the form and activity of the limb mesoderm cells. But in fact the genetic effects are apparent throughout homozygous mutant embryos and are not limited to mesodermal cells. The effect of the gene upon the ectoderm has become most evident in recent studies (EDE and FLINT, in preparation) on the developing brain in normal and talpid^3 embryos. We have found that it is a normal feature of stage 19 chick embryos that cracks appear in the neural tube wall on the ridge between ventricles. These appear to be formed as a result of mechanical distortions produced by the morphogenetic changes in shape of the originally tubular neural tube. They appear as tumour-like excrescences of neural cells, and in normal embryos they heal and disappear by about stage 22. In talpid^3 embryos, on the other hand, they appear as in the normal, but become more numerous and obvious as development progresses. The internal surface of the brain of talpid^3 embryo at stage 23 usually shows many of these tumour-like excrescences of loose cells.

The reason for this failure to produce a smooth internal brain surface in the mutant is probably related to the disordered arrangement of the neuroectoderm cells. In the normal brain at these stages they are arranged as a palisade layer, with the nuclei at approximately the same levels and with the very attenuated cytoplasmic cell bodies stretching directly from inner to outer neural surface without much intermingling with neighbours (Fig. 13). But in the mutant they are jumbled, with nuclei at different levels and the cytoplasm of neighbouring cells twisted together (Fig. 14).

This disorderly arrangement of the neuroectoderm cells appears to reflect a general effect of the talpid^3 gene upon the cell surface, which has been described in detail for the limb mesenchyme cell (EDE, 1976) and which produces there the disordered arrangement of the cartilage cells in the skeletal rudiments. The mutant cells are not polarized as normal cells are, and connect with their neighbours by filopodia produced all over the cytoplasmic surface. This produces in the limb ectoderm a disturbance of the normal palisade arrangement of the cells and a much tighter bonding between the cells of the basal layer (Fig. 15 , 16) which has been described in TEM studies by EDE, BELLAIRS and BANCROFT (1974).

This tighter bonding between the limb ectoderm cells may be expected to alter the mechanical properties of the ectodermal covering of the limb bud. It is a possibility that the characteristic modification of limb outgrowth in this mutant, producing a fan-shaped limb bud with polydactyly, might be produced by mechanical restrictions imposed by the altered ectodermal jacket. Experiments by SHAMSLAHIDJANI and EDE (Ms in preparation) have been designed to test this possibility by making reciprocal exchanges of normal talpid^3 ectoderm/mesoderm in limb buds grafted to normal hosts, using both mutant mesoderms and dissociated mesoderm cells packed back into ectodermal jackets.

For technical reasons the mesodermal component in these grafts is from stage 19 - 20 embryos, the ectoderm from stage 22 embryos. Resulting grafts were removed at total age of 10 - 11 days. The result show that when ectoderm and mesoderm are from the same genotype the characteristic form of the normal and mutant limbs are produced (Fig. 17 , 18). When normal whole mesoderm is cultured in a talpid^3 jacket all of the normal proximodistal sequence of skeletal elements is produced (though with reduction of elements in the antero-posterior axis), but they are bent back from the carpals or tarsals. Talpid³ mesoderm in normal jackets show the usual proximo-distal sequence (Fig. 19, 21), and no bending back (Fig. 20, 22). Normal elements are not shortened, and talpid³ elements are not lengthened. It appears that the ectoderm has had no effect on the early growth of the limbs in either case, but that the mutant ectoderm has had a restriction on the outward extension of the distal elements, causing them to be bent backwards. In those cases where the mesoderm has been dissociated (Fig. 23 - 26) even this bending back is not seen. The resulting limbs clearly express the genotype of the mesoderm, the ectoderm in this case having had no effect. Presumably the dissociated mesoderm has not grown so vigorously as the whole mesoderm, and the confining effect of the jacket has not been felt even at the late stages. We conclude that the characteristic abnormalities of the talpid³ limb are of mesodermal origin and that the effect of the epidermal basal layer disorganization is very slight.

ACKNOWLEDGEMENT

I wish to thank the SRC for financial support in this work.

REFERENCES

Amprino, R., 1977, Experimental study on the morphogenetic relationship between ectoderm and mesoderm in the developing chick embryo limb bud, Acta Embryol. Exp., 1, 51 - 70.

Amprino, R., Ambrosi, G., 1973, Experimental analysis of the chick embryo limb bud growth, Arch. Biol. (Bruxelles), 84, 35 - 86.

Ede, D.A., 1976, Cell interactions in vertebrate limb development, in: "The Cell Surface in Animal Development", (G. Poste, G. Nicolson, eds.), pp. 495 - 543, North-Holland Publ. Co., Amsterdam.

Ede, D.A, Bellairs, R., Bancroft, M., 1974, A scanning electron microscope study of the early limb bud in normal and talpid³ mutant chick embryos, J. Embryol. exp. Morph., 31, 761 - 785.

Hummel, K.P., 1958, The inheritance and expression of Disorganization, an unusual mutation in the mouse, J. exp. Zool., 137, 389 - 424.

Hummel, K.P., 1959, Developmental anomalies in mice resulting from action of the gene Disorganization, a semi-dominant lethal, Pediatrics, 23, 212 - 221.

Meredith, R., 1965, Genetic and embryological studies of some congenital malformations in the mouse, Institute of Biology, Thesis for full membership.

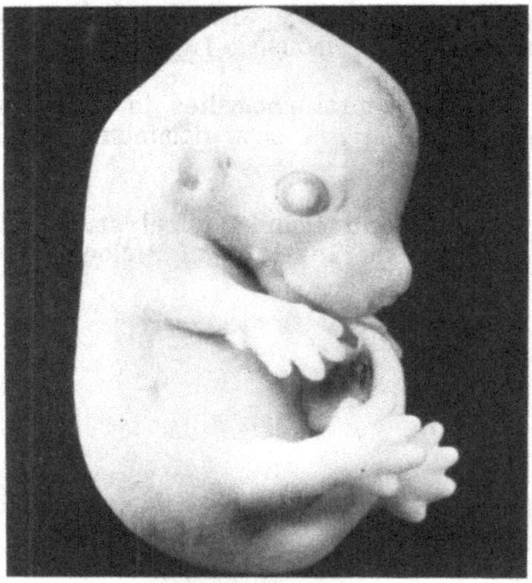

Fig. 1: Normal (+/+) mouse embryo, 15 days.

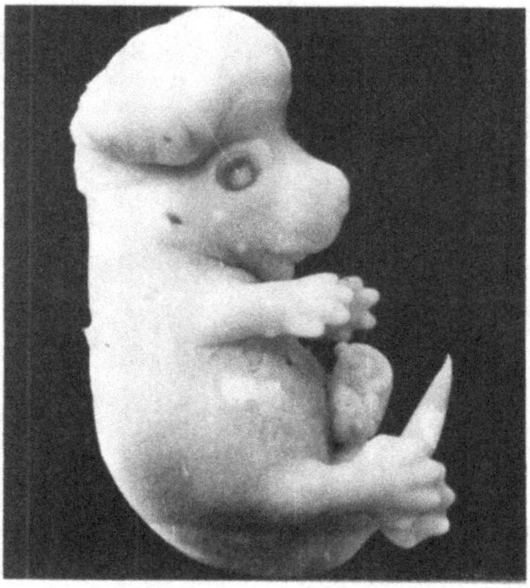

Fig. 2: Disorganization (Ds/+) mouse embryo, 15 days.

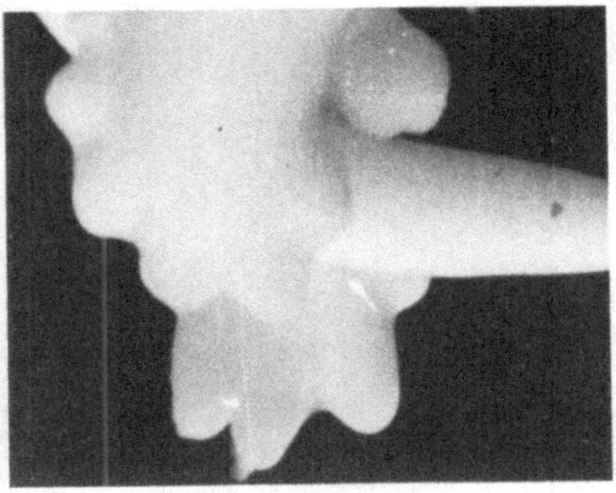

Fig. 3: Hind region of +/+ 15-d embryo, showing normal hind limb.

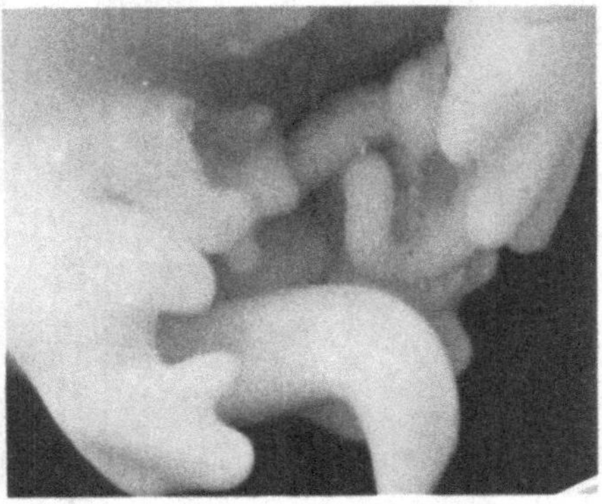

Fig. 4: Hind region of Ds/+ 15-d embryo showing limb-like projection at base of hind limb.

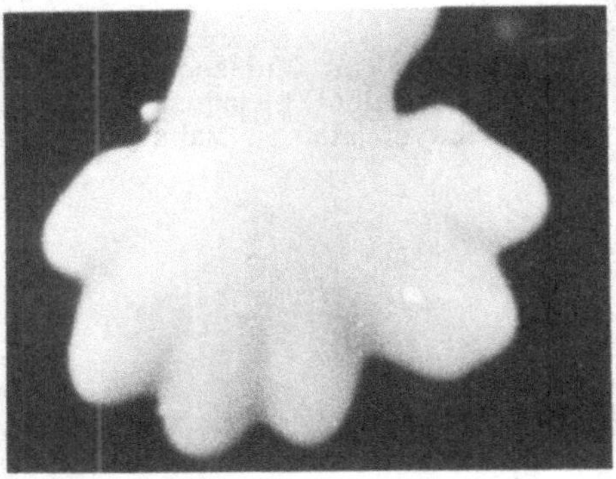

Fig. 5: Hind limb of Ds/+ 15-d embryo, showing pre-axial polydactyly.

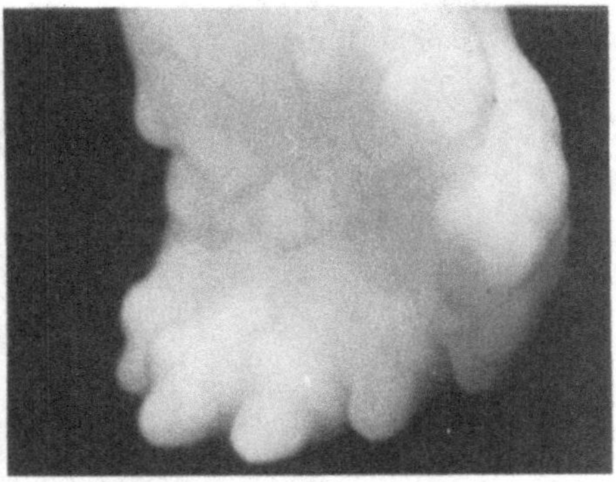

Fig. 6: Hind limb of Ds/+ 18-d embryo, with doubling of digit number.

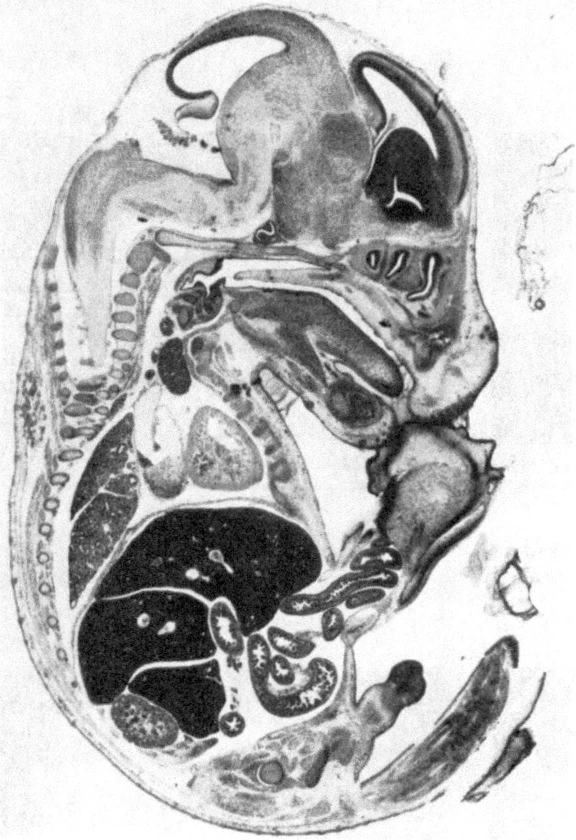

Fig. 7: Mid-sagittal section o
normal (+/+) mouse embryo, 16
days, stained Mallory.

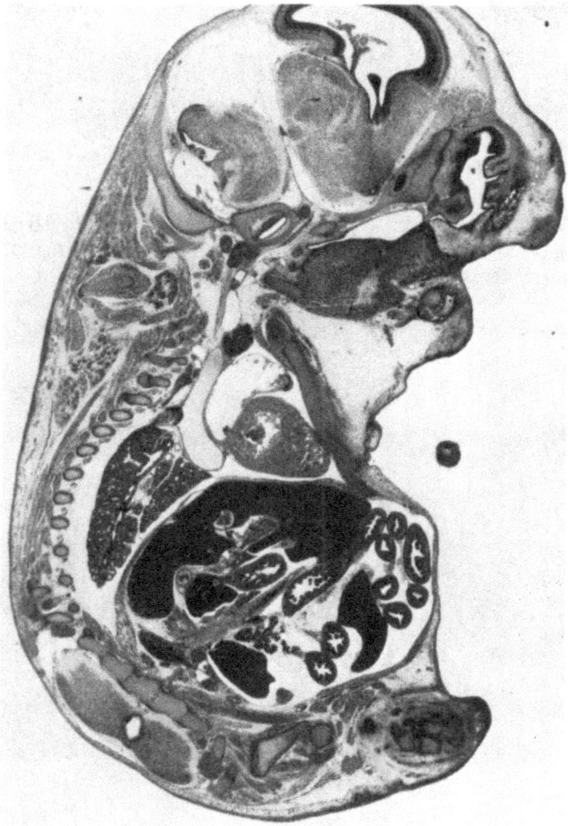

Fig. 8: Mid-sagittal section o
pupoid foetus (pf/pf) mouse em
bryo, 16 days, stained Mallory

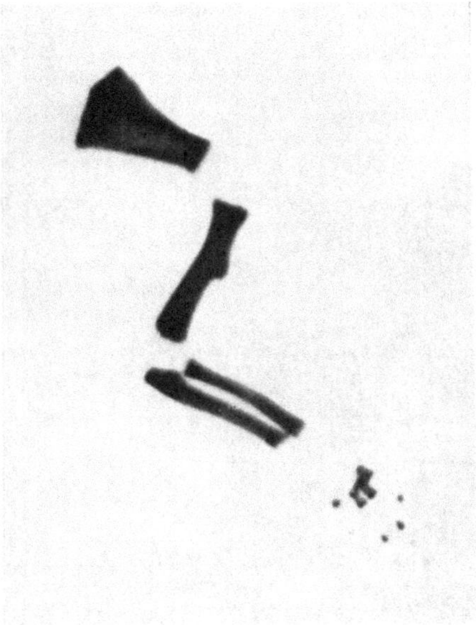

Fig. 9: Fore-limb of +/+ full term embryo, stained Alizarin Red-S to show bones.

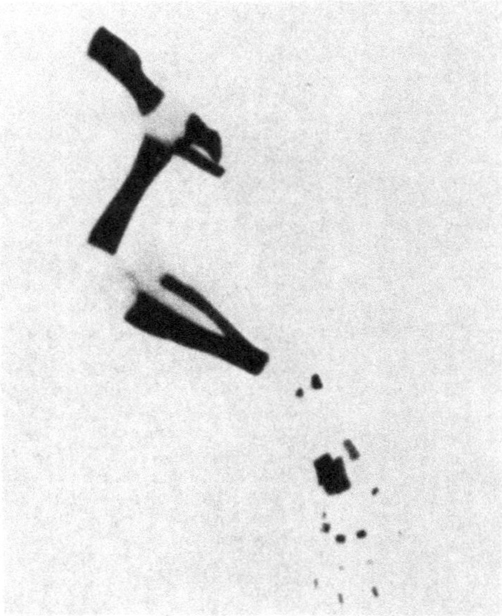

Fig. 10: Hind-limb of +/+ full term embryo.

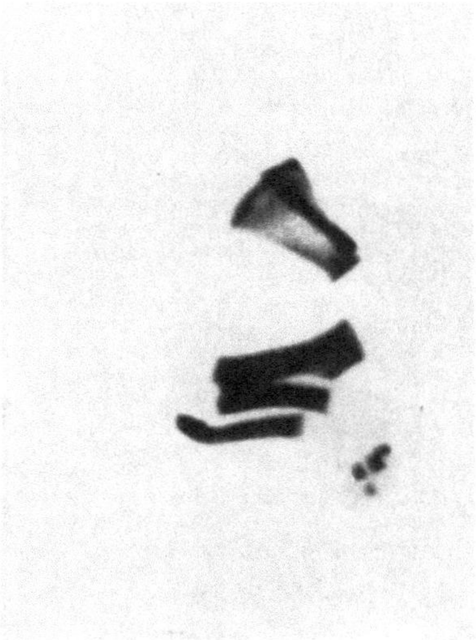

Fig. 11: Fore-limb of pf/pf full-term embryo.

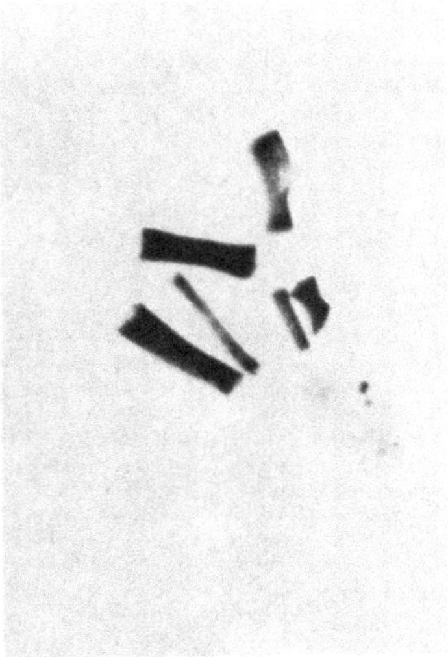

Fig. 12: Hind-limb of pf/pf full-term embryo.

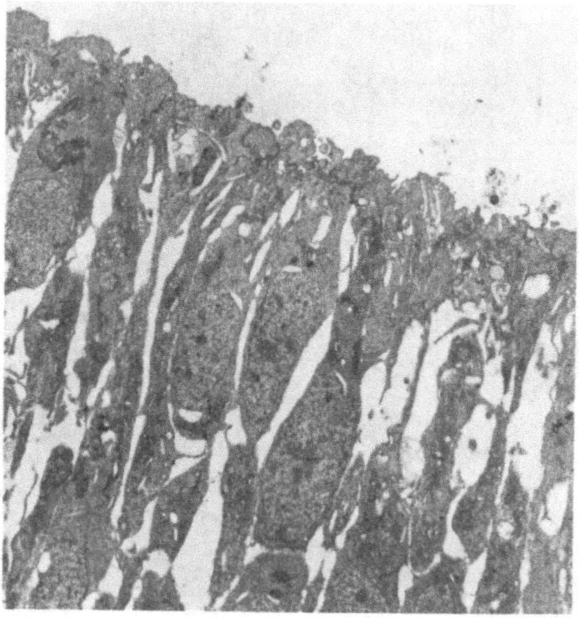

Fig. 13: TEM view of neural ectoderm in brain region of normal fowl embryo, stage 22. x 2 500.

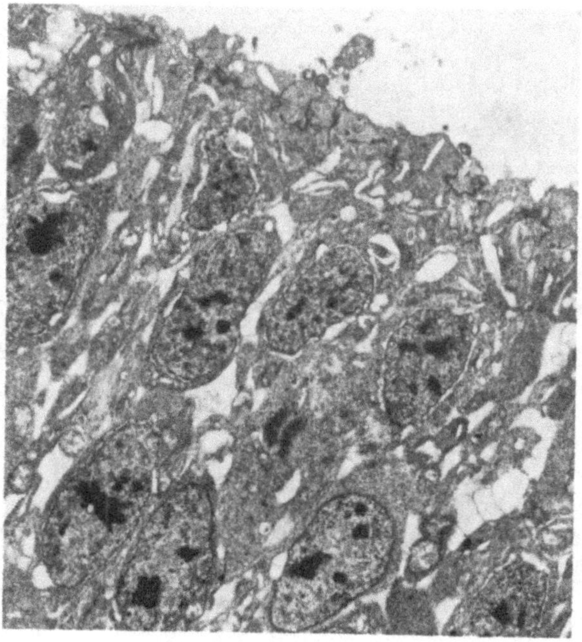

Fig. 14: TEM view of neural ectoderm in brain region of talpid[3] (ta^3/ta^3) fowl embryo, stage 22. x 2 500.

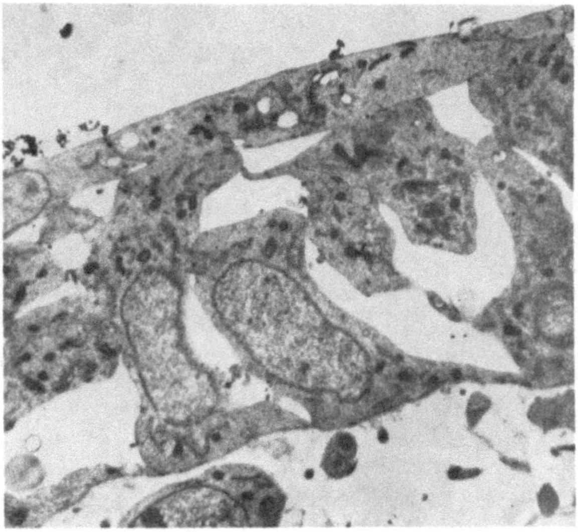

Fig. 15: TEM view of ectoderm from limb bud of normal fowl embryo, stage 25. x 9 000.

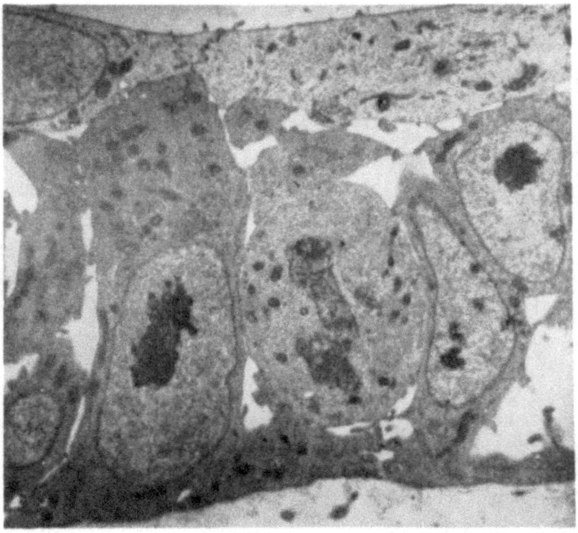

Fig. 16: TEM view of ectoderm from limb bud of talpid[3] (ta^3/ta^3) fowl embryo, stage 25. x 9 000.

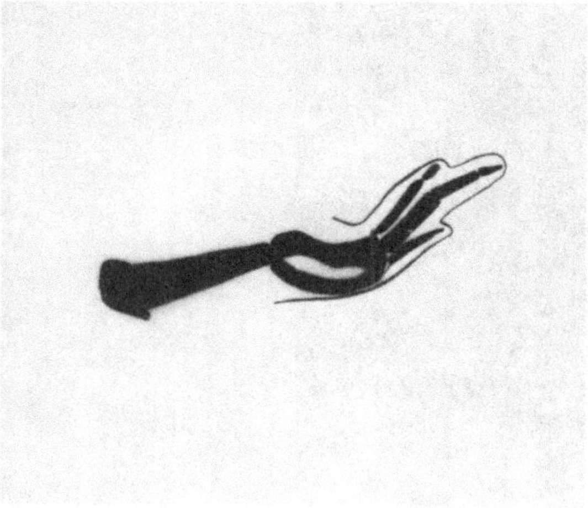

Fig. 17: Grafted wing from intact normal mesoderm in normal ectodermal jacket. Stained Alcian Blue.

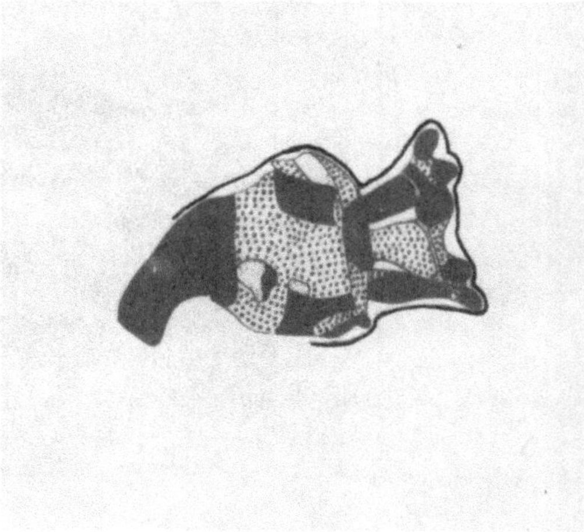

Fig. 18: Grafted wing from intact talpid3 mesoderm in talpid3 ectodermal jacket.

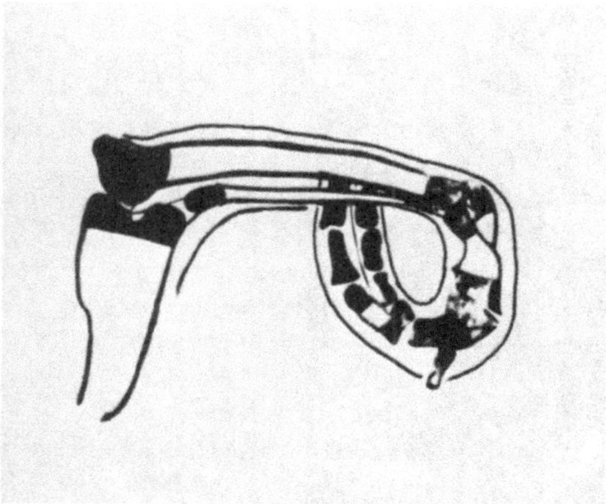

Fig. 19: Grafted leg from intact normal mesoderm in talpid3 ectodermal jacket.

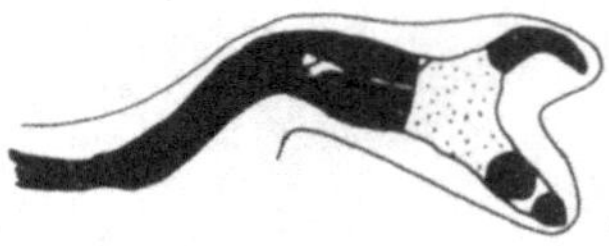

Fig. 20: Grafted leg from intact talpid3 mesoderm in normal ectodermal jacket.

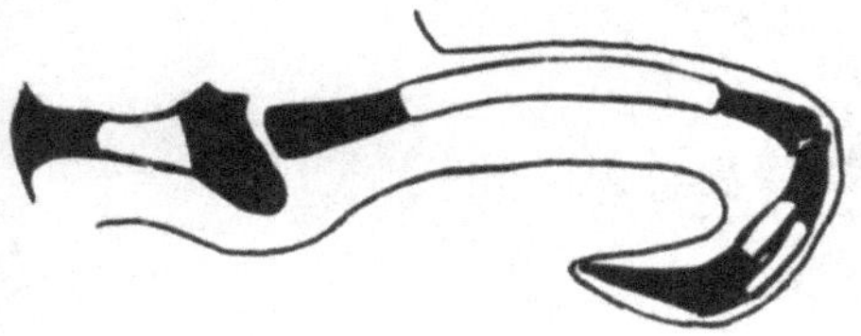

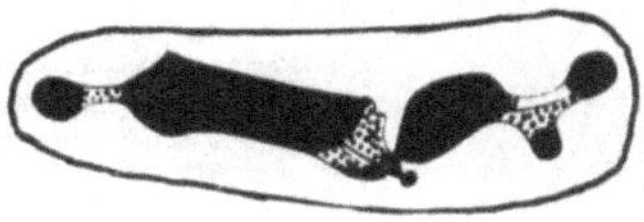

Fig. 21: Grafted wing from intact normal mesoderm in *talpid*^{3} ectodermal jacket.

Fig. 22: Grafted wing from intact *talpid*^{3} mesoderm in normal ectodermal jacket.

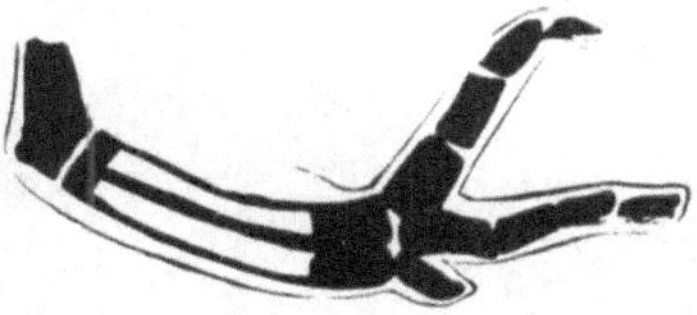

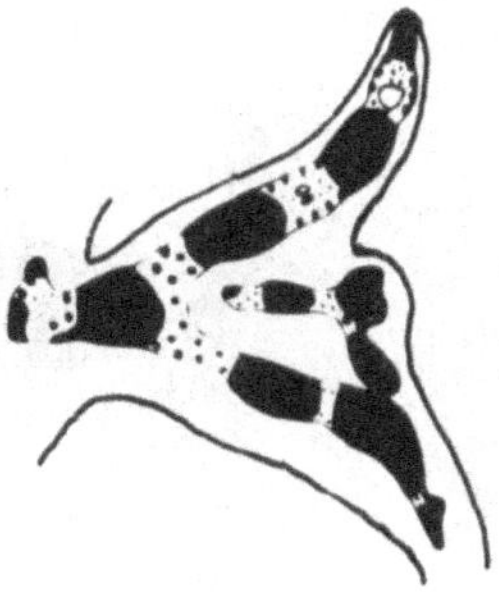

Fig. 23: Grafted leg from dissociated normal mesoderm in normal ectodermal jacket.

Fig. 24: Grafted leg from dissociated *talpid*^{3} mesoderm in *talpid*^{3} ectodermal jacket.

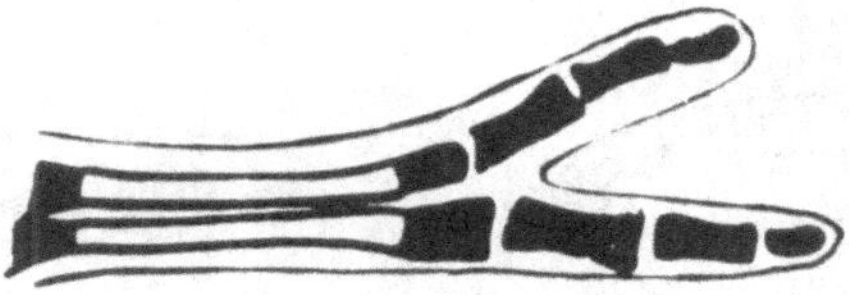

Fig. 25: Grafted leg from dissociated normal mesoderm in talpid^3 ectodermal jacket.

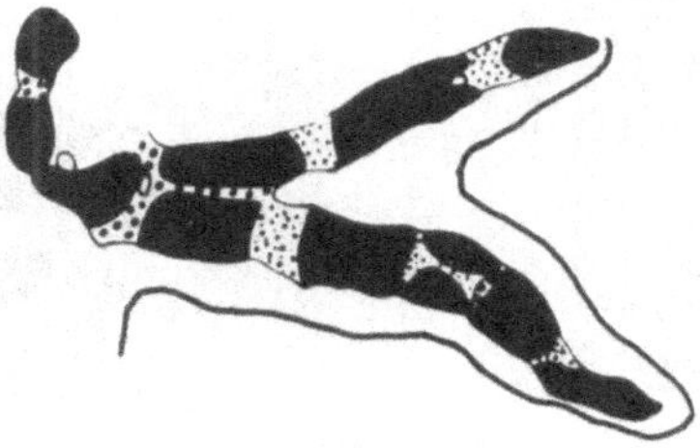

Fig. 26: Grafted leg from dissociated talpid^3 mesoderm in normal ectodermal jacket.

Origin, Distribution and Determination of Chick Limb Mesenchymal Cells

B. Christ and H. J. Jacob

Ruhr-Universität Bochum, Institut für Anatomie, Arbeitsgruppe für Experimentelle Embryologie
Universitätsstraße 150, D-4630 Bochum 1

During the third day of chick development the limb buds appear as thickenings of the lateral body wall. They are covered by the ectoderm and demarcated from the coelomic cavity by an epithelium representing the prospective serous membrane. Between the epithelial layers a mass of still undifferentiated mesenchymal cells can be observed (Fig. 1).

This early limb bud mesenchyme gives rise to several different tissues like muscles, cartilage, soft connective tissue and tendons which all can be found arranged in a characteristic spatial pattern at a later stage. Various aspects of cellular diversification as well as pattern formation have been investigated during the last few years (cf. CAPLAN and KOUTROUPAS, 1973; DIENSTMAN et al., 1974; TICKLE et al., 1975; WILBY and EDE, 1975; NEWMAN, 1977, 1980).

Our approach to the problem of early limb bud mesenchyme development had led to the following two questions: from which sources do the limb bud mesenchymal cells arise and does the early limb bud mesenchyme represent a uniform and pluripotent cell population?

Whereas it is generally accepted that the somatopleure gives rise to the limb bud mesenchyme, the role of the somites remained a matter of controversy (FISCHEL, 1895; MURRAY, 1927; SAUNDERS, 1948; STRAUS and RAWLES, 1953; PINOT, 1970; HAMBURGER, 1938, 1939). GRIM (1970) and GUMPEL-PINOT (1974) found that somite cells participate in wing development. Since these observations did not permit conclusions concerning the developmental fate of somite cells within the wing, we used the quail-chick marker system advocated by LE DOUARIN and BARQ (1969) to further investigate this problem. Owing to the distinctive structures of quail and chick interphase nuclei it is possible to identify the two cell types in quail-chick chimaeras and to observe their migration and development for long periods of time.

In our first series of experiments chick somite mesoderm from the wing or leg level was replaced by equivalent quail material before the development of secondary mesenchyme had taken place. Two to three days after grafting, numerous quail cells were found within the wing bud mesenchyme. Their occurrence was restricted to the myogenic zones and their numbers decreased in the proximo-distal direction (CHRIST et al., 1974, 1977 a,b).

After longer subsequent incubation periods, quail cells were observed to be limited to the muscle primordia which consisted of mixed populations of quail and chick cells (Fig. 2). Quail nuclei were found to be situated within myoblasts and myotubes whereas the fibroblasts of the muscular connective tissue and tendons exhibited nuclei of the chick type. Studies of CHEVALLIER et al. (1977 a,b, 1978) gave further evidence to support the somitic origin of limb musculature.

Teratology of the Limbs

In order to verify this concept we replaced the somatopleural epithelium of the prospective wing or leg region of chick hosts by somatopleure of quail embryos. Two to three days after grafting, a mixed population of chick and quail cells was found in the myogenic zones of limb anlagen, whereas the dermis as well as the chondrogenic area were exclusively made up of quail cells (CHRIST et al., 1977a). After further development within all parts of the limbs, chimaeric muscle organs could be seen in which the myotubes contain chick nuclei while the fibroblasts of endomysium, epimysium as well as of the tendons were regularly of quail origin (Fig. 3). Hybrid myotubes could not be found (CHRIST and JACOB, 1978 a; CHRIST et al., 1977 a,b, 1979 b).

The results mentioned clearly show that in avian embryos mesenchymal limb bud cells originate from two sources; cells which differentiate into muscle cells derive from the somites, whereas cells which later make up cartilage and connective tissues are of somatopleural origin.

We then investigated, from which part of the somites myogenic cells originate and on which pathways they reach their later position. As was first pointed out by GRIM (1970) myoblasts already differentiated within the myotome did not participate in wing myogenesis. However, the same author described cells lacking myogenesis coming from the ventral edges of the brachial dermatomes, which later were integrated into the wing mesenchyme where they could no longer be distinguished from the somatopleural cells.

Detachment and migration of somite cells at the wing level begins to take place at stage 14 (according to HAMBURGER and HAMILTON, 1951) when all brachial somites have been formed (CHRIST et al., 1977 a; JACOB et al., 1978). The wing buds are not yet distinguishable. Embryos at stages 15 and 16 show numerous transversally oriented cells between brachial somites and the wing region and, in stage 17-embryos when wing bud outgrowth has started, the cells continue to migrate. It should be mentioned that these myogenic cells exclusively originate from the dermatome at its lateral edges (JACOB et al., 1978; CHRIST and JACOB, 1978 b). The conclusion that the limb musculature mainly originates from the myotome (CHEVALLIER et al., 1977 b) can therefore not be supported.

Possible causes for the directional movement of these cells remain to be discussed. Although this process is basically not yet understood, environmental factors as well as cell behaviour must be involved. When migration of myogenic cells begins, an extracellular fibrillar network can be found within the space between somites and somatopleure (JACOB et al., 1978, 1979). The fibrils are mainly transversally oriented and sometimes show faint crossbands, which allow the assumption that they consist of collagen. The elongated cells which previously have broken through the incomplete basal membrane are regularly polarized in a medio-lateral direction (Fig. 4). Their laterally directed leading ends branch into thin processes which contact the surrounding fibrils. These cell processes contain many microfilaments which are arranged parallel to their long axis and are especially dense among those parts of the cell membrane, which are in contact with extracellular fibrils. In thicker cell processes microtubuli are found. The Golgi-field is seen to be situated in the medial part of the cells which, according to TRELSTAD et al. (1967), can therefore be considered as the trailing end of a migrating cell. Migration processes at the wing and leg levels do not fundamentally differ except for the fact that at the leg level migration starts at stage 16 and that the migrating cells are often found to be arranged in a chain-like manner (JACOB et al., 1979). According to numerous papers dealing with ultrastructural features and behaviour of migrating cells (cf. WEISS, 1961; EBENDAL, 1976, 1977; MARKWALD et al., 1977), myogenic cells use the alignment of the fibrillar substratum for orientation in the sense of contact guidance.

The question arises whether the concept of somitic contribution to limb development as studied in avian embryos may be applied to mammalian embryos. As shown by MILAIRE (1976) and HOUBEN (1976) somitic cells similarly participate in leg development of the mouse embryo. The migration modalities of these cells seem to resemble those observed in the avian embryo. Recent studies on human embryos (CHRIST and WACHTLER, unpublished data) show cells between somites and limb bud somatopleure which may correspond to the described migrating cells in avian embryos (Fig. 5). Because the contributions of somitic cells to limb bud development are quite similar in avian and mammalian embryos, basic differences do not seem to exist between embryos of higher vertebrates in regard to the developmental fate of these cells.

Reconsidering the above mentioned second problem it may be asked: are the mesenchymal cells of the early limb bud already determined by their different origin or does their determination depend on their position in the limb bud as suggested by ZWILLING (1966); SEARLS and JANNERS (1969) and CAPLAN and KOUTROUPAS (1973).

In order to test the differentiating abilities of somatopleural cells, wing or leg parts of the somatopleural mesoderm which had not yet been invaded by somitic cells, were isolated from quail donors and then grafted into the coelomic cavity or onto the chorioallantoic membrane of chick hosts. About 100 grafts were examined 2 to 12 days after the operation. Histological examinations of the developed structures showed that skeletal elements as well as the dermis were found well developed in their normal position. In the distal parts of the heterotopically grown limbs, tendons could be found (CHRIST et al., 1979 a,b). The rudimentary blood vessels within these grafts were composed of an endothelial layer which mainly consisted of chick cells and a tunica media made up of quail cells. From this it may be concluded that somatopleural cells are able to differentiate into smooth muscle cells. However, these grafts were always characterized by a total absence of skeletal musculature (Fig. 6). Between cartilage elements and dermis loosely arranged mesenchymal cells could be seen. Sometimes demarcated areas developed which showed numerous blood vessels. During further development these areas were found to differentiate into adipose tissue (CHRIST et al., 1979 b).

Summarizing the result of this grafting series it can be stated that somatopleural cells are able to differentiate into skeletal elements, smooth muscle tissue, tendons and soft connective tissue. No indication could be found that somatopleural cells can undergo muscular differentiation. Skeletal muscle cells were only found in those grafts which have grown within the coelomic cavity and which were found to be attached to the inner surface of the lateral body wall. Myotubes of these grafts showed, without exception, nuclei of the chick type (CHRIST, unpublished results). Therefore it must be assumed that the grafts were invaded by somitic cells of the host embryo.

Our findings that somatopleural cells had a limited ability for differentiation are in agreement with observations on clonal cell cultures of limb bud mesenchymal cells (DIENSTMAN et al., 1974; NEWMAN, 1977, 1980) and were recently confirmed by experimental studies on the development of the pectoralis major muscle in the avian embryo (BERESFORD et al., 1978). This, however, was questioned by CHEVALLIER et al. (1977 a,b) and by

McLACHLAN and HORNBRUCH (1979). Although both groups agree that during normal development the limb musculature originates from the somites, they suggest that under experimental conditions somatopleural cells may be able to compensate for the lack of somite myogenic cells.

McLACHLAN and HORNBRUCH (1979) base their conclusion on 34 retrieved grafts of wing somatopleure into the coelomic cavity. Fifteen of these had been isolated from quail donors at stages 14 to 20 and therefore may have already been invaded by somitic cells. Eight further grafts had been taken from embryos at stages 10 and 11, in which a clear separation between somitic and lateral plate mesoderm at the prospective wing level was not yet possible. Considering that eleven grafts remained and that five grafts did not show any musculature, the statement by the authors should be regarded with caution. The assumption of CHEVALLIER et al. (1977 a, b,) was based on two observations. After grafting somites from chick to quail, limb buds contained myotubes exhibiting chick and quail nuclei. Furthermore, in somatopleural parts of quail grown in place of a portion of the neural tube in chick host, muscle cells differentiated which were found to be of quail and chick origin. On the other hand, the same group has shown that after the destruction of brachial and adjacent somite mesoderm, muscleless wings developed (CHEVALLIER et al., 1978). In this case, however, somatopleural cells did not realize the assumed muscle-forming potential. Since the quail-to-chick somite grafting experiments by these authors failed to prove a participation of somatopleural cells in muscular differentiation the results are difficult to be interpreted.

Finally we would like to describe experiments begun by WACHTLER in our laboratory which were aimed at the determination state of those early limb bud mesenchymal cells which belong to the somitic lineage.

In two-stage grafting procedures quail-to-chick replacements of brachial somites were performed. After a subsequent incubation period of about 2 days the operated embryos (then at stages 19 - 22) were used as donors in the second step of the experiment, in which mesenchyme pieces containing myogenic somite cells of the quail graft were isolated from the wing bud and then grafted in place of a portion of the chondrogenic limb bud zone of chick host at the same stage. After a further incubation period of 2 - 7 days the distribution and differentiation of quail cells within the wing buds was studied. The results can be summarized as follows: although having been grafted into a central limb bud position, the vast majority of quail cells was found to have reached their normal position within the myogenic zone and have undergone muscular differentiation within normally situated muscles found distally of the implantation site (Fig. 7). Cartilage and soft connective tissue were normally distributed.

The problems of the origin, distribution and determination of early limb bud mesenchymal cells can be summarized as follows:

1.) Limb bud mesenchymal cells originate from the somatopleure and from the somites. These two cell lineages express different terminal phenotypes.

2.) Somatopleural cells differentiate into cartilage, smooth muscle tissue, soft connective tissue and tendons. Somite cells which immigrate in an undifferentiated state undergo muscular differentiation.

3.) From their origin onwards cells of both subpopulations are committed to either the myogenic or the non-myogenic lineage.

ACKNOWLEDGEMENTS

We would like to thank U. Ritenberg, I. Schaeben, I. Burks and H. Hake for expert technical assistance. Research supported by Grants Ch 44/2,3,4 from the Deutsche Forschungsgemeinschaft.

REFERENCES

Beresford, B., Le Lievre, C., Rathbone, M.P., 1978, Chimaera studies of the origin and formation of the pectoral musculature of the avian embryo, J. exp. Zool., 205, 321 - 326.

Caplan, A.J., Koutroupas, J., 1973, The control of muscle and cartilage development in the chick limb: the role of differential vascularisation, J. Embryol. exp. Morph., 29, 571 - 583.

Chevallier, A., Kieny, M., Mauger, A., 1977 a, Limb-somite relationship: origin of the limb musculature, J. Embryol. exp. Morph., 41, 245 - 258.

Chevallier, A., Kieny, M., Mauger, A., 1978, Limb-somite relationship: effect of removal of somitic mesoderm on the wing musculature, J. Embryol. exp. Morph., 43, 263 - 278.

Chevallier, A., Kieny, M., Mauger, A., Sengel, P., 1977 b, Developmental fate of the somitic mesoderm in the chick embryo, in: "Vertebrate Limb and Somite Morphogenesis", Brit. Soc. Devl. Biol. 3rd Symposium, (D.A. Ede, J.R. Hinchliffe and M. Balls, eds.), pp. 421 - 432, Cambridge University Press.

Christ, B., Jacob, H.J., 1978 a, Transplantationsexperimente mit Hühner- und Wachtelembryonen zur Frage der Herkunft der Extremitätenmuskulatur, in: "XIXth Morphological Congress Symposia, Charles University, Prague 1976" (E. Klika, ed.), pp. 109 - 117, Univerzita Karlova, Praha.

Christ, B., Jacob, H.J., 1978 b, Über die Entwicklung der Gliedmaßenmuskulatur, Medizin in unserer Zeit, 6, 166 - 176.

Christ, B., Jacob, H.J., Jacob, M., 1974, Über den Ursprung der Flügelmuskulatur. Experimentelle Untersuchungen mit Wachtel- und Hühnerembryonen, Experientia (Basel), 30, 1446 - 1448.

Christ, B., Jacob, H.J., Jacob, M., 1977 a, Experimental analysis of the origin of the wing musculature in avian embryos, Anat. Embryol., 150, 171 - 186.

Christ, B., Jacob, H.J., Jacob, M., 1977 b, Experimentelle Befunde zur Muskelentwicklung in den Extremitäten von Hühnerembryonen, Verh. Anat. Ges., 71, 1231 - 1237.

Christ, B., Jacob, H.J., Jacob, M., 1979 b, Differentiating abilities of avian somatopleural mesoderm, Experientia (Basel), 35, 1376 - 1378.

Christ, B., Hirschberg, M., Jacob, H.J., Jacob, M., 1979 a, Experimentelle Befunde zur Entwicklung der distalen Extremitätenmuskulatur, Verh. Anat. Ges., 73, 519 - 525.

Dienstman, S.R., Biehl, J., Holtzer, S., Holtzer, H., 1974, Myogenic and chondrogenic lineages in developing limb buds grown in vitro, Devl. Biol., 39, 83 - 95.

Ebendal, T., 1976, The relative roles of contact inhibition and contact guidance in orientation of axons extending on aligned collagen fibrils in vitro, Exp. Cell Res., 98, 159 - 169.

Ebendal, T., 1977, Extracellular matrix fibrils, and cell contacts in the chick embryo. Possible roles in orientation of cell migration and axon extension, Cell Tissue Res., 175, 439 - 458.

Fischel, A., 1895, Zur Entwicklung der vertebralen Rumpf- und der Extremitätenmuskulatur der Vögel und Säugetiere, Morph. Jb., 23, 544 - 561.

Grim, M., 1970, Differentiation of myoblasts and the relationship between somites and the wing bud of the chick embryo, Z. Anat. Entwickl. -Gesch., 132, 260 - 271.

Gumpel-Pinot, M., 1974, Contribution des mésoderme somitique a la genèse du membre chez l'embryon d'Oiseau, C. r. hedb. Séanc Acad. Sci., Paris, D 279, 1305 - 1308.

Hamburger, V., 1938, Morphogenetic and axial self-differentiation of transplanted limb primordia of 2-day chick embryos, J. exp. Zool., 77, 379 - 399.

Hamburger, V., 1939, The development and innervation of transplanted limb primordia of chick embryos, J. exp. Zool., 80, 347 - 389.

Hamburger, V., Hamilton, H.L., 1951, A series of normal stages in the development of the chick embryo, J. Morph., 88, 49 - 92.

Houben, J.-J.G., 1976, Aspects ultrastructuraux de la migration de cellules somitiques dans les bourgeons de membres postérieurs de souris, Arch. Biol. (Bruxelles), 87, 345 - 365.

Jacob, M., Christ, B., Jacob, H.J., 1978, On the migration of myogenic stem cells into the prospective wing region of chick embryos. A scanning and transmission electron microscope study, Anat. Embryol., 153, 179 - 193.

Jacob, M., Christ, B., Jacob, H.J., 1979, The migration of myogenic cells from the somites into the leg region of avian embryos, Anat. Embryol., 157, 291 - 309.

Le Douarin, N., Barq, G., 1969, Sur l'utilisation des cellules de la caille japonaise comme "marqueurs bilogiques" en embryologie expérimentale, C. r. hedb. Séanc. Acad. Sci., Paris, D 269, 1543 - 1546.

Markwald, R.R., Fitzharris, T.P., Manasek, F.J., 1977, Structural development of endocardial cushions, Am. J. Anat., 148, 85 - 120.

McLachlan, J.C., Hornbruch, A., 1979, Muscle-forming potential of the non-somitic cells of the early avian limb bud, J. Embryol. exp. Morph., 54, 209 - 217.

Milaire, J., 1976, Contribution cellulaire des somites a la genèse des bourgeons de membres postérieurs chez la souris, Arch. Biol. (Bruxelles), 87, 315 - 343.

Murray, P.D.F., 1927, Chorioallantoic grafts of fragments of two-day chick with special references to development of the limbs, intestine and skin, Australian J. exp. Biol. med. Sci., 4, 237 - 256.

Newman, S.A., 1977, Lineage and pattern in the developing wing bud, in: "Vertebrate Limb and Somite Morphogenesis", Brit. Soc. Devl. Biol. 3rd Symposium, (D.A. Ede, J.R. Hinchliffe, M. Balls, eds.), pp. 181 - 197.

Newman, S.A., 1980, Fibroblast progenitor cells of the embryonic chick limb, J. Embryol. exp. Morph., 56, 191 - 200.

Pinot, M., 1970, Le role du mésoderme somitique dans la morphogenèse précoce des membres de l'embryon de poulet, J. Embryol. exp. Morph., 23, 109 - 151.

Saunders, J.W., 1948, Do the somites contribute to the formation of the chick wing? Anat. Rec., 100, 756.

Searls, R.L., Janners, M.Y., 1969, The stabilisation of cartilage properties in the cartilage forming mesenchyme of the embryonic chick limb, J. exp. Zool., 170, 365 - 376.

Straus, W.L., Rawles, M.E., 1953, An experimental study of the origin of the trunk musculature and ribs in the chick, Am. J. Anat., 92, 471 - 509.

Tickle, C., Summerbell, D., Wolpert, L., 1975, Positional signalling and specification of digits in chick limb morphogenesis, Nature, 254, 199 - 202.

Trelstad, R.L., Hay, E.D., Revel, J.-P., 1967, Cell contact during early morphogenesis in the chick embryo, Devl. Biol., 16, 78 - 106.

Weiss, P., 1961, Guiding principles in cell locomotion and cell aggregation, Exp. Cell Res. (Supp.), 8, 260 - 281.

Wilby, O.K., Ede, D.A., 1975, A model generating the pattern of cartilage skeletal elements in the embryonic chick limb, J. theor. Biol., 50, 199 - 217.

Zwilling, E., 1966, Cartilage formation from so-called myogenic tissue of chick embryo limb buds, Annls. Med. exp. Biol. Fenn., 44, 134 - 139.

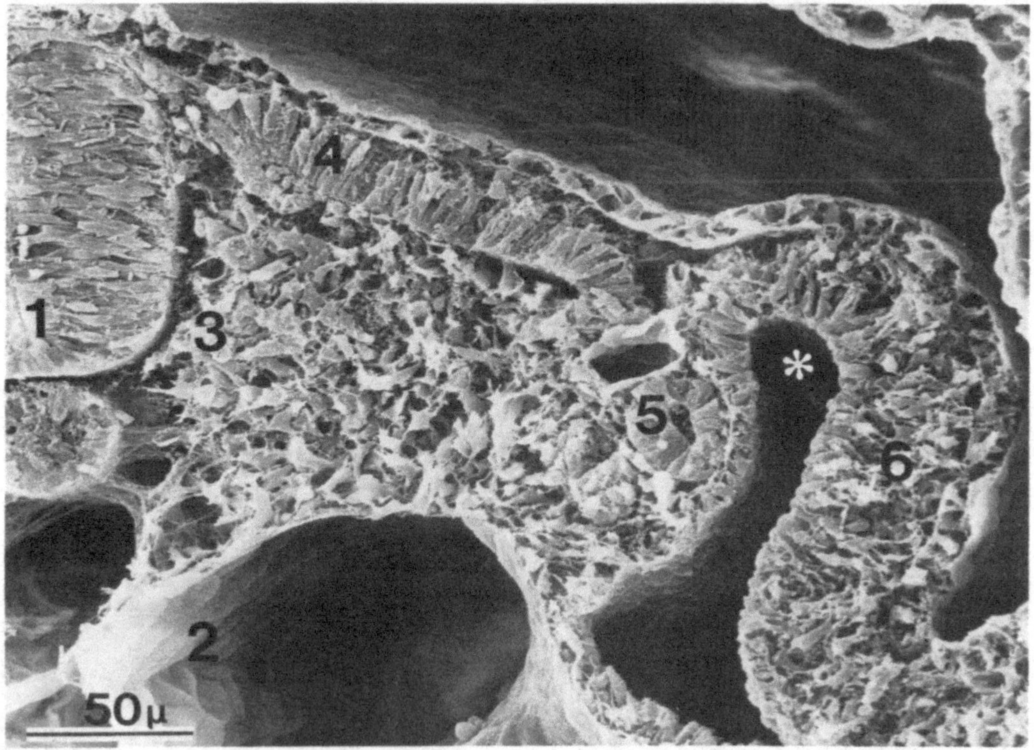

Fig. 1: SEM micrograph of a transverse section of a stage 16 chick embryo at the wing level. 1 neural tube, 2 aorta, 3 sclerotome, 4 dermatome, 5 Wolffian duct, 6 somatopleure; asterisk: coelomic cavity.

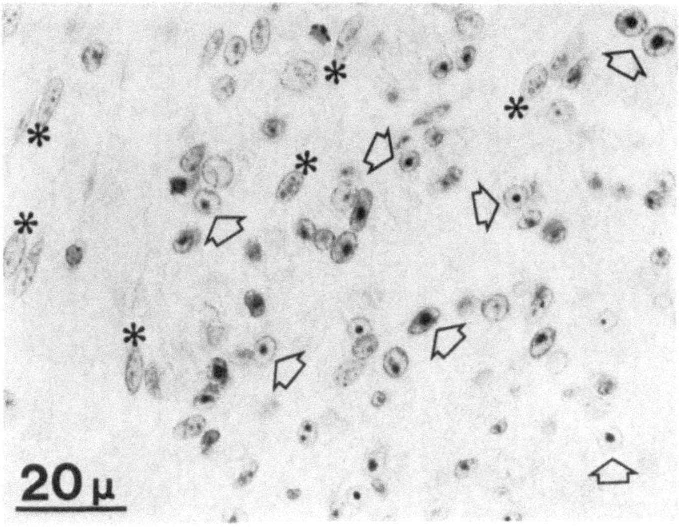

Fig. 2: Muscle blastema with adjacent epimysium of the autopodium eight days after replacement of brachial somites. Arrows: quail cells within the muscle; asterisks: chick cells of connective tissue.

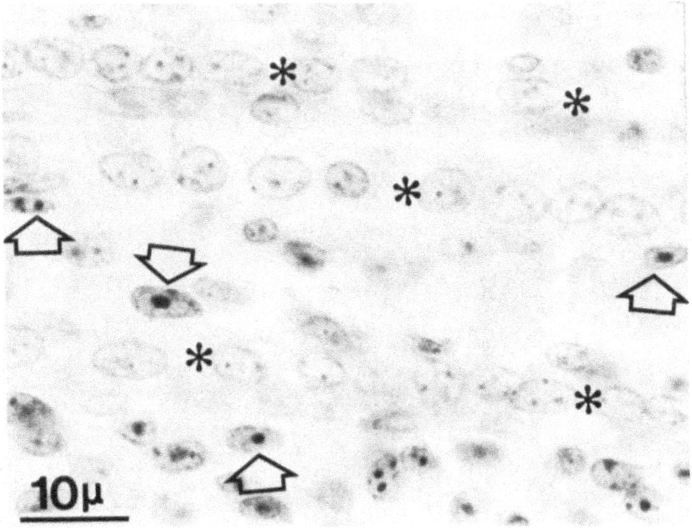

Fig. 3: Muscle blastema at the upper leg level seven days after replacement of somatopleure. Asterisks: myotubes containing chick nuclei; arrows: fibroblasts of quail origin.

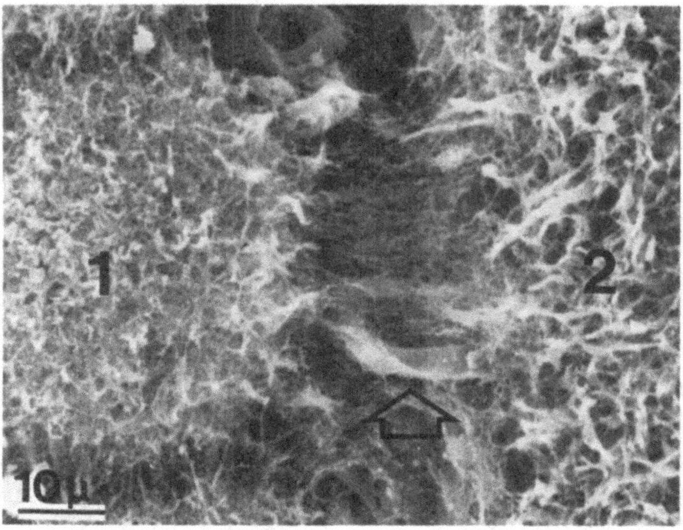

Fig. 4: SEM micrograph of the dorsal side of a stage 14 embryo at the wing level after removal of the ectoderm. Note the network of fibrils between the somite (1) and the somatopleure (2), arrow: transversally oriented cell.

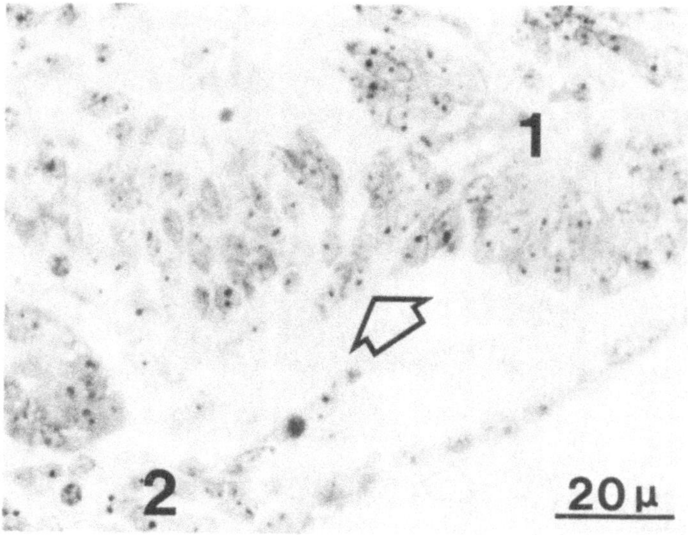

Fig. 5: Transverse section of a 4 mm human embryo at the leg level. Arrow: elongated cells between somite (1) and somatopleure (2). The courtesy of Dr. F. Wachtler, who supplied this illustration, is gratefully acknowledged.

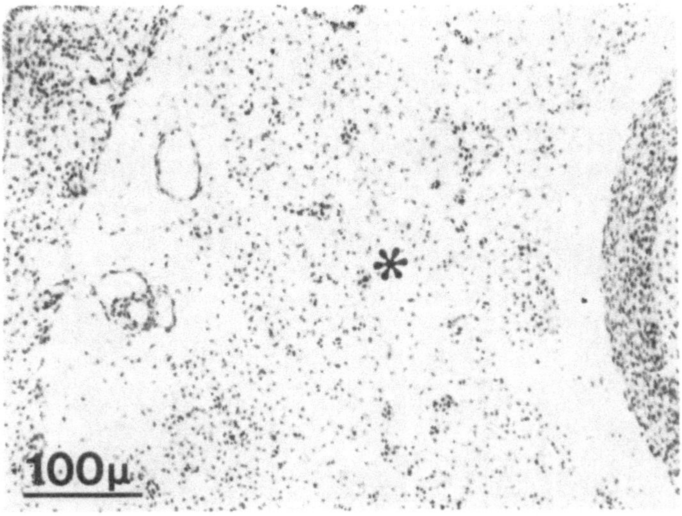

Fig. 6: Transverse section of a quail leg grown in 9 days in the coelomic cavity. Asterisk: myogenic area without musculature.

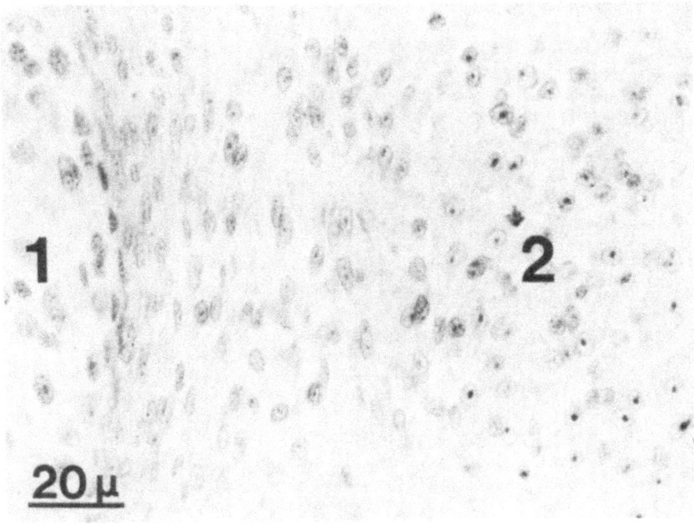

Fig. 7: Zeugopodium five days after second step of two-stage grafting procedure (see text for details). 1 radius (chick cells); 2 muscle blastema (quail cells).

The Concept of a Myogenic Cell Line in Developing Avian Limb Buds

Madeleine Kieny

Laboratoire de Zoologie et Biologie animale, Université scientifique et médicale de Grenoble BP53X F-38041 Grenoble Cédex, France

Use has been made of heterospecific chick/quail recombinations to demonstrate that, in the developing limb, the skeletal muscle cells are of somitic origin, whereas dermis, cartilage, smooth muscles, tendons, epi- and perimuscular connective tissues are all of somatopleural origin (CHRIST et al., 1974, 1977; CHEVALLIER et al., 1976, 1977; KIENY et al., 1979). Hence, the idea that the cells which leave the somites to enter the limb anlagen constitute a distinct cell line. This concept has been tested by various experiments which are based on two features of myogenic cells, namely their migratory capacity and their exclusive differentiation into striated muscle cells.

1. Retention of the migratory capacity of myoblasts (MAUGER and KIENY, 1980 a, b)

The migratory capacity of muscle cells at different stages of differentiation has been tested in heterochronic chick/quail recombinants. The somitic mesoderm adjacent to the limb anlage of 2-day chick embryos was replaced by quail muscle tissues, which were taken from 4- to 5-day limb premuscular masses, or from 12-day embryonic, or 4-day postnatal limb muscles. The implantation of quail premuscular mesenchyme containing muscle cells in the myoblast state resulted in the participation of quail cells in truncal and appendicular tissues. In the trunk the quail cells were found intermingled with chick cells in all mesodermal tissues except cartilage (loose connective tissue, dermis, tendons, muscle envelopes, myotubes, blood vessel walls, and nerve envelopes). However, within the experimental limb the quail cells contributed predominantly to myotubes and sporadically to nerve envelopes and blood vessel walls. They were absent from the tendons and muscle envelopes. The pattern of the limb musculature always developed appropriately to the experimental limb skeleton whatever the origin (wing or leg) of the mesenchymal graft. Unlike the muscle cells in the myoblast state, the already differentiated muscle cells, when replacing the somitic mesoderm at the limb level, did not invade the limb bud. Their migratory performance was limited to the immediate truncal vicinity.

The results of the implantation of premuscular mesenchyme indicate that only two kinds of cells are capable of extended migration: myoblasts and connective tissue cells that become incorporated into blood vessel walls and nerve envelopes. As, in the premuscular mesenchyme, the skeletal muscle cells are associated with connective tissue cells, it was necessary to ascertain the developmental origin of the migratory cells expressing myogenic potentialities. Therefore we replaced the somitic mesoderm adjacent to the limb anlage by a piece of bispecific premuscular muscle mass in which the myoblasts were of quail origin and the connective tissue cells of chick origin (Fig. 1). The bispecific masses were obtained according to the usual procedure of ortho- or heteropic somite-exchange between a quail donor and a chick host. The quail myoblasts and/or their offspring were found exclusively in muscles, namely in some truncal muscles at the operation site and in all intrinsic muscles of the limb, where they formed multinucleated unispecific quail or bispecific chick/quail myotubes (Fig. 2 - 5).

These results show that the cells which are able to enter a new somite-somatopleure migratory phase and participate in the de novo formation of myotubes are those which originate from the somitic mesoderm. Thus, myogenic cells at least up to the myoblast state still display developmental potentialities equivalent to those of the somitic myogenic stem cells. Myogenic cells express only the myogenic phenotype and represent a distinct myogenic cell lineage. These experiments support the lineage view proposed by DIENSTMANN et al. (1974).

2. Retention of differentiation properties

There is a considerable body of evidence suggesting an idea opposite to the lineage view, namely that of the multipotency of the limb bud cells, not only at early stages (ZWILLING, 1966; SEARLS and JANNERS, 1969; CAPLAN and KOUTROUPAS, 1973), but also at later ones, when the differentiation is presumed to be terminal (NATHANSON et al., 1978). In order to clarify this controversy, we investigated the following two questions using the chick/quail marker system:

1. Are other mesoderm-derived cells endowed with the capacity to express myogenic potentialities?

2. Are somite-derived myogenic cells able to give rise to appendicular cartilage?

a.) Myogenic potentialities of somatopleural mesoderm The possibility exists that, although limb muscle cells are usually of somitic origin, somatopleural cells can also give rise to striated muscle cells under certain conditions which are the following:

1. When quail somatopleural mesoderm was grafted ectopically into the flank or in place of the neural tube of the chick, the multinucleated myotubes contained quail nuclei or a mixture of quail and chick (host) nuclei in 24% of the resulting limbs (KIENY et al., 1978; MAUGER et al., 1980) (Fig. 6 - 8). It was made certain that no somitic material was included in the quail graft and, moreover, the somatopleural graft was taken at a stage before its invasion by the quail endogenous somitic cells (Fig. 6).

2. When quail limb primordia were explanted to the chick extra-embryonic coelom at stages before the invasion of endogenous somitic cells, 74% of the resulting patternless structures contained multinucleated quail myotubes (McLACHLAN and HORNBRUCH, 1979).

These experiments show that in the absence of somite-derived muscle cells, somatopleural cells of the limb anlage can give rise to muscle, which normally does not happen. Since somatopleural mesoderm consists of a mixed population of chondrogenic and fibroblastic stem cells, it is not possible to know the precise developmental history of the shunted cells.

b.) Modulation of the myogenic phenotype, In regard to the differentiation of myogenic and chondrogenic phenotypes, our group investigated the controversial alternative of an early and rigidly committed cell line versus a labile cell population whose differentiation into muscle or cartilage is liable to be modulated by the environment.

As skeletal muscle tissue is composed of muscle cells associated with connective tissue cells, cartilage can arise from either of these sources. In order to ascertain the possibility of a presumptive myogenic cell to differentiate into a chondrocyte, it was essential to be able to distinguish between cells of myogenic origin and others. Therefore, at first, we (KIENY, PAUTOU and CHEVALLIER, in preparation) created a bispecific limb bud, in which, as usual, only the somite derived cells of the myogenic line were quail cells, the other limb cells being chick cells. Secondly, the mesodermal cores of a number of bispecific limbs were pooled two days later (HAMBURGER-HAMILTON stages 23 - 24), enzymatically dissociated and reaggregated. Then, a limb-bud shaped piece of reaggregated mesoderm, in which the relative position of quail cells among chick cells was fortuituous, was stuffed into a chick limb bud ectodermal hull and the recombined limb bud grown as a graft on a chick host (Fig. 9). In the resulting experimental limbs, the quail cells were mainly concentrated in the intermediate zone of the appendage between the integumentary periphery and the cartilaginous centre shere they gave rise to multinucleated myotubes (Fig. 10 a). However, in each developing limb, numerous quail cells were found outside the muscular areas, particularly in the cartilaginous elements (Fig. 10). In 7-day limbs, no predominant distribution in perichondrium or hyaline cartilage could be detected. Moreover, some scattered quail cells took part in the dermis.

These results show that cells derived from the myogenic line, although they tend to congregate into normal muscle masses where they differentiate into myocytes, are nonetheless able to give rise to chondrocytes and fibroblasts, if their final position falls outside the muscle masses.

IN CONCLUSION,
in normal development somitic cells do not contribute to the limb cartilaginous skeleton, and somatopleural cells do not contribute to muscle proper. Normal development seems to proceed via one-way pathways in which chondrogenic and myogenic lines do not have the same spatial origin. But the possibility of a developmental plasticity among differentiating mesenchymal cells is not precluded.

REFERENCES

Caplan, A.I., Koutroupas, J., 1973, The control of muscle and cartilage development in the chick limb: the role of differential vascularization, J. Embryol. exp. Morph., 29, 571 - 583.

Chevallier, A., Kieny, M., Mauger, A., 1976, Sur l'origine de la musculature de l'aile chez les Oiseaux, C. R. Acad. Sci., Paris, série D, 282, 309 - 311.

Chevallier, A., Kieny, M., Mauger, A., 1977, Limb-somite relationship: origin of the limb musculature, J. Embryol. exp. Morph., 41, 245 - 258.

Christ, B., Jacob, H.J., Jacob, M., 1974, Über den Ursprung der Flügelmuskulatur. Experimentelle Untersuchungen mit Wachtel- und Hühnerembryonen, Experientia, 30, 1446 - 1448.

Christ, B., Jacob, H.J., Jacob, M., 1977, Experimental analysis of the origin of the wing musculature in avian embryos, Anat. Embryol., 150, 171 - 186.

Dienstmann, S.R., Biehl, J., Holtzer, S., Holtzer, H., 1974, Myogenic and chondrogenic cell lineages in developing limb buds grown in vitro, Develop. Biol., 39, 83 - 95.

Kieny, M., Chevallier, A., Mauger, A., 1978, Sur l'existence de myotubes bispécifiques contenant à la fois des noyaux de caille et des noyaux de poulet, Arch. Anat micr. Morph. exp., 67, 99 - 105.

Kieny, M., Mauger, A., Chevallier, A., Sengel, P., 1979, Origine embryologique des muscles lisses cutanés chez les oiseaux, Arch. Anat. micr. Morph. exp., 68, 283 - 290.

McLachlan, J.C., Hornbruch, A., 1979, Muscle-forming potential of the non-somitic cells of the early avian limb bud, J. Embryol. exp. Morph., 54, 209 - 217.

Mauger, A., Kieny, M., 1980 a, Sur les potentialités des cellules myogènes contenues dans les masses prémusculaires des membres des Oiseaux, C. R. Acad. Sci., Paris, série D, 290, 779 - 781.

Mauger, A., Kieny, M., 1980 b, Migratory and organogenetic capacities of muscle cells in bird embryos, W. Roux's Arch., (in press).

Mauger, A., Kieny, M., Chevallier, A., 1980, Limb-somite relationship: myogenic potentialities of somatopleural mesoderm, Arch. Anat. micr. Morph. exp., (in press).

Nathanson, M.A., Hilfer, S.R., Searls, R.L., 1978, Formation of cartilage by non-chondrogenic cell types, Develop. Biol., 64, 99 - 117.

Searls, R.L., Janners, M., 1969, The stabilisation of cartilage properties in the cartilage-forming mesenchyme of the embryonic chick limb, J. exp. Zool., 170, 365 - 376.

Zwilling, E., 1966, Cartilage formation from so-called myogenic tissue of chick embryo limb buds, Annl. Med. exp. Biol. Fenn., 44, 134 - 139.

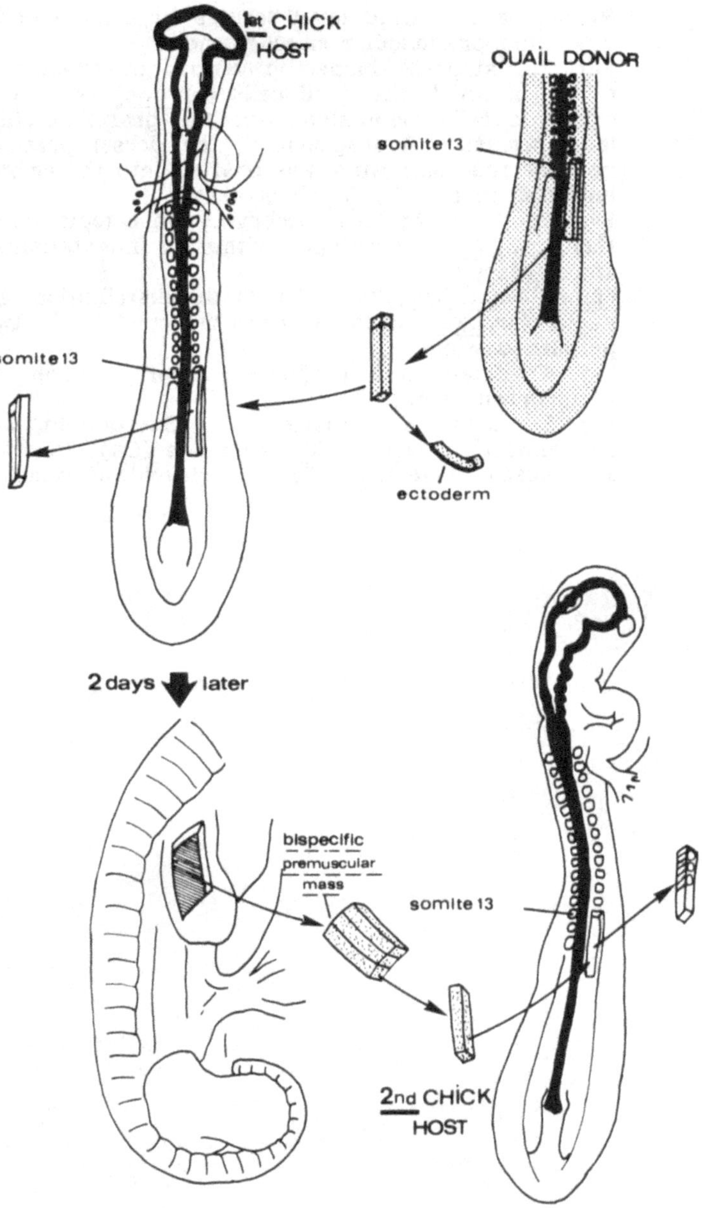

Fig. 1: Two-step replacement of chick somitic mesoderm of the wing level by a fragment of dorsal bispecific premuscular mass in which the myogenic cells are quail cells.

Figures 2 to 5: Replacement of wing level somites by a piece of bispecific wing premuscular mesenchyme.

Fig. 2: stage-24 bispecific ventral premuscular mass (VM), in which the quail cells (arrows) represent the myogenic cells originated from the grafted quail wing level somites. A fragment of the dorsal premuscular mass of the same wing was grafted into the embryo illustrated in Fig. 5; C, chick cells.

Fig. 3: 9-day operated embryo. An ectopic wing feather tract (FT) developed within an indentation of the spinal pteryla.

(Figs. 4 and 5): illustration of the distribution of quail nuclei (arrows) in the forearm musculature in two experimental wings;

Fig. 4: detail of a tendino-muscular junction in the wing shown in Fig. 3;

Fig. 5: detail of a muscle bulk. Surrounding muscular connective tissue (CT), cartilage (Ca), tendon (T), and muscle envelopes (E), are devoid of quail cells.

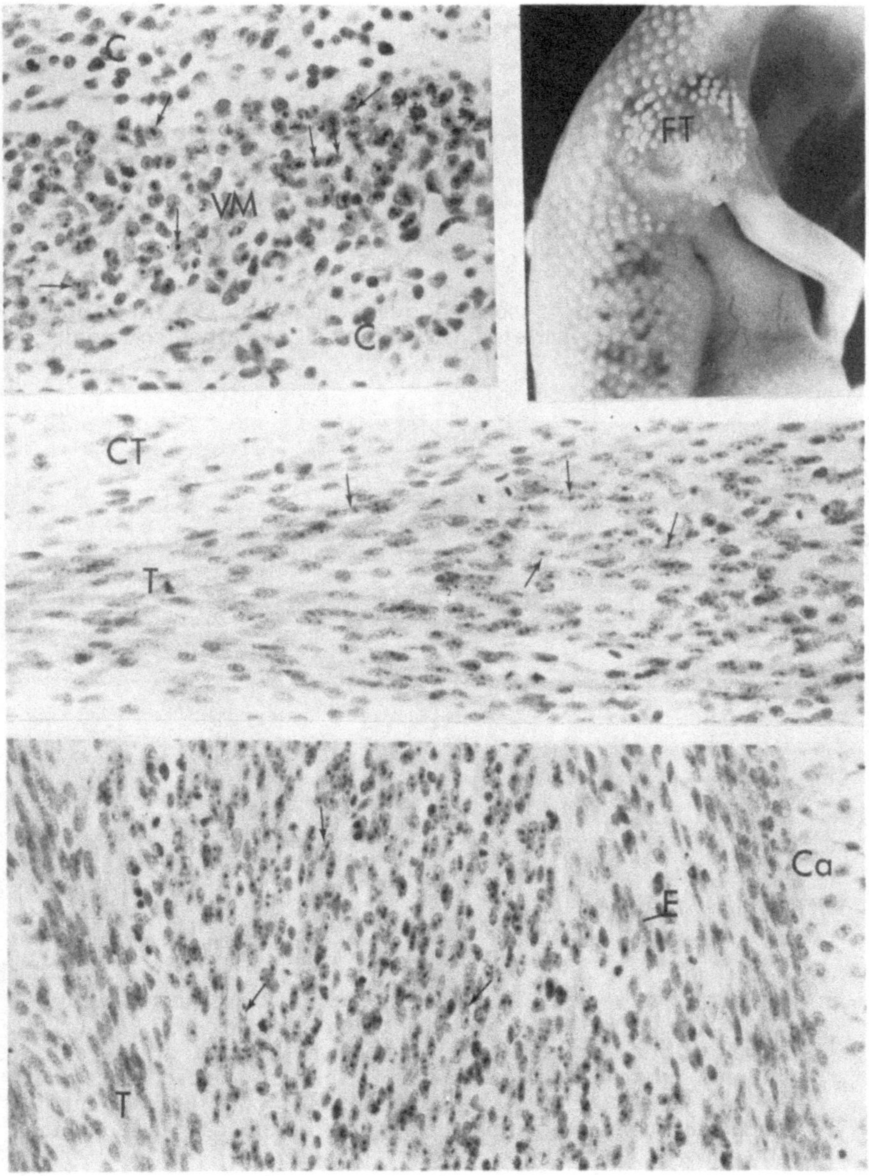
C
VM
C
FT
CT
T
Ca
E
T

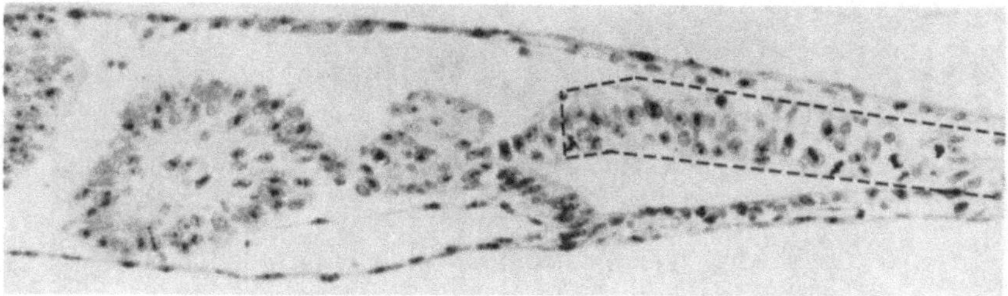

Fig. 6: Somite 14 of 17-pair of somites quail embryo. The interrupted line represents the limits of the ectopically grafted somatopleural mesoderm.

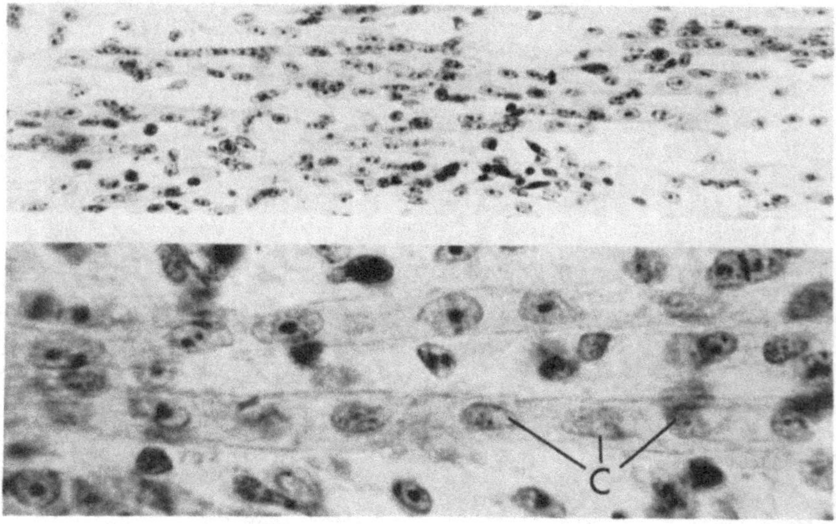

Figs. 7 - 8: General view and detail of forearm muscles in an ectopic wing resulting from the implantation of a piece of 17-pair of somites quail somatopleural mesoderm in place of the chick neural tube. The myotubes are either of monospecific quail (Figs. 7, 8) or bispecific chick/quail constitution. Intramuscular connective tissue cells are of quail type. C, chick nucleus.

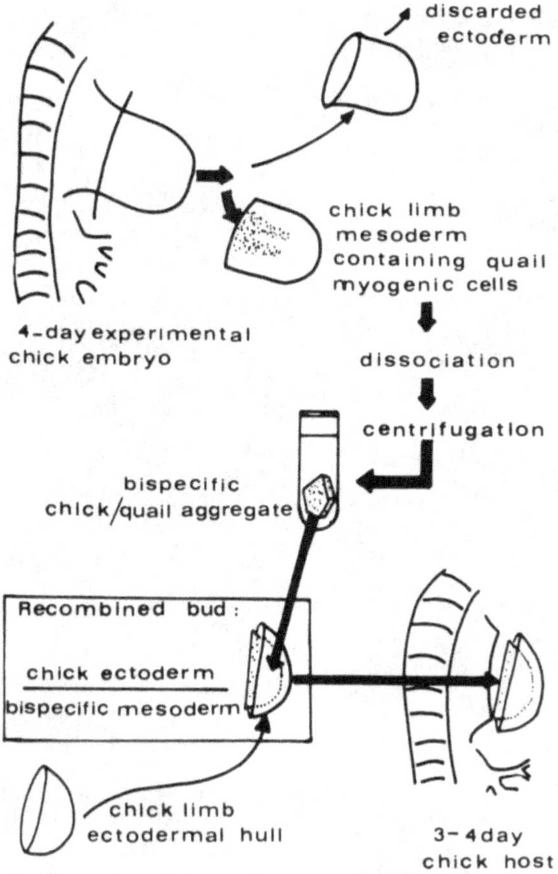

Fig. 9: Diagram illustrating the second step of the fabrication of a recombined limb bud, whose quail myogenic cells have been haphazardly redistributed among the chick limb cells.

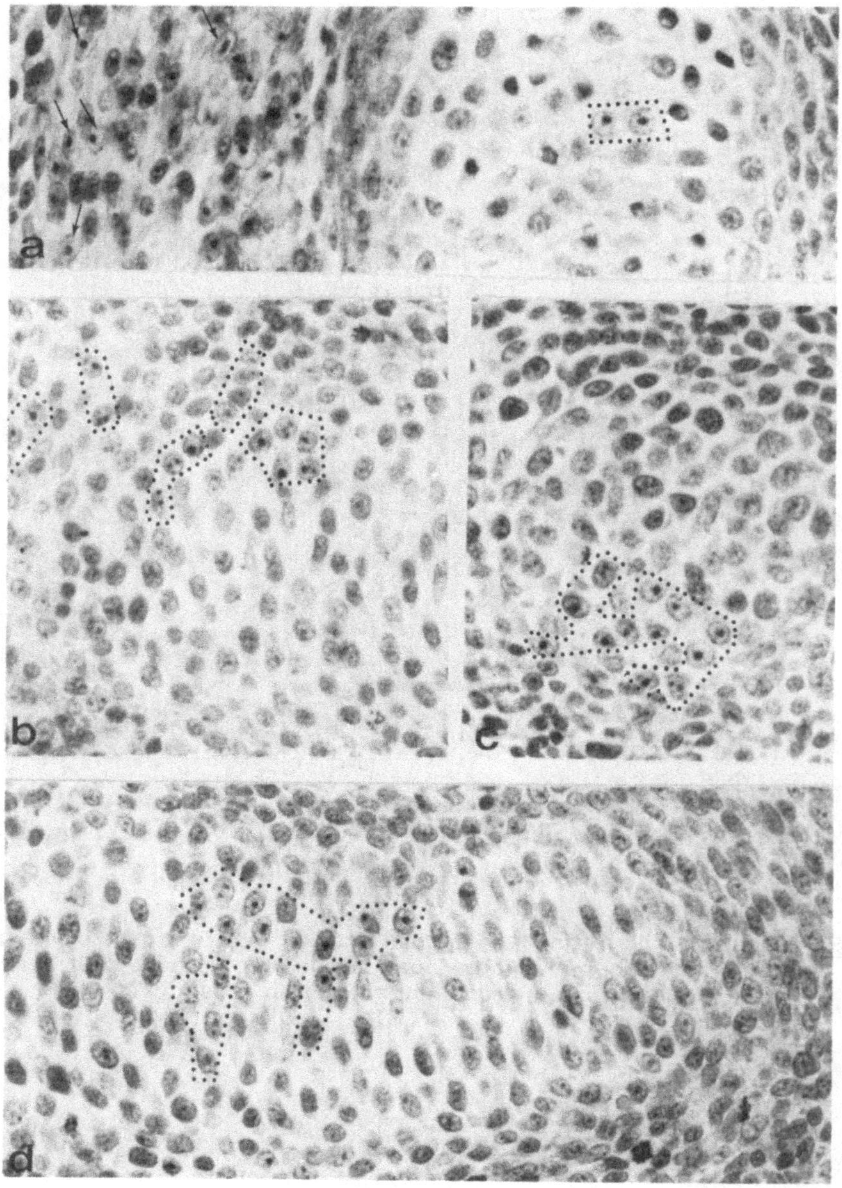

Fig. 10: Cartilaginous elements of 4 wings which developed from reaggregated bispecific mesoderm (see Fig. 9). Most of the quail cells are concentrated in the myogenic area (a), but numerous quail cells (delimited areas) are intermingled with the chick chondrocytes (a, b, c, d). Arrow, quail myocyte.

On the Formation of Muscular Pattern in the Chick Limb

H. J. Jacob and B. Christ

Ruhr-Universität Bochum, Institut für Anatomie, Arbeitsgruppe für Experimentelle Embryologie
Universitätsstraße 150, D-4630 Bochum 1

The process of muscle individuation in the avian limb bud is accompanied by the splitting up and the subdivision of previously undivided muscle blastemata. These appear in the so-called myogenic zone. The factors that control this splitting up are still a matter of controversy.

WORTHAM (1948) concluded that in the leg of the chick the spinal nerves will determine the muscle pattern. Recently CIHAK et al. (1978) arrived at similar conclusions. On the contrary, CAREY (1921) and SULLIVAN (1962), felt that the elongation of the limbs would influence this developmental process. Studying this question in human embryos, BLECHSCHMIDT (1960), concluded that muscle individuation was the result of the growth of cartilage which was farther than the growth of the skin. These concepts have been challenged by SHELLSWELL and WOLPERT (1977) who proposed that the spitting up of muscles was an autonomous process involving muscle blastemata only.

In order to clarify these controversial problems, the following experiments have been performed:

1) Nerveless limbs have been obtained to study the influence of innervation on muscle individuation.

2) Arrangement of connective tissue has been studied in muscleless limbs.

3) Somites from various levels have been allowed to contribute to limb development and vice versa in order to study their influence on the formation of the muscular pattern.

4) The somatopleure from the leg anlage has been replaced by somatopleure from the flank to study the muscle pattern under such conditions.

1.) If the neural tube from neck and thoracic levels was removed during the second day of incubation, the embryos exhibited no spinal nerves in the regions which were operated on. Limbs, however, were found to develop quite orderly after two days (Fig. 1). Up to eight days after this manipulation the muscles of the wing region and thoracic body wall showed a regular pattern on both sides (Fig. 2). After further reincubation, the muscles deprived of nerves degenerated, myoblasts and myotubes swelled, their nuclei disappeared and later on became homogeneous eosinophile bodies (CHRIST et al., 1979 a).

From these experiments it may be concluded, that spinal nerves are not necessary for the process of muscle individuation, but are necessary to maintain intact muscles. These findings agree with the results of SHELLSWELL (1977) who treated chick embryos with the nicotinamide analogue 3-acetylpyridine and observed a normal muscular pattern in nerve-free wings.

Teratology of the Limbs

It is difficult to imagine that external forces like tensions as postulated by CAREY (1921), SULLIVAN (1962), or BLECHSCHMIDT (1960) are responsible for individual muscle development, since SHELLSWELL and WOLPERT (1977) observed that the splitting up of the muscle anlagen occurs before the tendons of these muscles have developed distally.

2.) Up to now it has been assumed that mesenchyme of the early limb bud consists of a uniform and pluripotent cell population. Based on this premise special models have been established to explain the diversification of cells and pattern formation within the limbs (CAPLAN and KOUTROUPAS (1973); WOLPERT (1971); WILBY and EDE (1975); HINCHLIFFE and THOROGOOD (1974). From the studies of CHRIST et al. (1974, 1977 a), CHEVALLIER et al. (1977) and DIENSTMANN et al. (1974) it is evident that muscle pattern formation in the avian limbs involves two populations of cells of different origin: the myogenic cell lineage is of somitic origin whereas the cells giving rise to tendons and connective tissue originate from the somatopleure.

Prospective quail limb anlagen were grafted into the coelomic cavity or onto the chorioallantoic membrane of a chick. The grafts had not yet been invaded by cells of somitic origin. Grafts showing a normal form and eutopic development, exhibited loosely packed connective tissue that sometimes imitated a muscle-like pattern. This was evoked by fibroblasts differentiating into fat cells found in the regions where muscles would be expected. Muscles of quail origin in such limbs were never found (Fig. 3).

Signs of cellular degeneration, like those occurring in the nerveless grown muscles, were never found. In the distal parts of these limbs, tendons of quail origin appeared, in spite of the lack of muscle development (Fig. 4). These results (CHRIST et al., 1979 b) were confirmed by KIENY and CHEVALLIER (1979) and agree with previous findings of SHELLSWELL and WOLPERT (1977) who reported that tendons develop autonomously in the distal parts of the limbs.

3.) In order to investigate a possible determinative influence inherent in the myogenic cell line itself, interspecific transplantations of somites of different levels into other body regions have been performed. For example, somites from the neck level have been grafted to the limb levels and vice versa. These results were independently obtained by CHEVALLIER et al., 1977, and our group. CHRIST et al. (1977 b, 1978) showed that after 6 days of subsequent reincubation following this type of operations normally developed muscle patterns were found both in the operated and in the normal limbs (see Figs. 5 - 8).

These results clearly show that the myogenic cells from the somites are not determinated in view of muscle pattern formation.

4.) Finally the morphogenetic influence of connective tissue on muscle pattern formation has been studied to elucidate whether connective tissue is able to evoke an "ortsgemäß" muscle pattern or not.

Leg level somatopleure in chick embryos has been replaced by flank somatopleure (somites 21 to 25) from quail embryos.

After such operations no leg development at the operated side was observed. We found quail cells in the body wall forming connectve tissue of the muscles, (epimysium and endomysium). In some cases, a piece of ectopic cartilage was found as well which apparently corresponded to the sternum anlage (CHEVALLIER, 1975). No striated muscles in such embryos were of quail origin. The form of the muscles and their pattern corresponded to the source of the graft (flank) and not to the position within the host (leg) (Fig. 9 - 10). This means that connective tissue and not myogenic tissue was determined to control the formation of muscle pattern. This was also shown to be the case during muscle individuation within the abdominal wall of the chick (JACOB et al., 1980). It seems noteworthy to point out that pattern formation in the abdominal musculature occurred through mesenchymal cells invading the muscle primordium.

Our findings presented here indicate that:

1. The spinal nerves exert no influence on the establishment of a specific regional muscular pattern in the avian limb.

2. The myogenic cell lineage, originating from the somites, does not determine the muscular pattern.

3. The regional muscle patterns are formed under the influence of the regional somatopleure.

In summary, we feel that the connective tissue of somatopleure origin causes the myogenic cells of somitic origin to establish a specific regional muscle pattern.

We must however, admit, that we are still far from understanding the mechanism of this process.

ACKNOWLEDGEMENTS

We would like to thank U. RITENBERG, I. SCHAEBEN, I. BURKS and H. HAKE for expert technical assistance and DR. F. WACHTLER for helping with the English translation. This work was supported by a Grant Ch 44/4 from the Deutsche Forschungsgemeinschaft.

REFERENCES

Blechschmidt, E., 1960, Die vorgeburtlichen Entwicklungsstadien des Menschen, (S. Karger, ed.) Basel - New York.

Caplan, A.J., Koutroupas, J., 1973, The control of muscle and cartilage development in the chick limb: the role of differential vascularisation, J. Embryol. exp. Morph., 29, 571 - 583.

Carey, E.J., 1921, Studies in the dynamics of histogenesis. IV. Tension of differential growth as a stimulus to myogenesis in the chick limb, Am. J. Anat., 29, 93 - 115.

Chevallier, A., 1975, Rôle du mésoderme somitique dans le développement de la cage thoracique de l'embryon d'oiseau. I. Origine du segment sternal et mécanismes de la différenciation des cotes, J. Embryol. exp. Morph., 33, 291 - 311.

Chevallier, A., Kieny, M., Mauger, A., 1977, Limb-somite relationship: origin of the limb musculature, J. Embryol. exp. Morph., 41, 245 - 258.

Christ, B., Jacob, H.J., Jacob, M., 1974, Über den Ursprung der Flügelmuskulatur. Experimentelle Untersuchungen mit Wachtel- und Hühnerembryonen, Experientia, Basel, 30, 1446 - 1448.

Christ, B., Jacob, H.J., Jacob, M., 1977 a, Experimental analysis of the origin of the wing musculature in avian embryos, Anat. Embryol., 150, 171 - 186.

Christ, B., Jacob, H.J., Jacob, M., 1977 b, Experimentelle Befunde zur Muskelentwicklung in den Extremitäten von Hühnerembryonen, Verh. Anat. Ges., 71, 1231 - 1237.

Christ, B., Jacob, H.J., Jacob, M., 1978, Zur Frage der regionalen Determination der frühembryonalen Muskelanlagen. Experimentelle Untersuchungen an Wachtel- und Hühnerembryonen, Verh. Anat. Ges., 72, 353 - 357.

Christ, B., Jacob, H.J., Jacob, M., 1979 a, Experimentelle Untersuchungen zum Problem der Muskelindividuation in den Extremitäten von Vogelembryonen, Verh. Anat. Ges., 73, 537 - 544.

Christ, B., Hirschberg, M., Jacob, H.J., Jacob, M., 1979 b, Experimentelle Befunde zur Entwicklung der distalen Extremitätenmuskulatur, Verh. Anat. Ges., 73, 519 - 525.

Cihák, R., Doskocil, M., Seichert, V., 1978, Some morphogenetic aspects of the aneurogenic and explanted limb primordia, in: "XIXth Morphological Congress Symposia, Charles Univ. Prague, 1976", (E. Klika, ed.), pp. 119 - 160, Univerzita Karlova, Praha.

Dienstmann, S.R., Biehl, J., Holtzer, S., Holtzer, H., 1974, Myogenic and chondrogenic lineages in developing limb buds grown in vitro, Develop. Biol., 39, 83 - 95.

Hinchliffe, J.R., Thorogood, P.V., 1974, Genetic inhibition of mesenchymal cell death and the development of form and skeletal pattern in the limbs of talpid^3 (ta^3) mutant chick embryos, J. Embryol. exp. Morph., 31, 747 - 760.

Jacob, M., Christ, B., Jacob, H.J., 1980, Über die Entwicklung der Bauchmuskulatur. II. Ultrastrukturelle Untersuchungen an Vogelembryonen, Verh. Anat. Ges., 75, (in press).

Kieny, M., Chevallier, A., 1979, Autonomy of tendon development in the embryonic chick wing, J. Embryol. exp. Morph., 49, 153 - 165.

Shellswell, G.B., 1977, The formation of discrete muscles from the chick wing dorsal and ventral muscle masses in the absence of nerves, J. Embryol. exp. Morph., 41, 269 - 277.

Shellswell, G.B., Wolpert, L., 1977, The pattern of muscle and tendon development in the chick wing, in: "Vertebrate Limb and Somite Morphogenesis", Brit. Soc. Develop. Biol., 3rd Symposium (D.A. Ede, J.R. Hinchliffe, M. Balls, eds.), pp. 71 - 86, Cambridge Univ. Press.

Sullivan, G.E., 1962, Anatomy and embryology of the wing musculature of the domestic fowl (Gallus), Aust. J. Zool., 10, 458 - 518.

Wilby, O.K., Ede, D.A., 1975, A model generating the pattern of cartilage skeletal elements in the embryonic chick limb, J. theor. Biol., 50, 199 - 217.

Wolpert, L., 1971, Positional information and pattern formation, in: "Current Topics in Developmental Biology", 6, pp 183 - 224.

Wortham, R.A., 1948, The development of the muscles and tendons in the lower leg and foot of chick embryos, J. Morph., 83, 105 - 148.

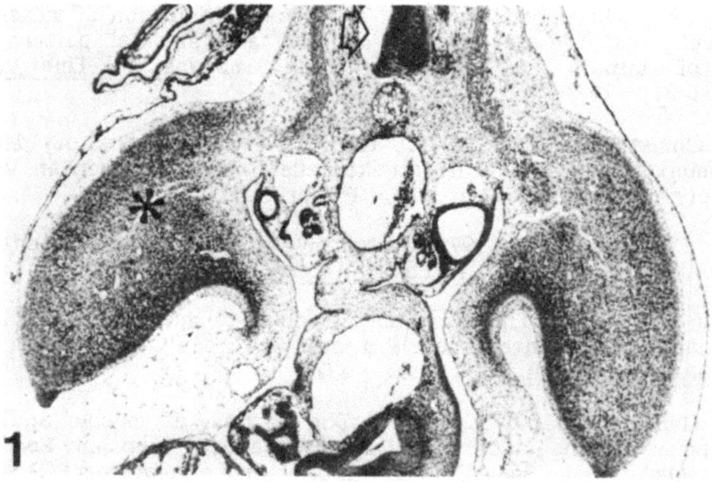

Fig. 1: Transverse section of an embryo after excision of one half of the neural tube, two days of reincubation. Arrow: neural tube; Asterisk: normally developed nerve free wing anlage.
Magn. approx.: 70 : 1

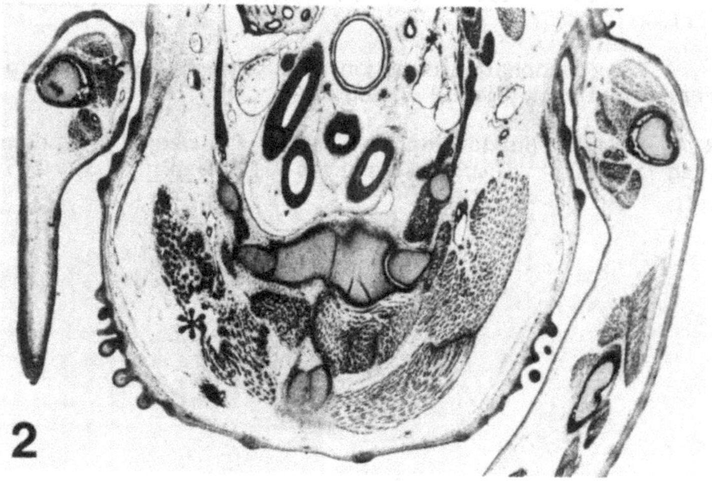

Fig. 2: Transverse section of an embryo after excision of one half of the neural tube after eight days of reincubation. The muscles of the wing and those of the pectoral region (asterisk) exhibit a normal pattern, despite the absence of spinal nerves.
Magn. approx.: 60 : 1

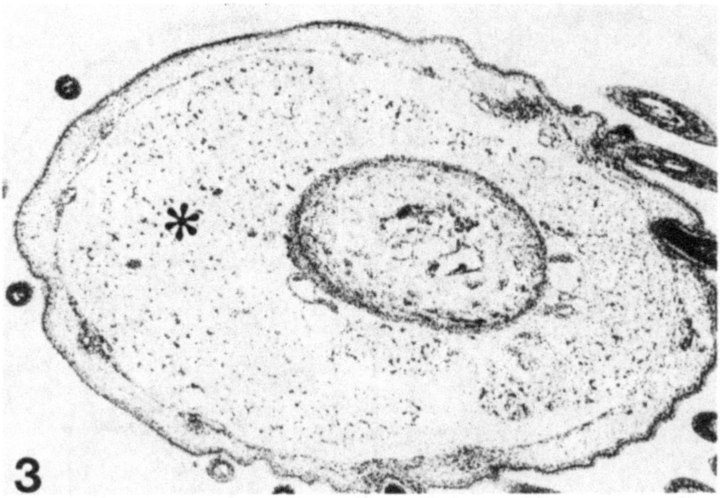

Fig. 3: Section of a muscle-free quail leg, grown in the coelomic cavity of a chick embryo. Asterisk: soft connective tissue instead of muscle "anlagen".
Magn. approx.: 50 : 1

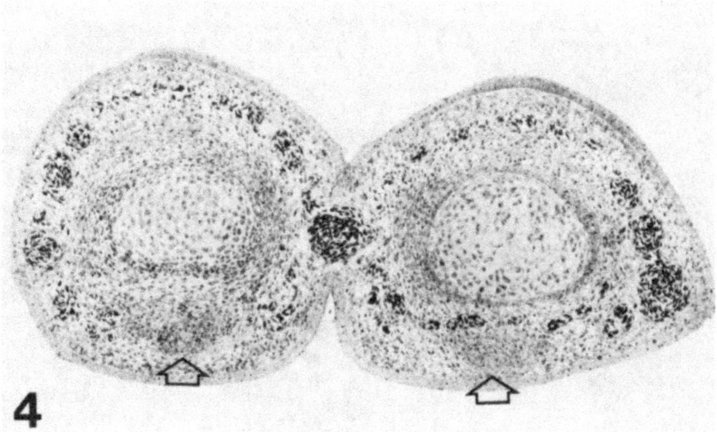

Fig. 4: Section of a muscle-free quail leg, grown on the chorioallantoic membrane. Tendons (arrows) are well developed in spite of the absence of muscles.
Magn. approx.: 100 : 1

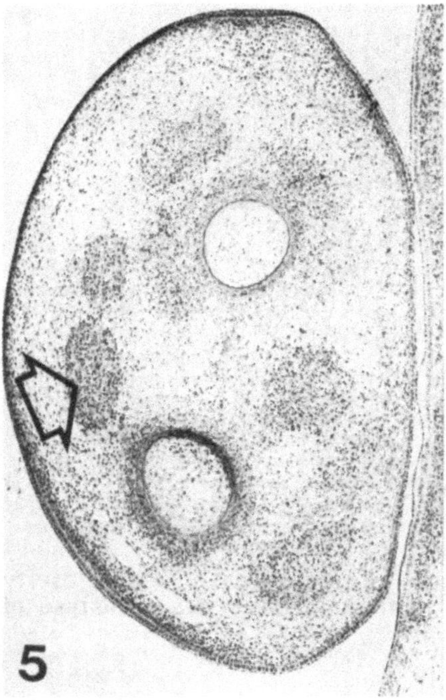

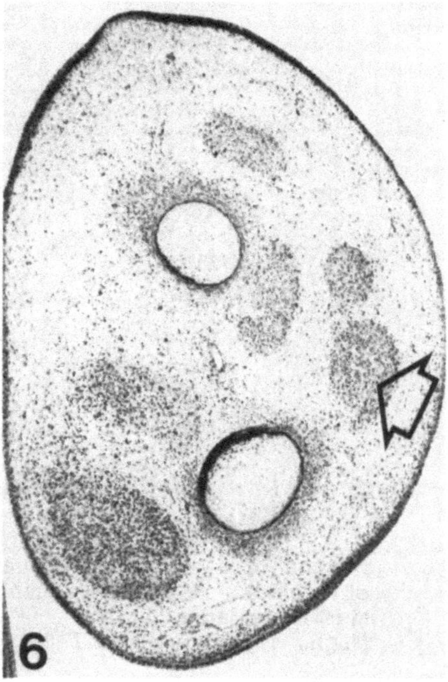

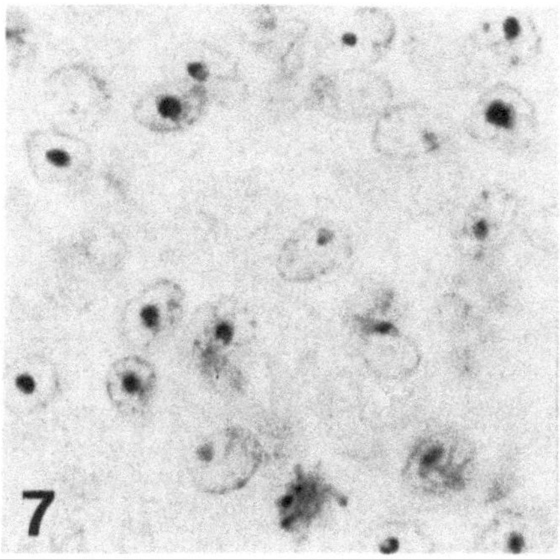

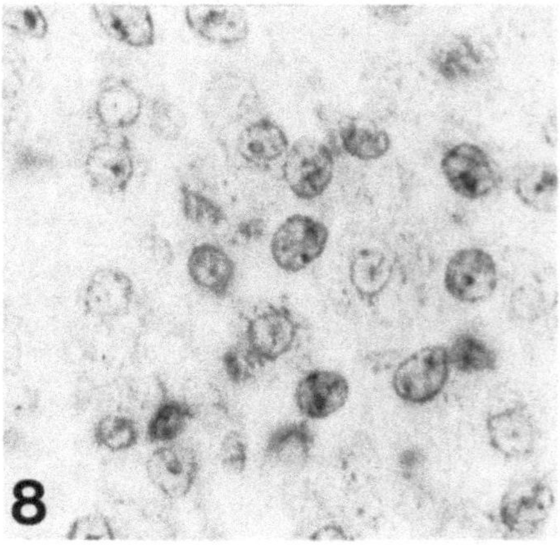

Fig. 5 and 6: Zeugopod from a chick embryo. Fig. 5: Neck somites had been allowed to contribute to the muscles. Fig. 6: Normal control of wing.
Magn. approx.: 50 : 1.

Fig. 7: Chimaeric muscle (see arros in Fig. 5). Magn. approx.: 1200 : 1.

Fig. 8: Normal muscle (see arrow in Fig. 6). Magn. approx.: 1200 : 1.

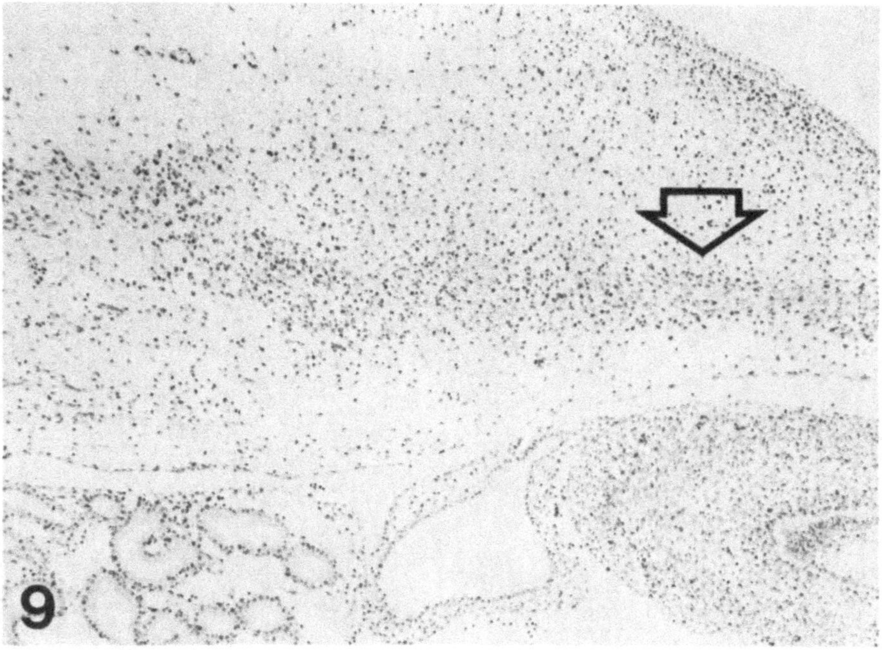

Fig. 9: Flank somatopleure in place of leg anlage, five days reincubated. Magn. approx.: 80 : 1.

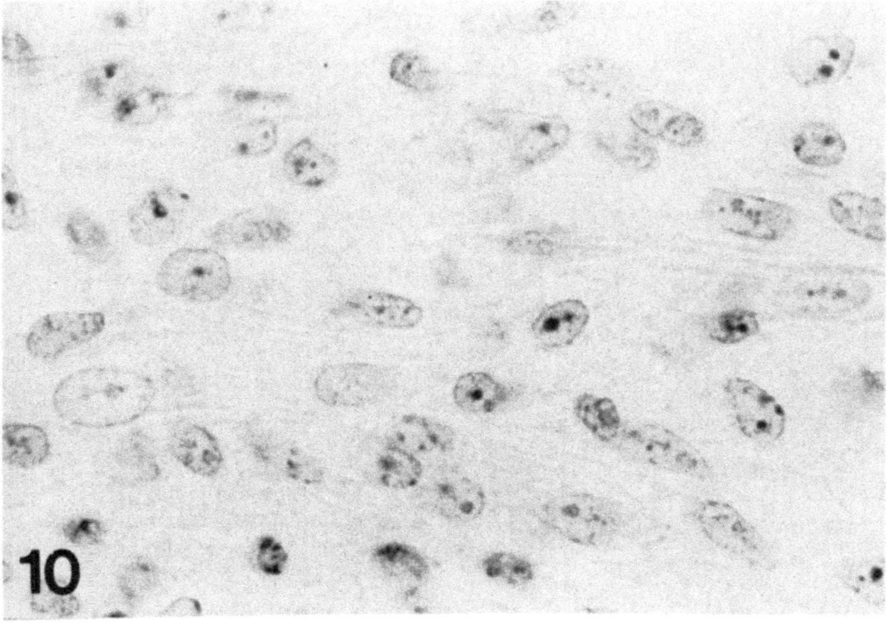

Fig. 10: Muscle blastema (see arrow in Fig. 9). Asterisks: chick myotubes; Arrows: quail cells in the interstitium. Magn. approx.: 1200 : 1.

Muscle Development during Normal and Disturbed Skelettogenesis

G. Bogusch
Institut für Anatomie, Freie Universität Berlin,
Königin-Luise-Straße 15, D-1000 Berlin 33

Most studies on the normal and experimentally altered development of limbs have been confined to the skeletal system. The muscular tissue has so far received only minor attention. This fact may, among others, be due to the easy stainability of the skeletal system in whole mounts, whereas the pattern of muscles is to be reconstructed from serial sections. It is a well known fact that myoblasts, myotubes, and early muscle fibres exhibit a high acetyl choline esterase activity (MUMENTHALER and ENGEL, 1961; FILOGAMO and GABELLA, 1967; FLUCK and STROHMAN, 1973; WAKE, 1976). In most cases, however, enzymatic activity is demonstrated in tissue sections. In whole mounts the staining of the muscles is not successful, because the penetration of the incubation medium is poor and the skin acts as a diffusion barrier. This difficulty is overcome by the following modified acetyl choline esterase staining technique.

MATERIALS and METHODS:

Forelegs from 11 to 18 day old mouse embryos and 19 to 21 day old rat embryos were fixed for 5 hours in a cold 4% paraformaldehyde - 0.1 M phosphate buffer solution (pH 7.2). After washing, a new step in the acetyl choline esterase staining procedure was introduced, as described elsewhere (BOGUSCH, 1980). In brief, the legs were incubated for 3 to 24 hours in a cold Ca-Mg-free HANKS salt solution containing 1% trypsin. Trypsin activity was stopped by replacement of this solution with cold HANKS salt solution containing 5% fetal calf serum. After treatment, the legs of the older embryos could easily be skinned with forceps. Staining of the skinned and unskinned whole legs was performed according to KARNOVSKY and ROOTS (1964) or to KOELLES original method modified by NAIK (1963). After staining and washing, the tissue was transferred in graded series of glycerin and stored in pure glycerin.

The skeletal system was stained according to WASSERSUG (1976).

RESUTS and DISCUSSION:

In the forelegs of 12 day old mouse embryos several muscle blastemata are seen (Fig. 1). At higher magnification, myotubes are clearly visible. The dorsal and the ventral muscle blastemata are separated by the developing skeletal tissue. Nerves innervating the muscle blastemata are also stained by the choline esterase technique. The development of the muscular pattern seems to be a rather rapid event. The forelegs of 13 day old embryos exhibit a muscular pattern, which already resembles that of adult animals (Fig. 2). The muscle bellies of the musculi extensores carpi radialis (longus and brevis are already discernible), the musculus extensor digitorum, the musculi extensores digitorum quarti and quinti, the musculus extensor carpi ulnaris and the musculi extensores pollicis are clearly

Teratology of the Limbs

separated from each other. The dotty appearance of the muscle fibres is due to the strong reaction in the perinuclear space of the myonuclei.

After formation of the muscular pattern the next remarkable event, which can be demonstrated with the choline esterase techniques, is the formation of motor end-plates. Figure 3 shows a skinned foreleg from a 15 day old mouse embryo. The motor end-plates appear in the middle of the muscle fibres and form characteristic bands in the fusiform and pennate muscles. At the myotendinous junctions a stronger choline esterase reaction may be observed.

In his study on the myoneuronal junction of skeletal muscles in embryonic chicken, WAKE (1976) pointed out that after the formation of myotendinous and myoneuronal junctions the acetyl-cholinesterase activity is restricted to these junctions, whereas the sarcoplasmic acetyl-cholinesterase is no longer detectable. In mice and rats, the decrease in extra-junctional acetyl-cholinesterase is much slower (Fig. 4). This figure shows an 18 day old mouse embryo. Although myotendinous and myoneuronal junctions exhibit the most intense reaction, the sarcoplasm is stained as well.

The staining of whole muscle fibres in older mouse embryos is not an artefact during the acetyl-cholinesterase staining procedure, because the staining is inhibited by 10^{-5} M physostigmine and is only slightly affected by 10^{-5} M iso-OMPA.

The contrast between the region of the motor end-plates and the residual muscle fibres is more enhanced after staining with the KOELLE method (Fig. 5). The demarcation of the individual muscles from each other is, however, not as clear as with the KARNOVSKY method. The KOELLE medium penetrates the tissue more easily than the KARNOVSKY medium. Therefore, the deep muscle fibres are stained as well. On the other hand, the KARNOVSKY medium only stains the superficial layer of the muscle fibres.

These better diffusion properties of the KOELLE medium allow the application of this medium in trypsin treated, but unskinned limbs from 12 to 16 day old mouse embryos (Fig. 6). Here the muscles are again clearly visible. This is especially important for the muscles of hands and feet, because these muscles are easily damaged during skinning. The same is true for the epifascial nerves (Fig. 6).

The muscular pattern of the rat is identical to that of the mouse (Fig. 7). However, in contrast to the mouse, tendons in the rat can also be stained with the choline esterase reaction (Figs. 7, 8). As is seen in higher magnifications, the nuclei of the fibroblasts in the tendons seem to be stained (Fig. 9). Enzymatic inhibitor studies indicate that this staining is due to an unspecific choline esterase.

The results obtained with the choline esterase staining methods in rats prompted us to investigate the behaviour of the muscular and tendinous patterns in forelegs with aplasia in the skeletal system. Rats were treated on day 12 of pregnancy with the metabolic inhibitor 6-mercaptopurine (i.p. 25 mg/kg; NEUBERT and BARRACH, 1977). The fetuses were investigated on day 19 of development.

The extent of aplasia is not uniform at a given embryological stage. However, all hands exhibit a drastic reduction of the skeletal elements (Fig. 9). As all extensor muscles insert at the metacarpal and phalangeal bones the question arises, what happens to muscles and tendons when insertions fail to occur? The result is a nearly normal development of the extensor muscles (Fig. 10). Tendons remain visible, but reductions in their distal parts are recognizable. The present findings seem to support the view that the development of muscles, tendons and skeletal system are independent processes. At this time we are investigating the problem whether these tendons have new, atypical insertions or whether they end freely in the connective tissue.

ACKNOWLEDGEMENTS

This work was supported by grants from the Deutsche Forschungsgemeinschaft awarded to Sonderforschungsbereich 29. -
The author wishes to express his appreciation to Mr. KRETSCHMER for his expert technical assistance.

REFERENCES

Bogusch, G., In situ staining of muscles during development with the choline esterase technique. Stain Technol., submitted for publication.

Filogamo, G., Gabella, G., 1967, The development of neuromuscular correlations in vertebrates, Arch. Biol., (Liege) 78, 9 - 60.

Fluck, R.A., Strohman, R.C., 1973, Acetyl-cholinesterase activity in developing skeletal muscle cells in vitro, Develop. Biol., 33, 417 - 428.

Karnovsky, M.J., Roots, L., 1964, A "direct coloring" thiocholine method for cholinesterase, J. Histochem. Cytochem., 12, 219 - 221.

Mumenthaler, M., Engel, W.K., 1961, Cytological localization of cholin-esterase in developing chick embryo skeletal muscle, Acta anat., (Basel), 47, 274 - 299.

Naik, N.T., 1963, Technical variations in Koelle's histochemical method for demonstrating cholinesterase activity, Quart. J. Micro. Sci., 104, 89 - 100.

Neubert, D., Barrach, H.-J., 1977, Organotropic effects and dose-response relationships in teratology, in: Methods in Prenatal Toxicology, Teratology Workshop, April, 1977, Berlin. (D. Neubert, H.-J. Merker, T.E. Kwasigroch, eds.), pp. 405 - 412, Georg Thieme Publ., Stuttgart.

Wake, K., 1976, Formation of myoneuronal and myotendinous junctions in the chick embryo. Role of acetyl-cholinesterase-rich granules in the developing muscle fibres, Cell Tiss. Res., 173, 383 - 400.

Wassersug, R.J., 1976, A procedure for differential staining of cartilage and bone in whole formalin-fixed vertebrates, Stain Technol., 51, 131 - 134.

LEGENDS

Abbreviations used in the legends:

1.) Extensor carpi radialis longus muscle
2.) Extensor carpi radialis brevis muscle
3.) Extensor pollicis muscles
4.) Extensor digitorum muscle
5.) Extensor indicis muscle
6.) Extensor digiti quarti and quinti muscles
7.) Extensor carpi ulnaris muscle
8.) Triceps brachii muscle, lateral head
9.) Epicondylus lateralis humeri
10.) Ulna

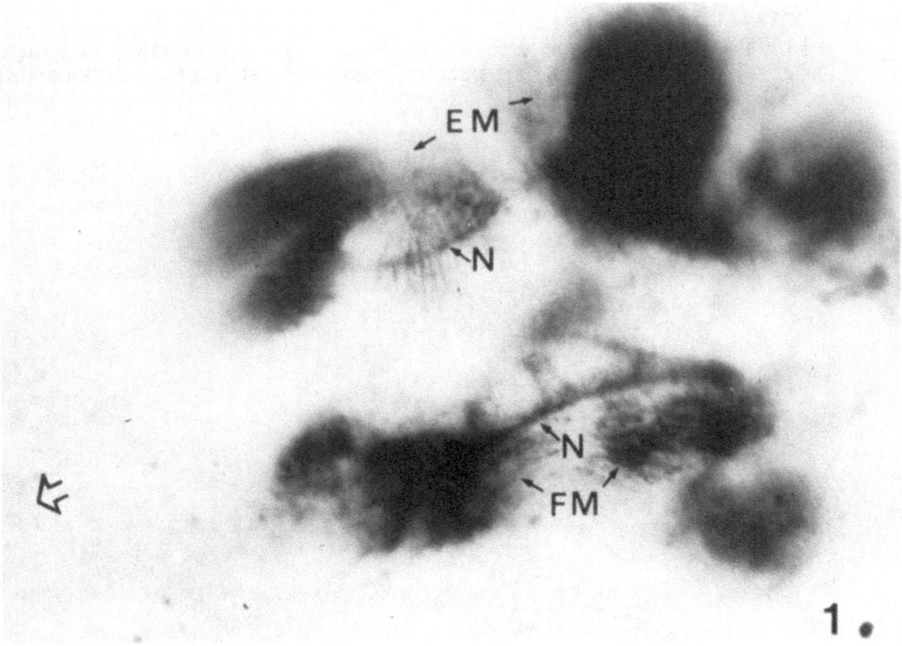

Fig. 1: 12 day old mouse embryo, unskinned foreleg. Karnovsky staining. Lateral view. The blastemata of the extensor (EM) and the flexor muscles (FM) are separated by the developing skeletal system. N = nerve, arrow = distal part of the limb bud. x 67.

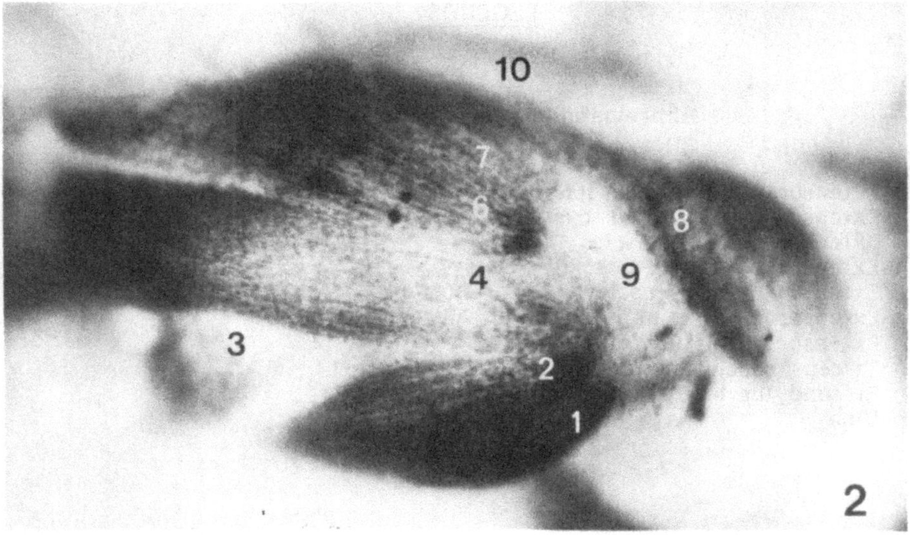

Fig. 2: 13 day old mouse embryo, skinned foreleg. Karnovsky staining. Dorsal view. The muscle pattern resembles that of adult animals. x 100.

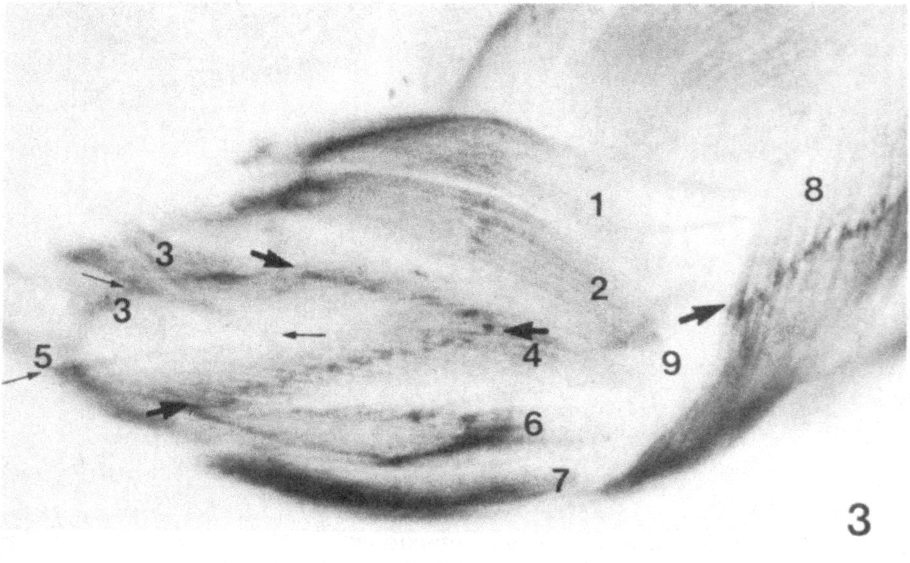

Fig. 3: 15 day old mouse embryo, skinned foreleg. Karnovsky staining. Dorsal view. The acetylcholinesterase reaction in the myoneuronal junctions (large arrows) and in the myotendinous junctions (small arrows) is enhanced.
x 48.

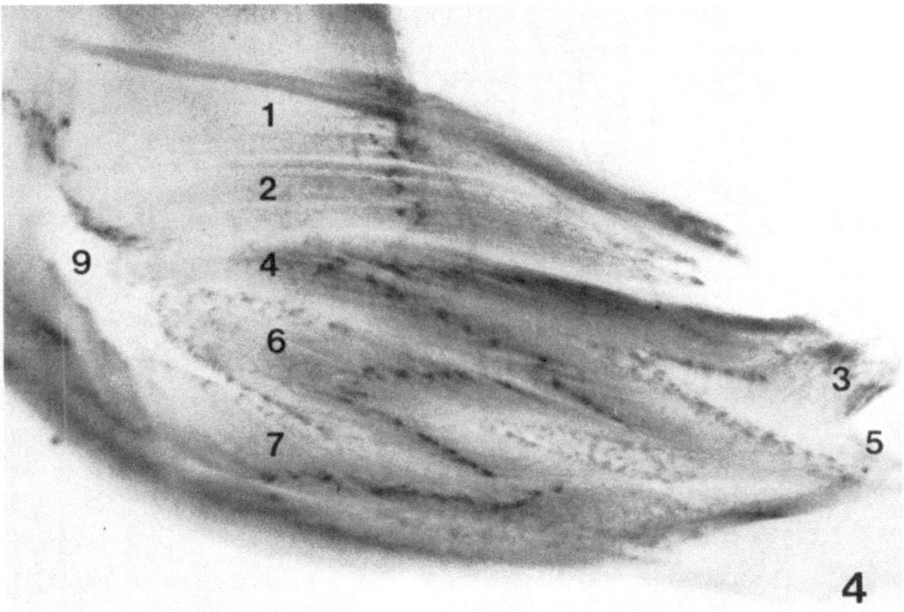

Fig. 4: 18 day old mouse embryo, skinned foreleg. Karnovsky staining. Dorsal view. The sarcoplasm still exhibits a high acetylcholinesterase reaction.
x 33.

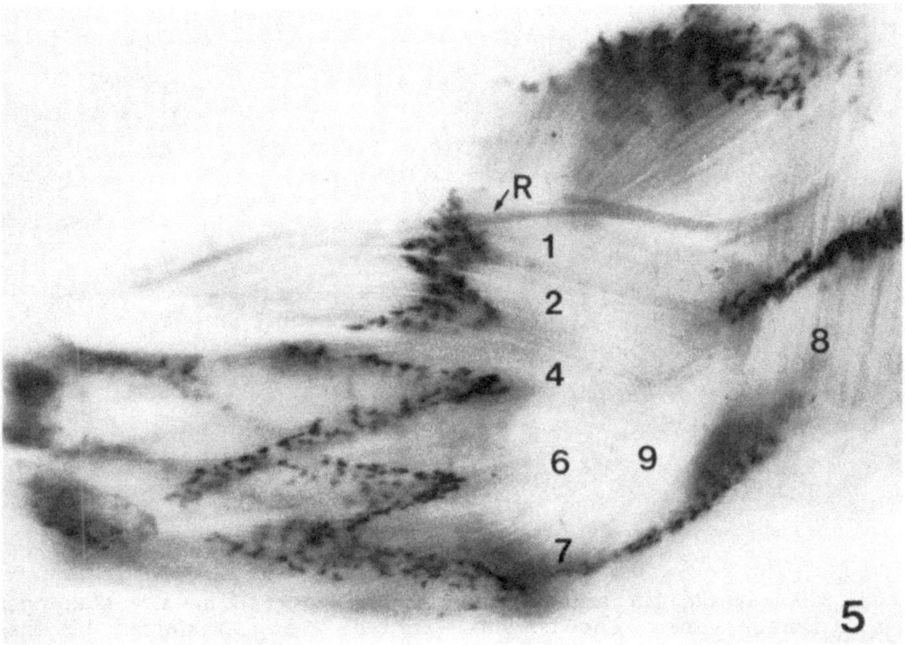

Fig. 5: 18 day old mouse embryo, skinned foreleg. Koelle staining. Dorsal view. In comparison with Fig. 4, the contrast between staining of the myoneuronal junctions and the residual sarcoplasm is more enhanced, but the demarcation of the individual muscles is poor. NR = radial nerve.
x 30.

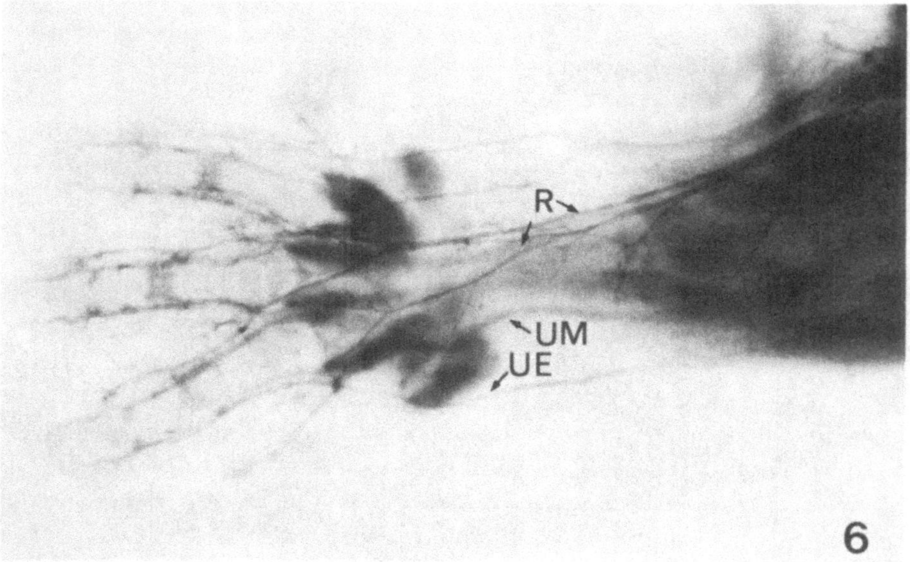

Fig. 6: 16 day old mouse embryo, unskinned foreleg. Koelle staining. Dorsal view. Muscles and nerves of the hand are completely stained. R = epifascial branches of the radial nerve, UE = epifascial branch of the ulnaris nerve, UM = motor branch of the ulnaris nerve.
x 30.

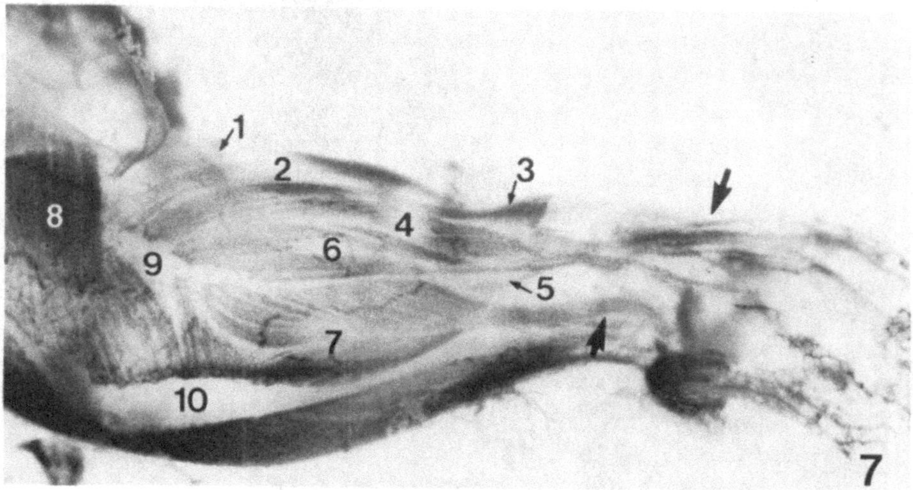

Fig. 7: 19 day old rat embryo, skinned foreleg. Karnovsky staining. Dorsal view. The tendons (arrows) are also stained by the cholinesterase reaction.
x 16.

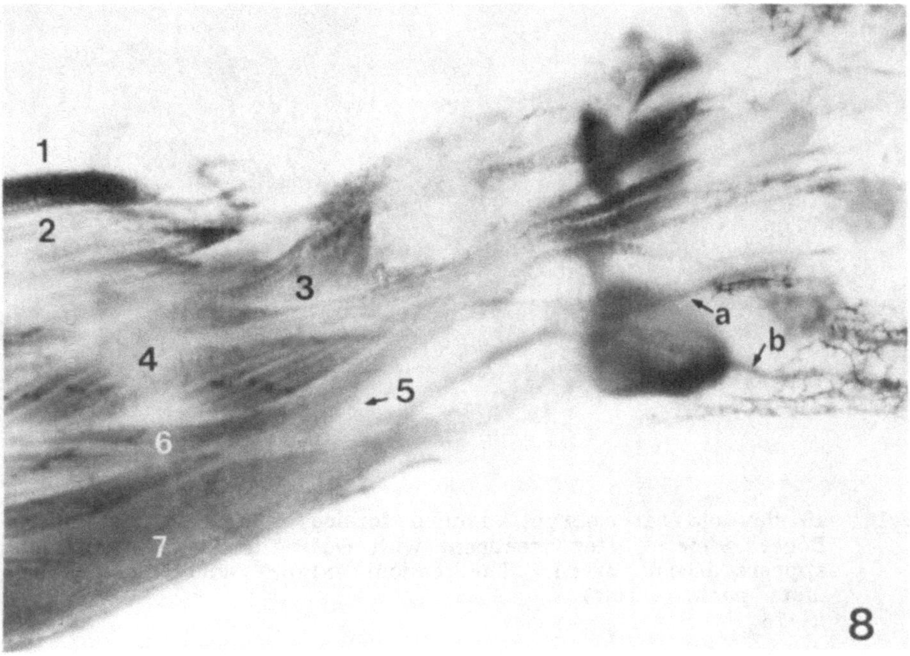

Fig. 8: 19 day old rat embryo, skinned foreleg. Karnovsky staining. Dorsal view. High magnification of the tendons from the extensor muscles. a) Tendon of the extensor digiti quarti muscle, b) tendon of the extensor digiti quinti muscle.
x 26.

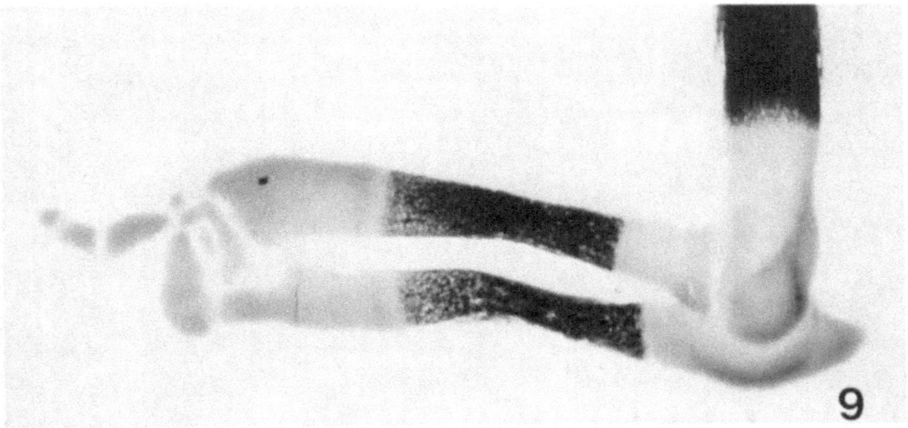

Fig. 9: 19 day old rat embryo. The skeletal elements of the hand show drastic reductions after treatment with 6-MP.
x 20.

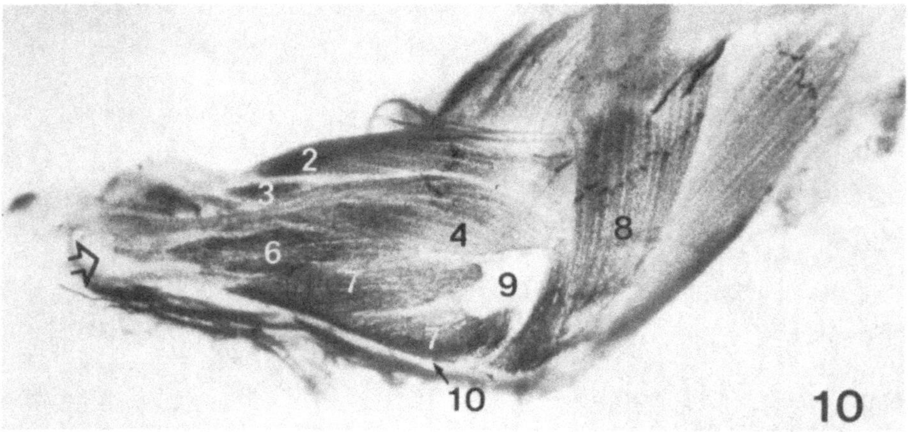

Fig. 10: 19 day old rat embryo, skinned foreleg. Karnovsky staining. Dorsal view. After treatment with 6-MP the muscular pattern appears almost normal. The tendons exhibit reductions in their distal parts (arrow).
x 16.

Developmental Properties of the Foot Integument in Avian Embryos

P. Sengel

Laboratoire de Zoologie et de Biologie animale,
Université scientifique et médicale de Grenoble, BP53X
F-38041 Grenoble Cédex, France

Birds, a taxinomic class of vertebrates, can be defined as feathered bipeds. This definition is based on the fact that feathers are their characteristic cutaneous appendages and that their forelimbs are transformed into wings. Feathers are believed to derive phylogenetically from reptilian scales, and may have served primitively the purpose of thermal insulation. On the wings and tail of most actual birds plumage has evolved into an apparatus adapted to air-borne locomotion. The feet of most birds, however, are covered by scales. Whether avian foot scales are phylogenetically related to reptilian scales or constitute a secondary acquisition is unknown. Therefore the question of their homology to feathers has been much debated (see review in LUCAS and STETTENHEIM, 1972, p. 344 - 346).

The problem is complicated by the fact that at least three types of scales can be distinguished on the feet of birds. For instance, in the chicken, there are: 1). large, more or less imbricated scutes (distally overlapping scuta, on the anterior face of tarsometatarsus and upper face of toes; proximally overlapping scutella, on the posterior face of the tarsometatarsus), and 2). non-overlapping tubercular reticula elsewhere.

Anatomical, genetic, biochemical, and embryological arguments support the idea that scutes and feathers are indeed homologous structures. Some species of birds (owls, grouses) have partially or completely feathered feet, so called ptilopody (DANFORTH, 1919). In fowl, many breeds are ptilopodous (for example, Brahmas, Faverolles, Silkies). The genetic trait is associated, in an unknown fashion, to brachydactyly; one of its phenotypic expressions is the replacement of scales by one or more rows of feathers along the fourth tarsometatarsus and digit IV (GOETINCK, 1967). Biochemically, feathers are typically made of keratin with a beta-type X-ray diffraction pattern, while interplumar epidermis produces alpha-type keratin. Likewise the outer face of scutes produces beta-keratin, while the inner face elaborates alpha-keratin (SAWYER, 1979). Accordingly, from the biosynthetical point of view, the outer face of scale and the feather may be considered as homologous structures, while the inner face of scale (actually the interscale hinge region) would correspond to interplumar skin. Furthermore, reticulate scales on the underside of the foot are made of alpha-keratin only (SAWYER and BORG, 1980), and for this reason may not be considered as cutaneous appendages at all.

The embryological arguments are derived from epidermal-dermal recombinations, which show that ectodermal epithelia from any body region or extra-embryonic area can be induced to form feathers or scales, depending on the type of dermal mesenchyme they are associated with, and that foot dermis is endowed with the capacity to induce feathers and/or scales, depending on the stage at which it is obtained.

Teratology of the Limbs

1. HETEROTOPIC RECOMBINANTS:

Heterotopic recombination experiments between dermis and epidermis from scale-forming and feather-forming regions have been performed in the chick or duck embryo at two different developmental stages of the integument:

A. Between 3 and 5 days of incubation in the limb bud, where the forerunners of dermis and epidermis (limb bud mesoderm and ectoderm) are exchanged long before skin tissues are histologically differentiated;

B. At a stage just prior to or concomitant with the initiation of cutaneous appendages in skin (between 6 and 9 days in back skin, and between 11 and 13 days in anterior tarsometatarsal (tmt) skin).

a. Limb bud recombinants: (SENGEL and PAUTOU, 1969). It is well known that the regional quality (wing or leg) of the limb skeleton and musculature is determined by the mesodermal component of the bud. In wings resulting from the combination of leg ectoderm and wing mesoderm, the cutaneous appendages are normally shaped and normally distributed feathers. The same is true for the stylopod and zeugopod of legs resulting from the association of wing ectoderm and leg mesoderm. In the latter legs, however, the cutaneous appendages are an abnormal and variegated superposition of more or less inhibited scales and more or less normal feathers, thus exhibiting the features of ptilopody (Fig. 1). The ectopic feathers tend to grow out of the distal rim of scales, and one or several feathers may be borne by one scute. In certain cases, and in certain zones of the foot, the scales are normal, while in others they are completely lacking and replaced by feathers. On the underside of the foot, tubercular scales may carry one feather each or be completely transformed into feathers. The distribution of these feathers is a typical scale pattern. The control homotopic recombinants of leg ectoderm and mesoderm always form legs with normally scaled feet, without any sign of ptilopody.

These results show that the ectoderm of the wing bud and that of the leg bud are not equivalent in respect to their morphogenetic capacity. Wing ectoderm is able to express feather-forming potentialities, in spite of the leg type induction imposed on it by the leg mesoderm. Leg ectoderm in the foot region does not express feather-forming ability, unless it is associated with wing mesoderm. Scale-forming information is not intrinsically contained in either wing or leg ectoderm, as neither ever produces scales unless combined with leg mesoderm.

b. Skin recombinants. When recombinants are grown in vitro or on the chick chorio-allantoic membrane for 5 to 8 days, the association of feather-forming epidermis and tmt scale-forming dermis leads to the formation of scales, while the reverse combination produces feathers, in accordance with the regional origin of the dermis (SENGEL, 1958; RAWLES, 1963). However, this clear-cut dermis-dependent morphogenesis is attained only if certain conditions of stage are fulfilled; otherwise, the predominance of feathers over scales again becomes evident. Only recombinants comprising 13-day tmt dermis form scales; and even some of these may bear abortive feathers at their distal rim. With 12-day tmt dermis, feathers are formed together with more or less retarded scales. With 11-day tmt dermis, only feathers develop (Fig. 2). These ectopic feathers are seemingly distributed in a typical scale pattern. It should be noted that control orthotopic recombinants of tmt epidermis with tmt dermis always form scales only, regardless of age. When similar experiments are perfomed in heterospecific chick/duck recombinations, the resulting feathers are chimeric: their macroscopical architecture is determined by the dermis and the structure of their barbules by the epidermis (DHOUAILLY, 1970). Thus the combination of 11-day tmt chick dermis with 9-day dorsal duck epidermis produces chick-type feathers with duck-type barbules. Likewise, the association of 12-day tmt duck dermis (developmentally equivalent to 11-day tmt chick dermis) with 7-day dorsal chick epidermis gives rise to duck-type feathers with chick-type barbules. When, on the contrary, the epidermis is tmt and the dermis dorsal, the resulting feathers again exhibit barbule morphology according to the specific origin of the epidermis, and gross anatomy in accordance with that of the dermis. In consequence, specific feather information is a property common to all regions of the skin, even those which normally form scales.

Quite similar results are obtained when tmt dermis is combined with extra-embryonic 8-day chick chorionic epithelium (FISHER and SAWYER, 1979). The latter has the capacity to transform into a typical epidermis when associated with dermis. Eleven-day tmt dermis induces feather-like structures (barb ridges) only; 12-day tmt dermis induces feather-like structures and scales; with 13-day tmt dermis, the chorionic epithelium forms scales only.

From the results of these and the previous limb bud experiments, the following conclusions can be drawn:

1.) Before 12 days, the prospective scale-forming dermis of the anterior tarsometatarsus is not endowed with scale-inducing capacity; apparently it transmits to the associated epidermis a species-specific "feather message", to which the feather-forming epidermis responds by forming feathers; this message, even though it causes the development of feathers, comprises instructions for the formation of a typical scale pattern.

2.) Unless in contact with tmt epidermis, tmt dermis does not acquire scale-inducing properties in isolation in vitro or on the chorioallantoic membrane. It may acquire them in vivo, however, when combined with wing bud ectoderm-derived epidermis, but then apparently it acquires them too late or too weakly to suppress all feather-forming properties.

3.) If in contact with tmt epidermis, tmt dermis acquires scale-inducing properties by 12 days of incubation.

4.) Dorsal prospective feather-forming epidermis - as well as feather-forming epidermis from other body regions, like the wing - and chorionic epithelium have an innate ability to form feathers and/or are able to respond to the feather-inducing message from the associated 11-day tmt dermis.

5.) Paradoxically, unlike epidermis from all other body regions and unlike chorionic epithelium, tmt epidermis (unless it originates experimentally from wing bud ectoderm) is unable to respond to the feather-forming message of early tmt dermis. The apparent contradiction resides in the fact that this epidermis is perfectly able to respond to feather-forming instructions originating from feather-forming regions. This leads to the conclusion that tmt feather message is different from that of, say, alar or dorsal feather message. One plausible explanation is that the feather message of tmt dermis is relatively weak and transient, while that of feather-forming regions is strong and more durable. Only epidermis with a bias towards feather formation is able to respond to the weak message. Epidermis from the scale-forming region, not being predestinated for feather formation, does not respond to this weak message, and must await the later and stronger scale message to undergo morphogenesis.

c. Region-specific keratin synthesis: Despite the peculiarities of foot integumentary tissues, the regional specificity of cutaneous appendages in birds on the whole, then, resides in the dermis. This is also strikingly illustrated at the biochemical level during keratin synthesis. Feathers and scales of birds differ in the composition of their keratin (KEMP and ROGERS, 1972). Feather keratin is characterized by a polygenic family of closely related beta-type polypeptides with molecular weights around 11,000 (ROGERS, 1978). The outer face of scales produces beta-type keratin polypeptides of about 14,000 M.W. Which of the two cutaneous tissues is responsible for the choice between these two types of keratin is shown by SDS-PAGE analysis of keratin proteins produced in heterotopic dorsal/tmt and tmt/dorsal recombinants of chick embryonic skin (DHOUAILLY et al., 1978). The answer is clear-cut: the dermis is the determinant tissue. Consequently, morphogenesis and keratin biosynthesis are, both in some coordinated fashion, under the control of the dermis. Whether the coordination operates at the genetic or at an epigenetic level is at present unknown.

2. GENETIC PTILOPODY:

A genetic switch is able to alter the situation of the normally non-feathered feet of fowl. This is the case of the mutation ptilopody, which was shown to affect both epidermis and dermis (GOETINCK, 1967). When ectodermal and mesodermal leg bud components are exchanged between normal and mutant embryos, the resulting composite legs all display the traits of ptilopody, whether it is the mesoderm or the ectoderm which originates from the mutant embryo. It is conceivable that the gene substitution lowers the level of response of the epidermis to dermal tmt feather induction and/or reinforces the feather-inducing capacity of the tmt dermis.

3. CHEMICAL PTILOPODY:

Finally, a simple molecule such as retinoic acid, when injected at an appropriate stage into the chick embryo, may bring about morphogenetic changes which mimic those obtained from heterotopic recombinations of scale-forming dermis with feather-forming epidermis. Intra-amniotic injection of 125 µg of retinoic acid at 10, 11, or 12 days causes the formation of feathered feet in a large proportion of the embryos (Fig. 3). This chemical ptilopody somewhat differs from that obtained in recombinants in that the formation of scales is not inhibited, but many, and sometimes all, scales bear feathers at their distal tip. Large scutes may carry two or more (up to four) feathers, while reticula form only one feather. In normal embryos, scales form in the foot integument in a precise time sequence, the large anterior tmt scuta appearing first, posterior scutella later, and reticula last. Correspondingly, only those scales which are at the beginning of their development on the day of injection and the following day are affected by the treatment, which means that scale primordia are sensitive to the drug during a limited period of their morphogenesis. This period actually corresponds, at least for anterior scutes, to the stage when tmt dermis exhibits feather-forming properties when confronted with feather-forming epidermis (DHOUAILLY et al., 1980).

Two possible mechanisms may be envisaged to explain the effect of retinoic acid. Either it reinforces the feather-forming induction of the tmt dermis, so that the tmt epidermis now becomes able to respond to it, or it enhances the sensitivity of the epidermis to the weak dermal feather-forming induction. Both mechanisms may be simultaneously valid. Heterotypic epidermal-dermal recombination experiments, where one of the two constituents originates from a retinoic acid-treated embryo, will have to clarify this point.

REFERENCES

Danforth, C.H., 1919, An hereditary complex in the domestic fowl, Genetics, 4, 587 - 596.

Dhouailly, D., 1970, Déterminisme de la différenciation spécifique des plumes néoptiles et téléoptiles chez le Poulet et le Canard, J. Embryol. exp. Morph., 24, 73 - 94.

Dhouailly, D., Hardy, M.H., Sengel, P., 1980, Formation of feathers on chick foot scales: a stage-dependent morphogenetic response to retinoic acid, J. Embryol. exp. Morph., 58, 63 - 78.

Dhouailly, D., Rogers, G.E., Sengel, P., 1978, The specification of feather and scale protein synthesis in epidermal-dermal recombinations, Develop. Biol., 65, 58 - 68.

Fisher, C., Sawyer, R.H., 1979, Response of the avian chorionic epithelium to presumptive scale-forming dermis, J. exp. Zool., 207, 505 - 512.

Goetinck, P.F., 1967, Tissue interactions in the development of ptilopody and brachydactyly in the chick embryo, J. exp. Zool., 165, 293 - 300.

Kemp, D.J., Rogers, G.E., 1972, Differentiation of avian keratinocytes. Characterization and relationships of the keratin proteins of adult and embryonic feathers and scales, Biochem., 11, 969 - 975.

Lucas, A.M., Stettenheim, P.R., 1972, Avian Anatomy. Integument. U.S. Agriculture Handbook, 362, Government Office, Washington, D.C.

Rawles, M.E., 1963, Tissue interactions in scale and feather development as studied in dermal-epidermal recombinants, J. Embryol. exp. Morph., 11, 765 - 789.

Rogers, G.E., 1978, Keratins viewed at the nucleic acid level, Trends biochem. Sci., 3, 131 - 133.

Sawyer, R.H., 1979, Avian scale development: effect of the scaleless gene on morphogenesis and histogenesis, Develop. Biol., 68, 1 - 15.

Sawyer, R.H., Borg, T.K., 1980, Avian scale development: VII. Normal keratinization follows abnormal morphogenesis of reticulate scales from the "scaleless" mutant, J. Morph., (in press).

Sengel, P., 1958, Recherches expérimentales sur la différenciation des germes plumaires et du pigment de la peau de l'embryon de poulet en culture in vitro, Ann. Sc. nat. Zool., 20, 431 - 514.

Sengel, P., Pautou, M.P., 1969, Experimental conditions in which feather morphogenesis predominates over scale morphogenesis, Nature, (London), 222, 693 - 694.

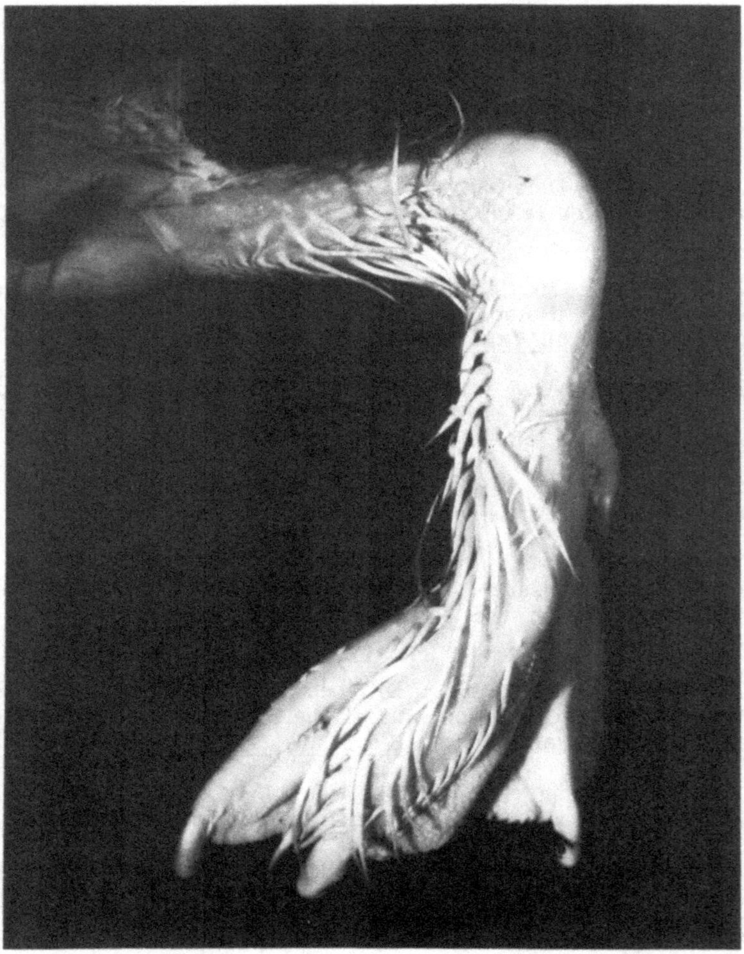

Fig. 1: Recombinational ptilopody (feathered foot) of an 18-day embryonic duck foot, which developed from the heterotopic recombination, at 4 days of incubation, of wing bud ectoderm and leg bud mesoderm. Note that many scales on digit III (digit I is on the right, digit IV on the left) are replaced by feather filaments, while others (on digit IV) bear short feather buds or filaments (SENGEL and PAUTOU, 1969).

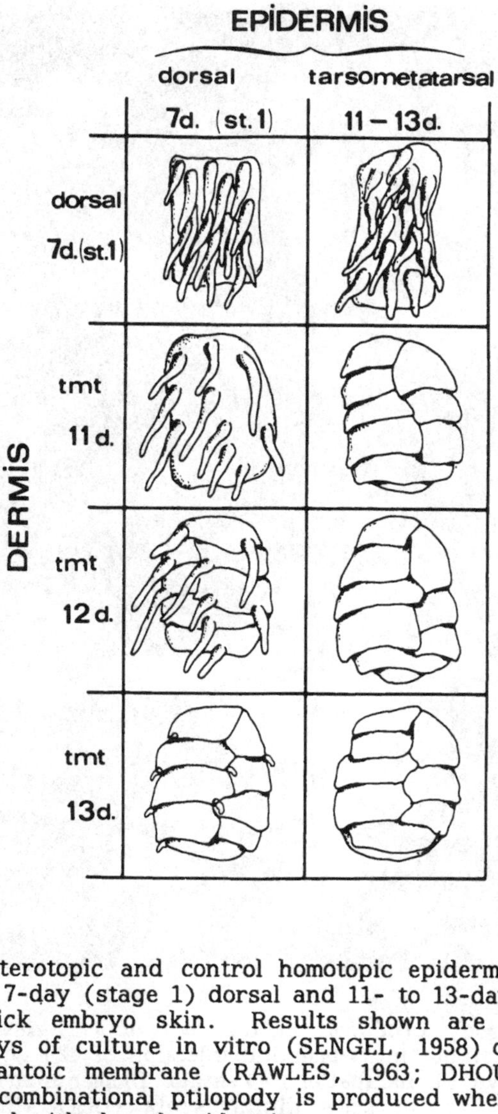

Fig. 2: Heterotopic and control homotopic epidermal-dermal recombinants of 7-day (stage 1) dorsal and 11- to 13-day tarsometatarsal (tmt) chick embryo skin. Results shown are obtained after 5 - 10 days of culture in vitro (SENGEL, 1958) or on the chick chorio-allantoic membrane (RAWLES, 1963; DHOUAILLY et al., 1978). Recombinational ptilopody is produced when tmt dermis is associated with dorsal epidermis.

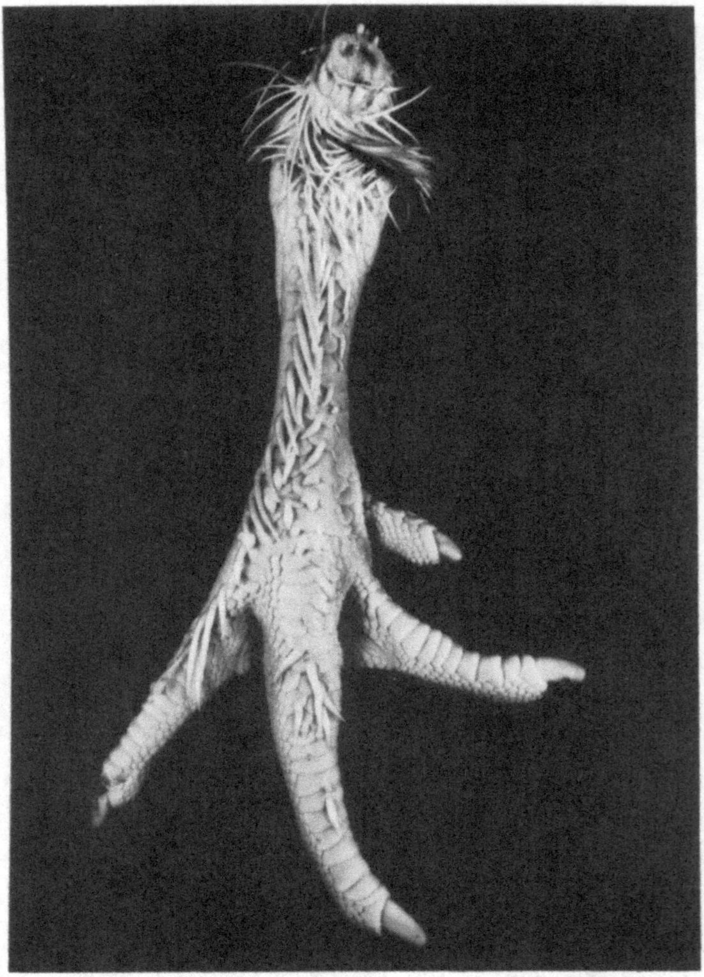

Fig. 3: Chemical ptilopody produced in the foot of a 17-day chick embryo, after a single intra-amniotic injection of 125 μg of retinoic acid at 10 days of incubation. Feather filaments are borne by all tmt scuta and by some digital scuta (DHOUAILLY et al., 1980).

The Contrast between Mouse and Ferret Limb Buds in Culture – Possible Advantages of Comparing Results from a Limb Culture System with Whole Embryo Explantation

F. Beck and A. P. Gulamhusein
Dept. of Anatomy, University of Leicester,
University Road, Leicester LE1 7RH, U.K.

Trowell (1954) based explantation of mouse limb bud cultures are now unremarkable standbys in the technology of any teratology laboratory interested in the direct effect of teratogenic agents upon embryonic tissues. The method was clearly described in relation to the effects of L-azetidine-2-carboxylic acid by AYDELOTTE and KOCHHAR (1972) and has since that time been extensively used in the laboratories of NEUBERT and MERKER (see Merker, 1975). More recently NEUBERT and BARRACH (1977) again using mice have developed a submerged culture system and described the advantages and disadvantages of their rotating culture with the standard Trowell technique. The differentiation of 43 somite mouse early limb buds in vitro to the point at which a cartilaginous skeleton of the paw has developed takes about 2 - 3 days while the same developmental stage is reached in about 6 days in vitro. Experience shows that no further differentiation will take place using the current techniques and attempts have been made with rabbits and rats (LESSMÖLLMANN, et al., 1976) to use other species in order - among other things - to extend the culture period. The limb buds have grown but differentiation of the paw skeleton is undoubtedly inferior to that obtained from mice. The present work describes the results obtained from growing ferret limb buds in a Trowell type culture. Differentiation, it was found, was comparable to that in the mouse and the culture period was extended to 18 days (equivalent to about 6 days of development in vivo).

Techniques for breeding and mating ferrets have been described (BECK 1975, BECK et al., 1976) as have the normal stages during ferret development (GULAMHUSEIN and BECK, in press). In the present investigation forelimb buds of ferret embryos at days 20, 21, 22, 23, and 24 of gestation were cultured (day of mating = day 0). The explanting procedure was similar to that of AYDELOTTE and KOCHHAR (1972) and the limbs were examined after 6, 12, 15 and 18 days. The culture medium was changed every 3 days. On harvesting the limb buds were examined by Methylene blue staining and light microscopy.

Day 20 embryo limb buds (42 - 45 somites) when explanted for 12 days allowed of easy identification of the scapula and humerus only. Extension of the culture to 18 days allowed only a little further development and the paw skeleton remained poorly developed with patchy cartilage which on examination by light microscopy was shown to be separated by densely packed blastema cells (Fig. 1).

Day 21 limb buds (46 - 48 somites) had far more densely packed central blastema cells at the time of explantation. The explants grew better than those explanted on day 20 but even after 18 days (Fig. 2) the distal segments remained poorly developed especially in the paw.

On day 22 (50 somites) maximal development was achieved. By day 18 in vitro both proximal and distal skeletal elements were well developed. All the cartilages including those of the paw skeleton were easily recognizable (Fig. 3). Although it was easy to culture limb buds from day 23 and 24

Teratology of the Limbs

embryos it was found that chondrogenesis was already underway at the time of explantation, nevertheless the buds developed well and the paw skeleton was easily demonstrable (Fig. 4 and 5). We have not yet attempted to carry out submerged cultures with the ferret but there seems no a priori reason for believing that they would not be as successful as the Trowell set. It is possible therefore to obtain limb cultures from an animal other than the mouse. Culture of ferret limb buds will have two particular advantages. First the prolonged period of differentiation in culture allows prolonged testing of a potential teratogen (possibly in low doses) when such a procedure is not possible in the mouse. Of course, the prolonged culture period is likely to be more of a disadvantage than a help in the large number of cases when adequate results are obtained after 6 days (Fig. 6) and for this reason we do not advocate using this species as first choice. Secondly, it is perhaps important in some cases to obtain results from animals whose pharmacokinetics differ from those of the mouse. While not suggesting that the ferret (a mustelid carnivore) is expected to metabolize substrates more like man than the mouse is, there is nevertheless the possibility that differences between the two species may result from idiosyncratic behaviour of one (or both) vis-à-vis man and the results obtained would have to be viewed in that light. Conversely, when the results correspond they are more likely to be of general applicability.

Teratological studies repeatedly throw up the question of whether an agent acts primarily (a) on the mother (b) on the extraembryonic membranes or (c) directly upon the embryo. These are difficult questions to answer. The vascular clamping experiment of BRENT and his group (BRENT and FRANKLIN, 1960) allow for temporary isolation of the uterus during the action of a quickly metabolized or excreted potential teratogen (90 mins or 2 1/2 hours if the embryo is cooled). This method of isolating the feto-placental unit has the advantage that potentially it may be carried out at any stage of gestation though it has only been researched at the early stages when embryonic requirements are relatively small - possibly it will not be feasable when a fully developed chorio-allantoic placenta is present. The other extreme of investigating this phenomenon is the limb bud culture system described above. Here the limitation is clearly whether the potential teratogen is ubiquitous or at least catholic enough to act upon the tissues of the limb bud in such a way as to interfere with growth or chondrification. Obviously, this will involve only a proportion of teratogenic agents whose critical period coincides with limb formation (or indeed with the formation of other structures such as the palate; POURTOIS, 1966) for which methods have been developed. These agents must also act directly upon the embryo and in the case of limb bud culture affect the processes of growth and cartilage formation. A third, equally restricted line, is the culture of whole embryos by the method of NEW et al. (1976). It is now possible to grow mouse embryos quite as easily as rat embryos and it is therefore possible to test whether a teratogen acts upon the feto placental unit. The method is effectively restricted in the mouse to between 8 1/2 and 10 1/2 days and in the rat to between 9 1/2 and 11 1/2 days but nevertheless it has demonstrated a number of agents which almost certainly act upon the 'placental' unit which in this case is the inverted yolk sac. In our experiments rat embryos were explanted according to the method of NEW et al. (1976) at 9 1/2 days of gestation, i.e. at the head process stage, and then treated with a tripeptide, leupeptin which was dissolved in the culture serum. Leupeptin is a bacterial (Actinomycetes) product which specifically inhibits the lysosomal cathepsins B, L and H (AOYAGA and UMEZAWA, 1975). It seems unlikely that a molecule as big as leupeptin would penetrate the yolk sac and for this reason its site of action is almost certainly upon the lysosomes of the visceral yolk-sac epithelium. When present in the serum in dilutions as low as 1 µg/ml the mean protein content of embryos (n = 10) fell from control levels of 191.5 ± S.E. 3.39 to 142.8 ± S.E. 10.1. The general development of the embryo (n = 40) was retarded (Fig. 7) and there were a number of abnormalities of shape. At 2 µg/ml protein levels were still lower 194.5 ± S.E. 7.3 (control) against 98.37 ± S.E. 3.39 (experimental); more embryos were retarded or abnormal. At 4 µg/ml dramatic effects were observed. Protein values fell from 196.9 ± S.E. 10.02 to 50.9 ± S.E. 8.17 (n = 10) and the majority of the embryos were grossly abnormal, e.g. none had a closed neural tube compared with 100% among controls. Electron microscopy of the yolk sac showed all the signs of a storage disease (e.g. Figs. 8 and 9) though it is realised that protein storage diseases are incompatible with life.

Examination of an embryo and its fetal membranes at any stage before 11.00 days shows that a portion of the embryonic endoderm is exposed to the culture serum (Fig. 10). Therefore, theoretically it is possible that leupeptin may affect the embryo directly. To overcome this objection a series of embryos were cultured in which leupeptin was placed into the culture serum as late as 11.00 days. At this stage the embryo has become completely invaginated into its own yolk sac (Fig. 11) but unfortunately the time remaining for meaningful culture is restricted to 12 hours. In spite of this, addition of 10 µg/ml at this late stage still results in a significant fall in protein levels: 221.9 ± S.E. 6.6. (control) 143.5 ± S.E. 8.7 (experimental). There were also statistically significant changes ($p > 0.01$) in somite numbers and crown rump length.

An interesting variation of both the limb culture technique and the whole embryo culture technique is that they can be performed in the presence of serum from a treated rat. It is therefore possible to note the difference between the effects of a potential teratogen applied directly to the embryo and one which has first undergone possible biotransformation in the maternal tissues (see McGARRITY et al., in press).

DISCUSSION:

We have outlined methods whereby it is possible to test whether teratogenic agents are primarily active on maternal tissues (culture in serum from a treated mother, uterine clamping in a quickly metabolized drug) on embryonic tissues (limb culture, palate culture, etc.) or on the extraembryonic membranes (whole embryo culture in certain controlled circumstances). It is important to stress however, that these relatively sophisticated techniques are by no means comprehensive. Any experienced teratologist will appreciate that (a) the limb culture technique, though now no longer restricted in time to quite the same extent as before, is still applicable to only those relatively few agents that effect the tissues in culture, (b) the uterine clamping technique is available for the investigation of short lived rapidly metabolized materials and (c) the whole embryo culture technique spans a very short development period only.

Nevertheless, it is clear that an increasing battery of techniques are becoming available and an intelligent combination of these together with standard in vivo investigations are now necessary for the thorough experimental investigation of a given agent - i.e. for teratological experimentation <u>not</u> for simple drug screening. Thus it is clear that the application of leupeptin to the limb culture system is well worth doing because it may shed considerable light on the function of lysosomes in early limb morphogenesis and chondrogenesis.

ACKNOWLEDGEMENTS

The authors are grateful to the M.R.C. for a grant in aid of research. Dr. Madhu Gupta and Messrs. Lowy and Moore actively participated in the research work and we are also grateful to Mr. Chris Rigel D'Lacey and Mrs. S. Bulman for excellent technical assistance.

REFERENCES

Aoyaga, T., Umezawa, H., 1975, Structure and activities of protease inhibitors of microbial origin, in: "Proteases and Biological Control", (E. Reich et al., eds.). Cold Spring Harbor.

Aydelotte, M.B., Kochhar, D.M., 1972, Development of mouse limb buds in organ culture: chondrogenesis in the presence of a proline analog, L-azetidine-2-carboxylic acid, Devl. Biol. 21, 191 - 201.

Beck, F., 1975, The ferret as a teratological model, in: "New approaches to the evaluation of abnormal embryonic development", (D. Neubert, H.J. Merker,eds.). Georg Thieme Publ., Stuttgart.

Beck, F., Schön, H., Mould, G., Swidzinka, P., Curry, S., Grauwiler, J., 1976, Comparison of the teratogenic effects of mustine hydrochloride in rats and ferrets. The value of the ferret as an experimental animal in teratology, Teratology, 13, 151 - 166.

Brent, R.L., Franklin, J.B., 1960, Uterine vascular clamping: New procedure for the study of congenital malformations, Science, 132, 89 - 91.

Gulamhusein, A.P., Beck, F., Normal stages of ferret development, Bib. Anat. (in press).

Lessmöllmann, U., Hinz, N., Neubert, D., 1976, In vitro system for toxicological studies on development of mammalian limb buds in a chemically defined medium, Arch. Toxicol. 36, 169 - 176.

McGarrity, C., Samani, N.J., Beck, F., Gulamhusein, A.P., The effect of sodium salicylate on the rat embryo in culture : An in vitro model for the morphological assessment of teratogenicity (in press).

Merker, H.J., 1975, Significance of the limb bud culture system for investigations of teratogenic mechanisms, in: "New approaches to the evaluation of abnormal embryonic development" (D.Neubert, H.-J. Merker, eds.). pp. 161 - 199, Georg Thieme Publ., Stuttgart.

Neubert, D., Barrach, H.-J., 1977, Techniques applicable to study morphogenic differentiation of limb buds in organ culture, in: "Methods in Prenatal Toxicology", (D. Neubert, H.-J. Merker, T.E. Kwasigroch, eds.). pp. 241 - 251, Georg Thieme Publ., Stuttgart.

New, D.A.T., Coppola, P.T., Cockcroft, D., 1976, Improved development of rat head fold embryos in culture resulting from low oxygen and modification of culture serum, J. Reprod. Fert. 48, 219 - 222.

Pourtois, M., 1966, Onset of the acquired potentiality for fusion in the palatal shelves of rats, J. Embryol. exp. Morphol. 16, 171 - 182.

Trowell, O.A., 1954, The culture of mature organs in synthetic media, Exp. Cell Res. 16, 118 - 147.

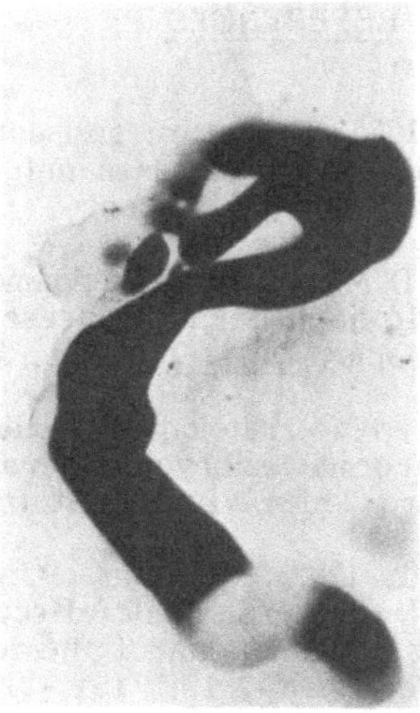

Fig. 1: Day 20 ferret limb bud cultured for 18 days. x 25

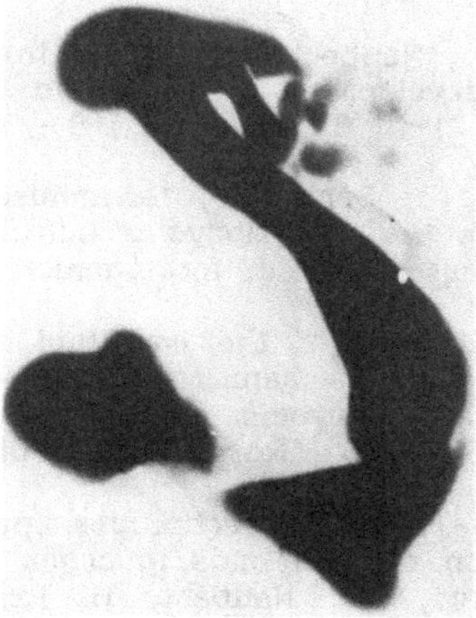

Fig. 2: Day 21 ferret embryo limb bud cultured for 18 days. x 25

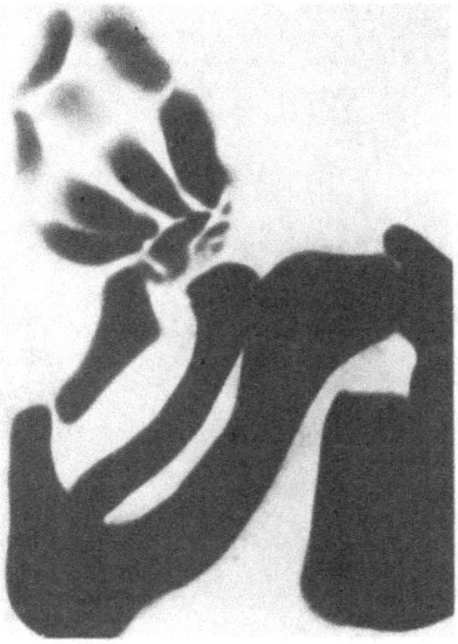

Fig. 3: 22 day ferret embryo limb bud cultured for 18 days. x 25

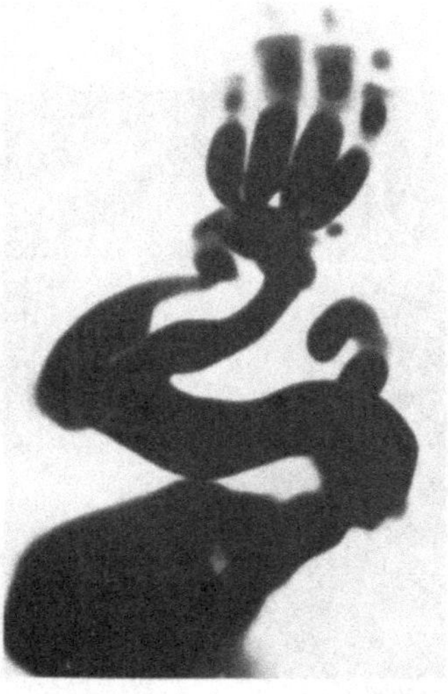

Fig. 4: 23 day ferret embryo limb bud cultured for 18 days. x 25

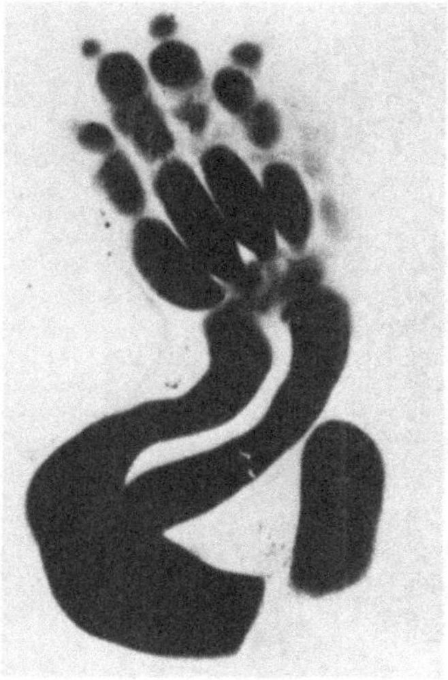

Fig. 5: Ferret 24 day limb bud cultured for 18 days. x 25

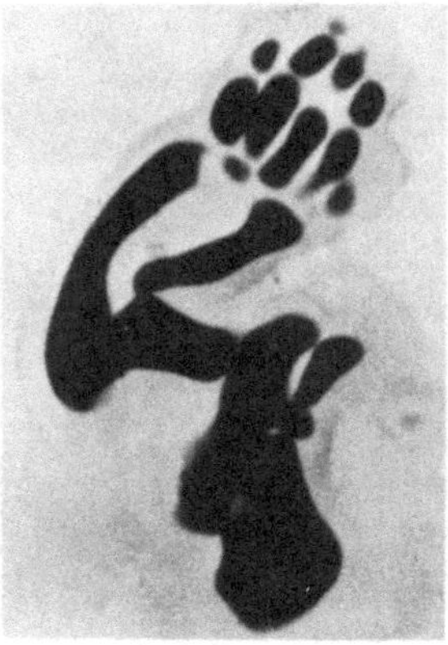

Fig. 6: 12 day mouse embryo limb bud cultured for 6 days. x 25

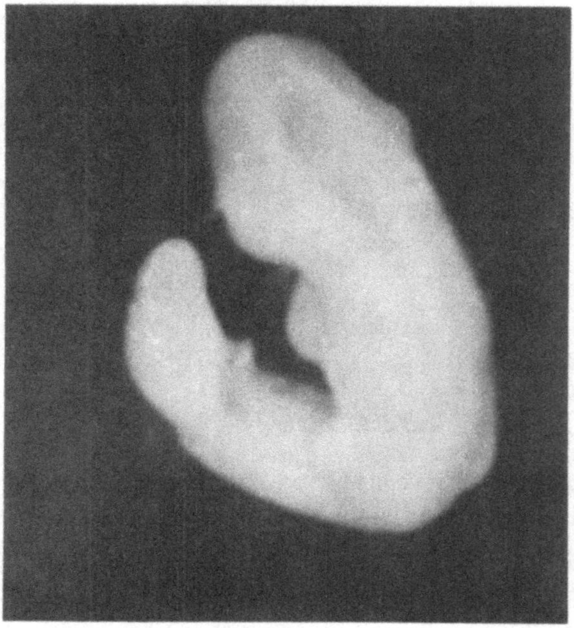

Fig. 7: Retarded 11 1/2 day rat embryo following culture by the NEW technique between 9 1/2 and 11 1/2 days in the presence of 1 µg/ml leupeptin in the serum. The tail is stunted and does not lie along the right side of the head as in normal embryos. x 25

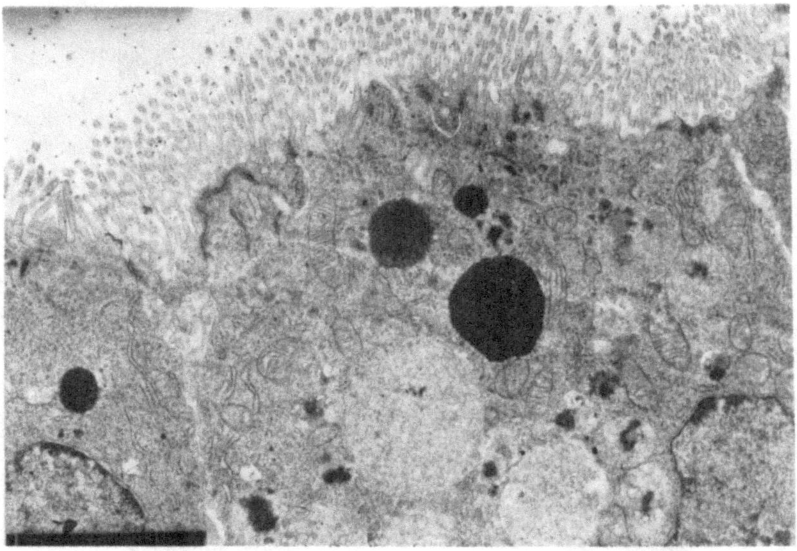

Fig. 8: Normal 9 1/2 day yolk sac. Note regular appearance and size of lysosomes. x 8 000

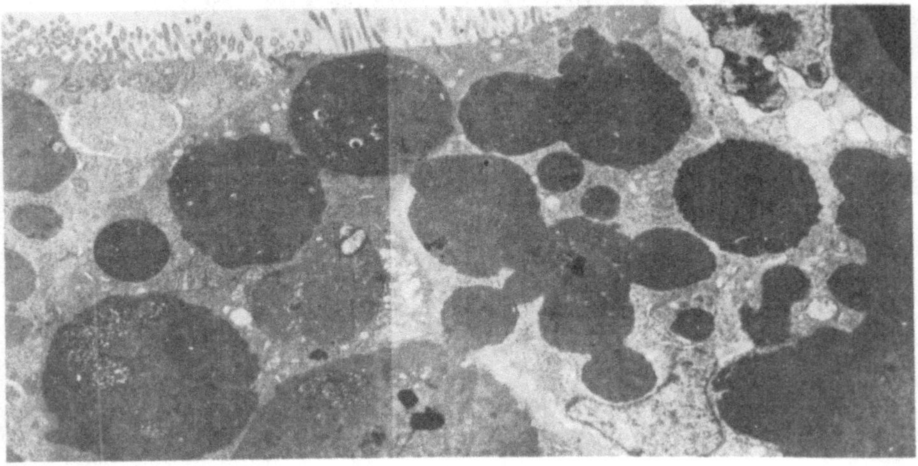

Fig. 9: Electron micrograph of abnormal yolk sac following culture in the presence of 4 µl/ml of leupeptin in the serum. Note the abnormal disposition of the secondary lysosomes. x 6 000

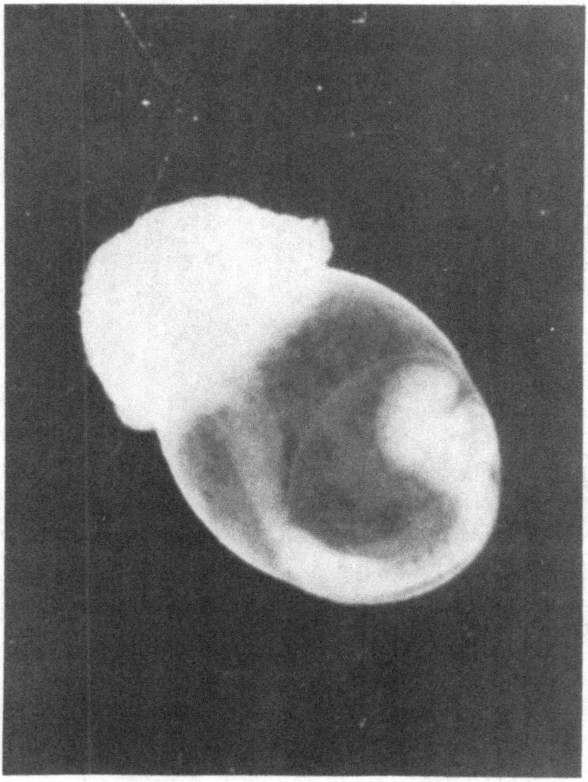

Fig. 10: Showing a 10.5 day rat embryo after 24 hours of culture. The endoderm is still exposed to the exterior in the convexity of the embryo. Note the amniotic membrane and the allantoic bud. The latter has grown towards the ectoplacental cone and fused with it. The portion of the specimen not enclosing amniotic fluid contains the extraembryonic coelom. x 25

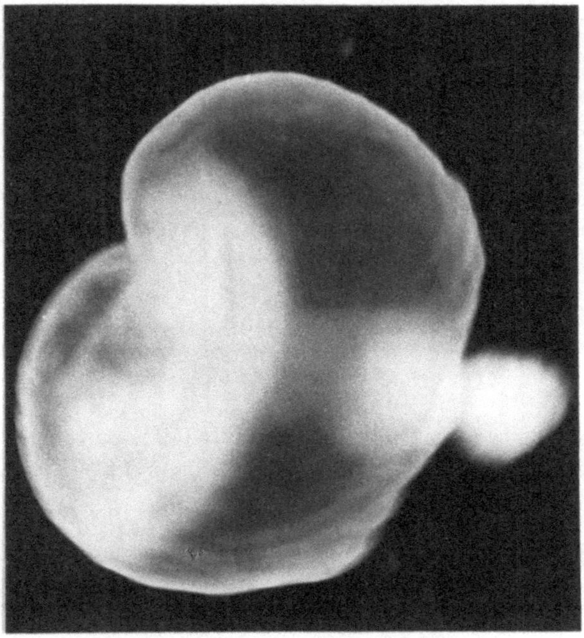

Fig. 11: Showing a rat embryo cultured for 36 hours (between 9 1/2 days and 11.0 days. Complete invagination of the embryo into the yolk sac has now occurred leaving just a small dimple at the site of inversion. Nothing can reach the embryo from this point onwards without first passing through the walls of the yolk sac. x 20

Transfilter Interaction of the Zone of Polarizing Activity with the Apical Ectodermal Ridge and the Distal Mesenchyme in the Chick Embryo Wing Bud in Ovo

Eero A. Kaprio

The Children's Hospital, University of Helsinki,
Stenbäckinkatu 11, SF-00290 Helsinki 29, Finland

INTRODUCTION:

According to the SAUNDERS-ZWILLING hypothesis the proximo-distal morphogenesis of the limb is controlled by a reciprocal interaction between the Apical Ectodermal Ridge (AER) and the limb bud mesenchyme. The AER has been found to be largely non-specific in its actions. According to the hypothesis the AER is elevated in form when morphogenetically active and flat when inactive (SAUNDERS, 1977).

A precisely located post-axial mesenchymal activity, that displays polarizing properties in limb morphogenesis has been named the Zone of Polarizing Activity (ZPA) (BALCUNS et al., 1970; MacCABE et al., 1973). This activity is tested by its transplantation to a pre-axial location. There it causes pre-axial changes, including AER elevation and pre-axial polydactyly. Though the presence of the AER is necessary for the polydactyly to develop (SUMMERBELL, 1974), it has been claimed, that the ZPA does not act directly on the AER (MacCABE and PARKER, 1979). The role of the ZPA in normal morphogenesis of the limb has been doubted for several reasons. Normal limb morphogenesis has been claimed after the removal of the ZPA (MacCABE et al., 1973; FALLON and CROSBY, 1975). Also tissues other than of limb bud origin, when placed in the pre-axial location, are able to induce pre-axial polydactyly, e.g. the flank of the chick embryo (SAUNDERS, 1977). However this raises the possibility, that the flank's ZPA-like-activity may induce the ZPA-freed limb bud to regenerate a new ZPA.

In order to circumvent this objection, barriers were placed anterior to the ZPA. Stage 20 HH (HAMBURGER and HAMILTON, 1951) right wing bud of the chick embryo was used. The ZPA maps of MacCABE et al. (1973) show, that the ZPA is, at this stage, to be found in the posterior third of the wing bud. The AER, on the other hand, overlies the middle third of the same stage wing bud (KAPRIO and TÄHKÄ, 1978). Thus the placing of a barrier anterior to the ZPA would leave the AER and most of the distal wing bud mesenchyme on the other side of the barrier. Four types of barriers were used. Cellophane was the impermeable barrier. The three others were Nuclepore filters with different pore sizes. Transfilter experiments with embryonic tissues (SAXÉN, 1980) have shown, that by selecting Nuclepore filters with 0.05 um, 1.0 um and 8.0 um pores, three types of transfilter communications are to be expected: diffusion, cell contact and cell penetration, respectively.

MATERIAL AND METHODS:

White Leghorn eggs were incubated for 3 1/4 days at 38° C. They were fenestrated, membranes cut and the embryos were kept moist with DULBECCO'S phosphate buffer. Only stage 20 HH (HAMBURGER and HAMILTON, 1951) embryos were used. A radial incision was made to separate the posterior third from the anterior two-thirds of the right wing bud. The controls had the incision made, but nothing inserted. Cellophane, Nuclepore filters with either 0.05 um (Np 0.05), 1.0 um (Np 1.0) or 8.0 um (Np 8.0) sized pores were inserted. The fenestration was sealed with tape and the egg returned to the incubator. The presence of the barrier was checked the next day - 13 to 32 hours later. The embryo was rejected, if the barrier had fallen off, or the wing bud showed signs of damage, e.g. opacity or haematomas. The embryos were allowed to develop to ten days of incubation. They were then fixed in TCA and the cartilage was stained with Alcian Green. Except for the control group (17 cases, with an average L/W of 0.31, see HAMBURGER and HAMILTON, 1951) all others were photographed immediately after barrier insertion (Tab. 1). Most of these were successfully rephotographed the next day (Tab. 2).

RESULTS:

The Length/Width (L/W) ratio for each group in Table 1 shows that the developmental stage was late 20 HH for all others, except for Np 8.0 group. No obvious differences were found in the average lengths of the barriers, the proportion of them within the wing bud, nor in the area of the wing bud anterior to the barrier. The outgrowth rates of the wing buds were of similar order of magnitude (Table 2). This indicates that they were equally viable. The wing buds overgrew the barriers at different rates. Cellophane and Np 1.0 were overgrown at a faster rate than the other two barriers. In other words they were retained more proximally.

In the sham operated control group six wing buds developed into normal wings without cartilage deletions. Seven others did not develop any deletions either, but had one of the digital rays distally pre-axially deviated, with cartilage deformation of the most distal part (Fig. 1). In the four remaining cases, of the seventeen, there were some digital cartilages missing.

In the four barrier groups not a single case of a deletion free skeleton developed. A high percentage of missing wrist cartilages was common to all barrier groups.

Of the twenty cases after cellophane insertion twelve wings developed only a humerus and a radius (Fig. 2). Three others had also an ulna. In the remaining cases single digital rays were deleted.

In the twenty cases after Np 0.05 insertion, eight had ulna and digital ray IV deletions. The remaining had mainly single digital ray deletions (Fig. 3), with only one case where all three digital rays failed to develop.

Of the sixteen cases with Np 1.0, fifteen had the ulna missing or very short and blunt ulnae. In thirteen cases the radius was deformed into a curve (Fig. 4). There were less digital cartilage deletions than in the Np 0.05 group, and those that were deleted were mainly ray IV (eight cases).

The deletion and deformation pattern of the seventeen cases after Np 8.0 insertion was intermediate to the patterns seen after Np 0.05 and Np 1.0 insertions.

DISCUSSION:

The sham operated wing buds developed wing skeletons with deletions only occasionally. In them the wound heals. This does not exclude the persisting barrier, irrespective of its permeability, from interfering at a local level, in the morphogenetic behaviour of the AER and the mesenchyme, e.g. through changes in the local micro-environment.

Removal of a short segment of the AER causes subsequent segmental distal deletions (SAUNDERS, 1948). At stage 20 HH the proximo-distal deletion level after total AER removal is the wrist (KAPRIO and TÄHKÄ, 1978; KAPRIO, 1979). The single digital ray deletions after barrier insertions could be explained simply by local AER damage. This would seem a probable explanation, as digital ray IV, the post-axial, was most often deleted.

When a barrier is placed into a stage 16 to 18 HH wing bud, so that it does not project out and the AER has not been cut, humerus deformations nevertheless occur (SUMMERBEL, 1979). In this study, two barriers, the Cellophane and Nuclepore 1.0 caused more ulnar deletions and deformations than the other two. Also in the former two groups the barriers remained more proximally. Thus the ulna deletions and deformations could be explained by local effects of the barrier on the mesenchyme.

The total removal of the AER causes distal deletion patterns in the limb (SAUNDERS, 1948; SUMMERBELL et al., 1973; KAPRIO and TÄHKÄ, 1978; KAPRIO, 1979). Disconnecting the ZPA by an impermeable membrane from the rest of the limb bud causes also a distal deletion defect limb to develop. The pattern is the same as if the AER had been removed, except for the added local effect of the barrier on the mesenchyme, i.e. missing ulna. Thus, this suggests that the ZPA is as necessary for normal limb morphogenesis as is the AER.

The interposed membranes used in the present study can be classified roughly into four categories: one preventing diffusion (Cellophane), the others allowing it, but preventing actual cell contacts (Np 0.05), or cell passage (Np 1.0), and finally the type most probably allowing passage of cells (Np 8.0). The fact, that the main differences in their biological consequences were observed between cellophane and Np 0.05 suggests that interference with a diffusible factor rather than with cell relations affected the development. MacCABE et al. (1977) have also suggested a diffusible factor with which the ZPA affects the morphogenetic characteristics of the pre-axial AER in vitro conditions. However they were careful not to claim that their in vitro evidence necessarily means that it is also so in vivo. The present filter experiments' results do suggest, that it may indeed be so, that their in vitro morphogen also functions in vivo.

ACKNOWLEDGEMENTS

The author wishes to thank Prof. LAURI SAXÉN for his helpful critisism during the course of this project. Financial support was received from the Aaltonen Foundation, Finnish Cultural Foundation and the Foundation for Paediatric Research, Finland.

Table 1:

Data from the photographs after barrier insertion. The average width (W) of the tip from flank base line over the length (L) along flank base line, ratio, of the wing bud. The area anterior to the barrier (Pre-aA) and the average lengths of the barriers (F mm.) in millimeters, and the portion of the barrier within the wing bud (F_{in} mm.) in millimeters for each group is shown.

	Cellophane	Np 0.05	Np 1.0	Np 8.0
No. cases	20	20	16	17
W/L	0.34	0.33	0.33	0.28
Pre-aA	71 %	70 %	68 %	74 %
F mm.	1.04	0.98	0.92	0.83
F_{in} mm.	0.48	0.50	0.49	0.46

Table 2:

Data from comparing photographs taken after barrier insertion and next day. Time interval varied from 13 to 32 hours. Outgrowth indicates average distal elongation rate in each group. The shortening rate of the barrier projecting out of the wing bud is indicated as an average for each group (F_{disapp}).

	Cellophane	Np 0.05	Np 1.0	Np 8.0
No. cases	14	19	6	10
outgrowth	28 u/hr	31 u/hr	28 u/hr	32 u/hr
F_{disapp}	17 u/hr	14 u/hr	16 u/hr	12 u/hr

REFERENCES

Balcuns, A., Gasseling, M.T., Saunders, J.W., Jr., 1970, Spatio-temporal distribution of a zone that controls anterior-posterior polarity in the limb bud of the chick and other bird embryos, Am. Zool., 10, 323 (abstract).

Fallon, J.F., Crosby, G.M., 1975, Normal development of the chick wing following removal of the polarizing zone, J. exp. Zool., 193, 449 - 455.

Hamburger, V., Hamilton, H.L., 1951, A series of normal stages in the development of the chick embryo, J. Morph., 88, 49 - 67.

Kaprio, E.A., 1979, Ultrastructural changes in the distal wing bud of the chick embryo after removal of the apical ectodermal ridge, Wilh. Roux's Arch., 185, 333 - 346.

Kaprio, E.A., Tähkä, S., 1978, Lack of correlation between mesenchymal cell death and morphogenesis after different extents of apical ectodermal ridge/rim ectoderm removal in the chick embryo wing bud, Med. Biol., 56, 321 - 327.

MacCabe, A.B., Gasseling, M.T., Saunders, J.W., Jr., 1973, Spatiotemporal distribution of mechanisms that control outgrowth and anterior-posterior polarization of the limb bud in the chick embryo, Mech. Age. Develop., 2, 1 - 12.

MacCabe, J.A., Parker, B.W., 1979, The target tissue of limb-bud polarizing activity in the induction of supernumerary structures, J. Embryol. exp. Morph., 53, 67 - 73.

MacCabe, J.A., Calandra, A.J., Parker, B.W., 1977, In-vitro analysis of the distribution and nature of a morphogenetic factor in the developing chick wing, in: "Vertebrate limb and somite morphogenesis", (D.A. Ede, J.R. Hinchliffe, M. Balls, eds.), Cambridge Univ. Press, Cambridge.

Saunders, J.W., Jr., 1948, Proximo-distal sequence of origin of the parts of the chick wing and the role of the ectoderm, J. exp. Zool., 108, 363 - 404.

Saunders, J.W., Jr., 1977, The experimental analysis of chick limb bud development, in: "Vertebrate limb and somite morphogenesis", (D.A. Ede, J.R. Hinchliffe, M. Balls, eds.), pp, 1 - 24, Cambridge Univ. Press, Cambridge.

Saxén, L., 1980, Mechanisms of morphogenetic tissue interactions: the message of transfilter experiments, in: "Results and problems in cell differentiation", (W. Beerman, W.J. Gehring, J.B. Gurdon, F.C. Kafatos, J. Reinert, eds.), Springer Verlag, Berlin.

Summerbell, D., 1974, Interaction between the proximo-distal and anterior-posterior co-ordinates of positional value during the specification of positional information in the early development of the chick limb-bud, J. Embryol. exp. Morph., 32, 227 - 237.

Summerbell, D., 1979, The zone of polarizing activity: evidence for a role in normal chick limb morphogenesis, J. Embryol. exp. Morph., 50, 217 - 233.

Summerbell, D., Lewis, J.H., Wolpert, L., 1973, Positional information in chick limb morphogenesis, Nature, London, 244, 492 - 496.

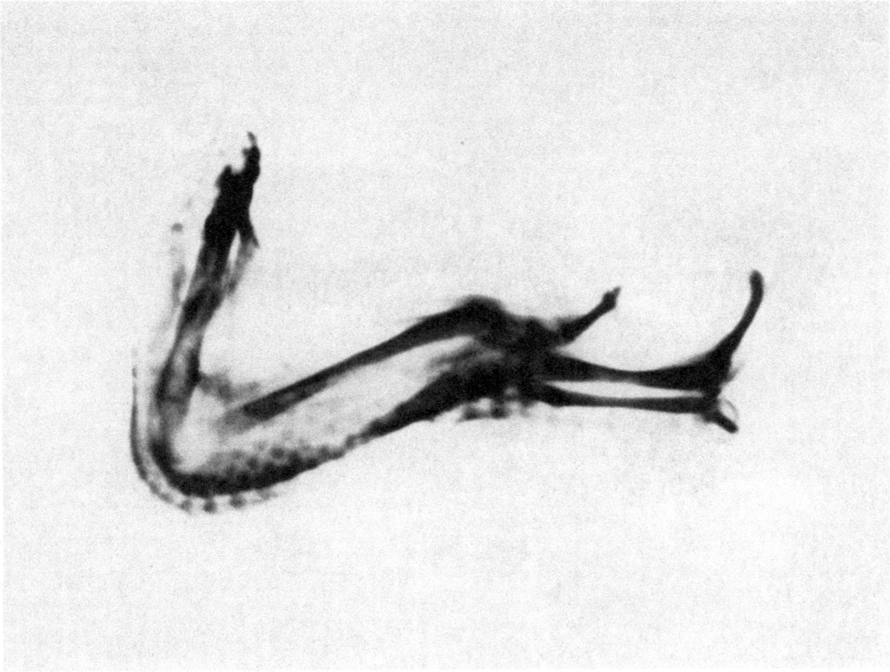

Fig. 1: A wing skeleton stained with Alcian Green after a sham operation (control) showing digital ray III pre-axial deviation.

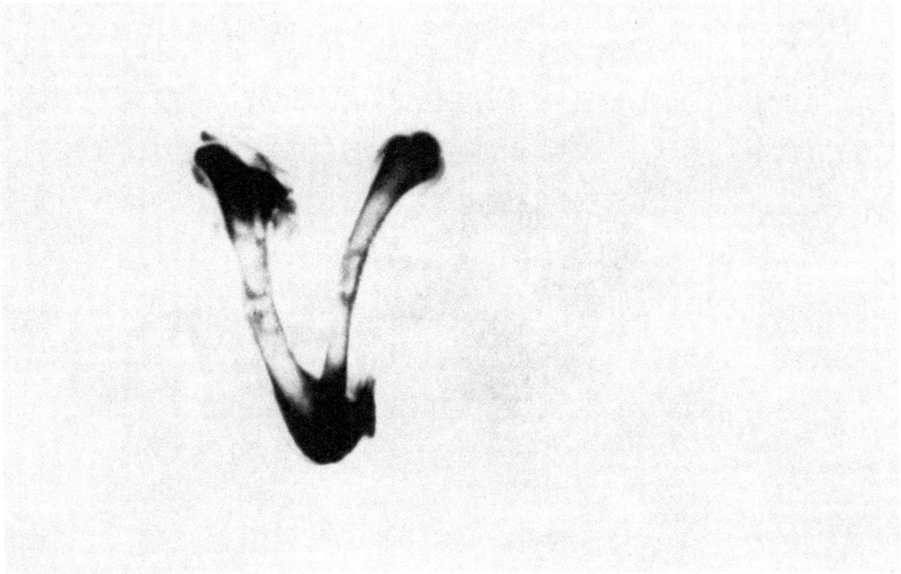

Fig. 2: A wing skeleton after cellophane insertion. Only humerus and radius have developed.

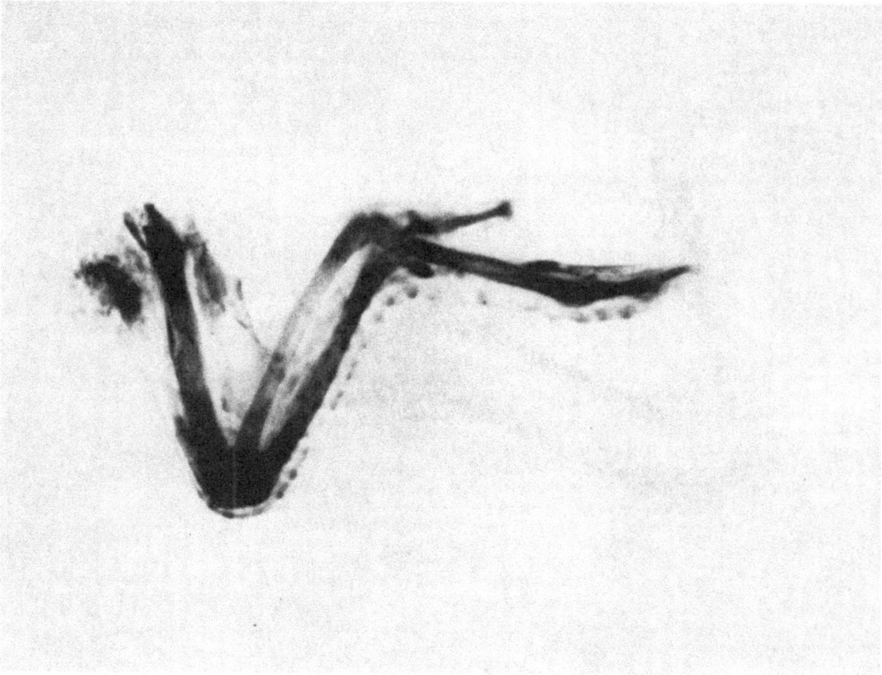

Fig. 3: A wing skeleton after Np 0.05 insertion. The digital ray IV cartilages are missing.

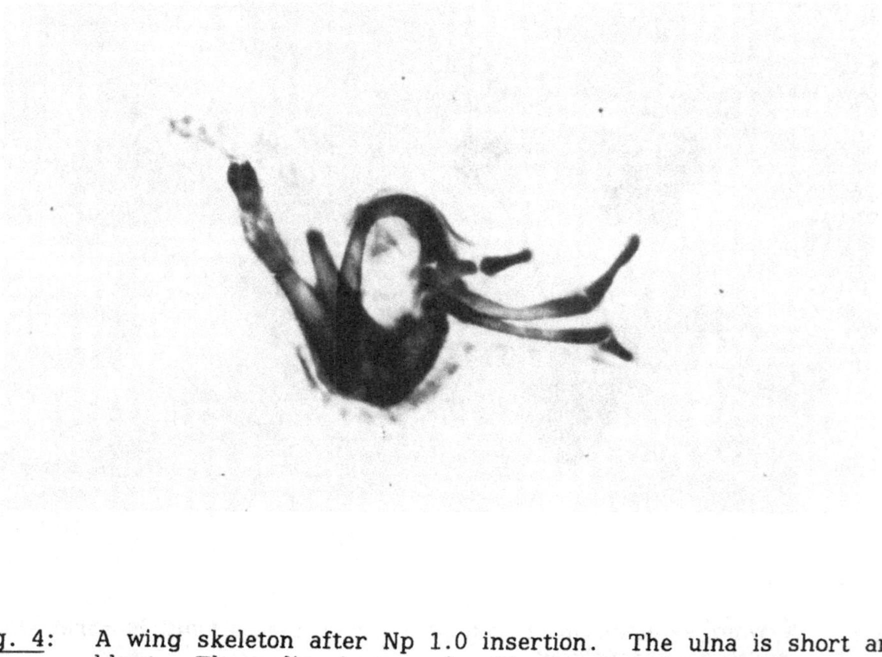

Fig. 4: A wing skeleton after Np 1.0 insertion. The ulna is short and blunt. The radius is curved. The humerus is split.

Simulation of Steps of Limb Skelettogenesis in Vitro

H.-J. Merker, B. Zimmermann, H.-J. Barrach, K. Grundmann, H. Ebel

Institut für Toxikologie und Embryonal-Pharmakologie, Freie Universität Berlin, Garystraße 9, D-1000 Berlin 33

The significance of in vitro methods for testing teratogenic effects has increased considerably during the last few years (BARRACH and NEUBERT, 1980; ZIMMERMANN et al., 1975; NEUBERT et al., 1974 a, b, 1976, 1980). To be able to make full use of the advantages in vitro techniques offer, the knowledge of methods available for these purposes is a prerequisite. In this connection those models are of special importance which simulate the morphogenetic processes organogenesis consists of.

The development of the limb skeleton starts with the formation of mesodermal structures (somite, somatopleure). From here cells migrate into the limb buds (migration), increase in number (proliferation), and form blastemata with a typical pattern. Subsequently, the central areas of the blastemata differentiate into cartilage cells and produce a cartilage-specific matrix. After a number of maturation stages the cartilage model is disaggregated and at the same time replaced by bones (chondral osteogenesis).

The sensitivity of these different steps to teratogenic effects varies greatly. Attempts to project the so-called critical or sensitive phases on the described limb bud development have shown that besides migration and proliferation it is especially blastema formation and the onset of cartilage differentiation which can be disturbed by teratogenic substances (MERKER, 1977). For a purposeful testing of teratogenic substances in vitro particularly those models seem to be suitable which simulate blastema formation and differentiation.

A number of culture techniques are already available for this purpose, among which organ cultures are of special importance (ABBOTT et al., 1972; AYDELOTTE and KOCHHAR, 1972; FLICKINGER, 1974; HALL, 1977; KOSHER, 1976; MERKER, 1975; NEUBERT et al., 1974 a, b).

For a number of reasons it also seems to be interesting to study the formation and differentiation of blastemata in cultures of isolated blastemal cells. The behaviour of these cells in vitro is dependent upon the cell density (HASSEL et al., 1978; MERKER et al., 1980; KARASAWA et al., 1979; SCHACTER, 1970; SOLURSH et al., 1978; UMANSKY, 1966). At low cell density fibroblast-like cells (FLC) develop, which produce collagen type I and III. At high cell density, however, blastemal cells differentiate into chondrocytes and synthesise a cartilage-specific matrix, i.e. collagen type II and chondroitin-sulphate-containing proteoglycans (MERKER et al., 1980). The triggering of cartilage differentiation at high cell density may be due to three mechanisms:

1. Differentiation is induced by cellular contacts;
2. The production of a morphogenic substance, which reaches a sufficient concentration at high cell density only;
3. Selection processes stimulate proliferation of certain cell types only.

Although some indications speak for a participation of cellular contacts in the triggering of differentiation (BELLAIRS et al., 1978; MERKER et al.,

1980; MOSCONA, 1957), the two other possibilities still require further investigations. Two models may be suitable in this respect:

1. The existence of a morphogenetic factor, which induces cartilage differentiation, presupposes a synthesis process. It probably does no longer proceed in isolated membrane fragments. Such membrane fragments, on the other hand, might simulate cellular contacts. Therefore we investigated the effect of isolated blastemal cell membranes on the behaviour of blastemal cells in monolayer culture at low cell density.

2. In order to exclude a participation of selection mechanisms in monolayer cultures we performed the following experiment: Isolated blastemal cells were first grown as FLC in monolayer culture, subsequently they were again isolated and grown at high cell density.

MATERIAL and METHODS:

1.) Isolation of blastemal cells.

The upper limb buds of day 11 or 12 mouse embryos were removed and incubated in 0.2% trypsin in Ca^{2+} - and Mg^{2+} - free balanced salt solution (for 25 min.) in a 37° C waterbath with moderate agitation. After incubation, trypsin was replaced by complete growth medium. Limb buds were dissociated in growth medium by repeatedly pipetting into single cells, washed once in growth medium and filtered through a nylon mesh of 20 µm pore size. This type of cell suspension was used in all experiments.
Growth medium: nutrient mixture Ham F12, supplemented with 15% fetal calf serum, 75 µm ascorbic acid/ml, 50 IU penicillin and 50 µg streptomycin/ml (Seromed, München, Germany).

2.) Monolayer culture.

The cell suspension was diluted to 2.5 - 5 x 10^5 cell /ml and seeded into Lux-plastic petri dishes with glass cover slips for light microscopy or with Thermanox cover slips for electron microscopy. The medium was changed after two or three days. The culture period lasted for up to 14 days.

3.) Mass culture.

The cell suspension was sedimented by centrifugation (50 x g). 10 µl of the sediment were placed in approximately 2 mm^3 holes in a silicone plate which was placed on a membrane filter (Sarsorius TM 11303). 10 µl of the sediment contained about 2 x 10^6 cells, which grew in a small volume on a membrane filter at the medium-air interface. Growth medium as in 1., but glucose increased up to 5 g/l.
For the cultivation of precultured monolayer cells in mass culture, confluent monolayer cultures were trypsinized, dissociated into single cells, washed in medium and filtered through a 20 µm nylon mesh before sedimentation.

4.) Isolation of cell membranes.

Limb buds from day 12 mouse embryos were collected and washed in HBSS. Homogenisation was performed by a DUALL-Homogenizer in 250 mM sucrose, 1 mM EDTA - 4 mM Tris, pH 7.6. Centrifugation of the homogenate was carried out at 700, 1 500, 10 000, 40 000 and 100 000 x g. Sediments of the 10 000 and 40 000 x g run were collected, re-homogenised and used for culture experiment in a 1 : 20 dilution.

5.) Light microscopy.

Cultures were fixed in 10% formalin for 30 min. and after thorough rinsing, stained in diluted Giemsa solution.

6.) Electron microscopy.

Cultures were fixed in 1% glutaraldehyde with 1% tannic acid in 0.1 M phosphate buffer, pH 7.4. Postfixation was carried out in 1% OsO_4 in phosphate buffer. Dehydration in acetone, embedding in Mikropal (Ferak, Berlin). Sections were prepared with an LKB-ultrotom. Electron microscopy utilized a Siemens EM 101.

7.) Immunofluorescence.

After isolation of collagen type I, II and pro-III, rabbit antibodies were prepared and purified over immunoadsorbent column chromatography (von der MARK et al., 1976). Indirect immunofluorescent staining was performed according to the sandwich technique with fluorescein (FITC) conjucated anti-rabbit g-globulins (GRUNDMANN et al., 1980). Fluorescence microscopy utilized a Zeiss H photomicroscope III, HBO 50 bulb, filter KP 490/500, barrier filter 560.

FINDINGS:

Trypsinized blastemal cells from the upper limb buds of 11- and 12-day old mouse embryos grow as FLC in monolayer culture at low cell density. These cells are flat and stretched and contain numerous cavities of the rough endoplasmic reticulum. In the intercellular spaces, particularly between the cells and the bottom of the culture dish, fibrillar bundles of collagen occur after approximately 24 hours. The single fibril is 200 - 300 Å thick and shows clear-cut cross-striation (Fig. 1). Using immunofluorescent optical techniques, it can be shown that fibres of collagen type I and pro-III are formed.

If these blastemal cells are, however, grown in a micro-mass culture at high cell density, numerous specific contacts (gap junctions) develop within a few hours (Fig. 2). On the third day differentiation starts and the cells produce a cartilage matrix, which consists of single irregularly running collagen filaments of 100 - 180 Å thickness without distinct cross-striation. Using special staining techniques (ruthenium red), cartilage-specific proteoglycans can be demonstrated as electron-dense granules (300 - 600 Å). The cartilage matrix reveals a clearly metachromatic behaviour (Fig. 3). Immunofluorescent optical techniques help demonstrate collagen type II.

If isolated cell membranes from blastemal cells are grown in monolayer culture at low density, morphologically reproducible effects are observed. In controls, FLC grow at even distribution, mainly in an isolated and only after 3 - 4 days in an increasingly confluent manner. After addition of cell membrane fragments, areas with densely packed cells (nodules) develop as early as after 24 hours. These nodules become more distinct within the next few days and start to produce a metachromatic matrix after approximately 6 days in vitro (Fig. 4). Electron microscopically, the cartilage-specific structures (irregularly running filaments without cross-striation and proteoglycan granules) can also be demonstrated.

In another experimental series, isolated blastemal cells were grown for 2 - 4 days in monolayer culture at low density, i.e. as FLC, isolated again by trypsinization and further grown in micro-mass culture. Under these culture conditions FLC change the direction of their differentiation. At high cell density they start to form cartilage tissue after three days in culture. While in monolayer culture, they produce collagen type I and pro-III. However, they do not produce cartilage-specific proteoglycans; they now synthesize collagen type II and proteoglycans. The morphology of the cells and the matrix also corresponds to that of cartilage tissue (Fig. 5). The cells adopt a round to polygonal shape, develop a large amount of membranes of the rough endoplasmic reticulum and a Golgi apparatus. In the intercellular spaces more and more irregularly running collagen filaments (100 - 180 Å) without cross-striation and ruthenium red-positive proteoglycan granules occur.

DISCUSSION:

The experiments described here were performed in order to define more precisely the reasons for the various courses of differentiation, which blastemal cells take in vitro at different cell densities. Three hypotheses, which might help explain this behaviour, had to be investigated:

1.) the formation of cellular contacts as inducing factor of cartilage differentiation;

2.) the occurrence of a cartilage-inducing substance, which reaches a sufficient concentration only at high cell density;

3.) the occurrence of selection processes.

On the basis of our findings the third hypothesis can clearly be rejected. Since isolation of limb bud cells not only yields actual blastemal cells, but other mesenchymal cells, myoblasts, endothelial cells, etc., it is not surprising that besides cartilage tissue also FLC and myotubes are detected in so-called high density cultures. Different adhesion tendencies or proliferation rates might lead to a selection of FLC under monolayer conditions at low cell density. However, the capability of up to four-day-old fibroblast-like blastemal cells from monolayer cultures to form again cartilaginous tissue under micro-mass culture conditions, makes this explanation rather unlikely. There exists, of course, the possibility that all or a large number of mesenchymal cell types form cartilaginous tissue at high cell density after trypsinization and cultivation. But this hypothesis cannot be verified when growing mixtures of different cell types (MERKER et al., 1980).

Much more difficult is the investigation of the second hypothesis, i.e. the possible formation of a morphogenic agent. The search for an experimental situation, where this factor is not present but where densely packed cellular contacts can be simulated, led to the use of isolated cell membrane fragments. However, these experiments did not yield the expected result. We failed to observe a direct transformation of blastemal cells into chondrocytes after the addition of membrane fragments in monolayer cultures at low cell density. When interpreting the findings, methodological problems have to be considered. In membrane fractions important substances can be removed during the different preparation steps, or vesicle formation occurs reversely from membrane fragments (inside - out). However, the purity of the fraction, which also constitutes a possible factor of uncertainty, could be confirmed electron microscopically. Treatment of monolayer cultures with these membrane fragments yielded another unexpected effect. Blastemal cells form densely packed nodules as early as after 24 hours. The cells of control cultures are however still loosely packed and regularly distributed. Hence, cell membrane fragments do not directly induce cartilage differentiation but first stimulate the migration of cells and the formation of blastema-like areas. This effect makes these experiments even more interesting. In vivo, too, similar migration processes participate in the formation of blastemal cells (EDE and AGERBAK, 1968; EDE and FLINT, 1975; THOROGOOD and HINCHLIFFE, 1975). Consequently, using this model it is possible to simulate blastema formation in vitro and to study this process experimentally. It is, however, not possible to make any definite statements as to the actual causes of cartilage differentiation with these experiments. Since under these conditions a blastema-like structure develops before the onset of cartilage differentiation, again only the significance of a dense cell packing and cellular contacts for cartilage formation is emphasized.

The significance of dense cell packing and/or cellular contacts for the induction of differentiation can also be observed in other in vitro models (EICHENBERGER-GLINZ, 1979; EKBLOM et al., 1979; MOSCONA et al., 1980; SAXÉN and LEHTONEN, 1978). An exact morphological analysis of the early stages of skelettogenesis in vivo also shows that cellular contacts are characteristic of the blastemal stage. A functional significance can therefore be assumed (BORCK, 1977; EDE and AGERBAK, 1968; GOULD et al., 1972; KELLEY and FALLON, 1978; LEWIS et al., 1978; MINKOFF and KUNTZ, 1978; THOROGOOD and HINCHLIFFE, 1975). This theory has been confirmed experimentally. Vitamin a, which inhibits chondrogenesis in vitro, considerably changes membrane properties (LEWIS et al., 1978). A number of considerations may help explain this phenomenon. First it has to be kept in mind that only a so-called specific adhesion is able to trigger the differentiation of blastemal cells. A mixture with other cell types at a ratio of 1 : 1 prevents this process (MERKER et al., 1980). A specific adhesion can be attributed to a receptor mechanism. As is known from other experiments, many membrane properties are influenced by a specific binding of substances to a receptor: for example, permeability, the activity of membrane-bound enzymes (adenyl-cyclase), the behaviour of the microfilamentary system, fluidity, turnover, etc. The significance of cyclic nucleotides as second messenger for the triggering and control of differentiation has been well established. The concentration of c-AMP is also supposed to be of great importance for the differentiation of blastemal cells into cartilage (AHRENS et al., 1977; KOSHER et al., 1979; MERKER and GÜNTHER, 1979; MILLER et al., 1979; RICHMOND and ELMER, 1980; SOLURSH et al., 1979). However, it must be kept in mind, that besides a specific adhesion isolated blastemal cells also form characteristic contacts (gap junctions). Their existence might play an important role in the processes of chondrogenesis. A cycle-specific alteration in the concentration of cyclic nucleotides is typical of proliferating cells. Cyclic nucleotides can be exchanged at gap junctions, whereby the different c-AMP levels in neighbouring cells are adjusted. Homogeneous concentration inhibits proliferation and stimulates differentiation. Morphological investigations of chondrogenesis in limb buds reveal a rapid differentiation of large blastemal areas. This phenomenon can be attributed to a communication in the blastema via gap junctions. Information necessary for cartilage differentiation is quickly passed on via these contacts. Thus cellular contacts are important not only for synchronous differentiation, but also for the size and shape of the developing cartilage pieces. The notion that chondrogenesis might start from a small point is very tempting.

Finally, the gradient theories have to be discussed briefly. In densely packed tissues, which have numerous gap junctions, the transcellular transport of fluids is facilitated, the intercellular one aggravated. In addition, the small size of the intercellular space makes an effective control by the cell membrane likely. If a certain concentration of a morphogenetically effective substance is important for the differentiation of the blastema or for pattern formation (CAPLAN and KOUTROUPAS, 1973; McCABE and PARKER, 1976; SUMMERBELL et al., 1973; WILBY and EDE, 1975; WOLPERT, 1978), cell density and contact behaviour are bound to influence their expansion.

Our findings, the similarity with other in vitro models, and the notions here discussed, suggest that the dense cell packing in the blastema and the occurrence of numerous gap junctions are a prerequisite or even the inducing factor for differentiation. Alterations in the cell density and membrane and contact behaviour therefore lead to disturbances in skelettogenesis. These processes should be considered as sensitive mechanisms when interpreting teratogenic effects.

ACKNOWLEDGEMENTS

The expert technical assistance of Mrs. U. KRÜGER and Mrs. H. SOMOGYI is gratefully acknowledged.

This work was supported by grants from the DFG awarded to Sfb 29.

REFERENCES

Abott, J., Mayne, R., Holtzer, H., 1972, Inhibition of cartilage development in organ cultures of chick somites by the thymidine analog 5-Bromo-2'-deoxynoidine, Develop. Biol., 28, 430.

Ahrens, P.B., Solursh, M., Reiter, R.S., 1977, Stage related capacity for limb chondrogenesis in cell culture, Develop. Biol., 60, 69 - 82.

Aydelotte, M.B., Kochhar, D.M., 1972, Development of mouse limb buds in organ culture: Chondrogenesis in the presence of a proline analog, L-Azetidine-2-carboxylic acid, Develop. Biol., 28, 191.

Barrach, H.-J., Neubert, D., 1980, Significance of organ culture techniques for evaluation of prenatal toxicity, Arch. Toxicol., 45, 161 - 187.

Bellairs, R., Curtis, A.S.G., Sanders, E.J., 1978, Cell adhesiveness and embryonic differentiation, J. Embryol. exp. Morph., 46, 207 - 213.

Borck, Ch., 1977, Elektronenmikroskopische Untersuchungen an Mäuseembryonen über die Differenzierung des Blastems in den Extremitäten zum embryonalen Vorknorpel, Acta Anat., 97, 423 - 434.

Caplan, A.J., Koutroupas, S., 1973, The control of muscle and cartilage development in the chick limb: The role of differential vascularization, J. Embryol. exp. Morph., 29, 571 - 583.

Ede, D.A., Agerbak, G.S., 1968, Cell adhesion and movement in relation to developing limb patterns in normal and talpid chick embryos, J. Embryol. exp. Morph., 20, 81 - 100.

Ede, D.A., Flint, O.P., 1975, Cell movement and adhesion in the developing chick wing bud: Studies on cultured mesenchyme cells from normal and talpid-3 mutant embryos, J. Cell Sci., 18, 301.

Eichenberger-Glinz, S., 1979, Intercellular junctions during development and in tissue cultures of drosophila melanogaster: An electron microscopic study, Roux's Arch., 186, 333 - 346.

Ekblom, P., Nordling, S., Saxén, L., Rasilo, M.-L., Renkonen, O., 1979, Cell interactions leading to kidney tubule determination are tunicamycin sensitive, Cell Diff., 8, 347.

Flickinger, R.A., 1974, Muscle and cartilage differentiation in small and large explants from the chick embryo limb bud, Develop. Biol., 41, 202.

Gould, R.P., Day, A., Wolpert, L., 1972, Mesenchymal condensation and cell contact in early morphogenesis of the chick limb, Exp. Cell Res., 72, 325 - 336.

Grundmann, K., Zimmermann, B., Barrach, H.-J., Merker, H.-J., 1980, Behaviour of epiphyseal mouse chondrocyte populations in monolayer culture, Virchow's Archiv, in press.

Hall, B.K., 1977, Adv. in Anat., Embryol. and Cell Biol., Vol. 53, Springer Verlag, Berlin, Heidelberg, New York.

Hassel, J.R., Pennypacker, J.P., Lewis, E.A., 1978, Chondrogenesis and cell proliferation in limb bud cell cultures treated with cytosine arabinoside and vitamin A, Exp. Cell Res., 112, 409.

Karasawa, K., Kimata, K., Ito, K., Kato, Y., Suzuki, S., 1979, Morphological and biochemical differentiation of limb bud cells cultured in chemically defined medium, Develop. Biol., 70, 287 - 305.

Kelley, R.O., Fallon, J.F., 1978, Identification and distribution of gap junctions in the mesoderm of developing chick limb bud, J. Embryol. exp. Morph., 46, 99 - 110.

Kosher, R.A., 1976, Inhibition of "spontaneous" notochord-induced and collagen-induced in vitro somite chondrogenesis by cyclic AMP derivatives and theophylline, Develop. Biol., 53, 265 - 275.

Kosher, R.A., Savage, M.P., Chan, S.-C., 1979, Cyclic-AMP derivatives stimulate the chondrogenic differentiation of the mesoderm subjacent to the apical ectodermal ridge of the chick limb bud, J. exp. Zool., 209, 221.

Lewis, C.A., Pratt, R.M., Pennypacker, J.P., Hassel, J.R., 1978, Inhibition of limb chondrogenesis in vitro by Vitamin A: Alterations in cell surface characteristics, Develop. Biol., 64, 31 - 47.

McCabe, J.A., Parker, B.W., 1976, Evidence for a gradient of a morphogenetic substance in the developing limb, Develop. Biol., 54, 297 - 303.

Merker, H.-J., 1975, Significance of limb bud culture system for investigations of teratogenic mechanisms, in: New approaces to the evaluation of abnormal embryonic development, (D. Neubert, H.-J. Merker, eds.), pp. 161 - 199, Thieme-Verlag, Stuttgart.

Merker, H.-J., 1977, Considerations on the problem of critical period during the development of limb skeleton, in: Birth defects: original article series, Vol XIII, (D. Bergsma, W. Lenz, eds.), pp. 179 - 202, Alan R. Liss, Inc.

Merker, H.-J., Günther, Th., 1979, The influence of insulin, c-AMP and the calcium ionophore x 537 A on the growth of cartilage anlagen of limb buds in vitro, Experientia, 35, 1307 - 1308.

Merker, H.-J., Zimmermann, B., Grundmann, K., 1980, Differentiation of isolated blastemal cells from limb buds into chondroblasts, in: Tissue culture in medical research (II), (R.J. Richards, K.T. Rajan, eds.), pp. 31 - 39, Pergamon Press, Oxford and New York.

Miller, R.P., Husain, M., Lohin, S., 1979, Long acting c-AMP analogues enhance sulfate incorporation into matrix proteoglycans and suppress cell division of fetal rat chondrocytes in monolayer culture, J. Cell Physiol., 100, 63.

Minkoff, R., Kuntz, A.J., 1978, Cell proliferation and cell density of mesenchyme in the maxillary process and adjacent regions during facial development in chick embryo, J. Embryol. exp. Morph., 46, 65 - 74.

Moscona, A., 1957, The development in vitro of chimeric aggregates of dissociated embryonic chick and mouse cells, Proc. Nat. Acad. Sci., USA, 43, 184 - 194.

Moscona, A.A., Moscona, M., Linser, P., 1980, Induction of glutamin-synthetase in embryonic neural retina: Role of cell interactions, in: Tissue culture in medical research (II), (R.J. Richards, K.T. Rajan, eds.), pp. 59 - 70, Pergamon Press, Oxford.

Neubert, D., Merker, H.-J., Tapken, S., 1974 a, Comparative studies on the prenatal development of mouse extremities in vitro and in organ culture, Naunyn-Schmied. Arch. Pharmacol., 286, 251 - 270.

Neubert, D., Tapken, S., Merker, H.-J., 1974 b, Induction in skeletal malformation in organ cultures of mammalian embryonic tissue, Naunyn-Schmied. Arch. Pharmacol., 286, 271 - 282.

Neubert, D., Merker, H.-J., Barrach, H.-J., Lessmöllmann, U., 1976, Biochemical and teratological aspects of mammalian limb bud development in vitro, in: Tests of teratogenicity in vitro, (J.D. Ebert, M. Marois, eds.), pp. 335, North-Holland Publ. Co., Amsterdam.

Neubert, D., Barrach, H.-J., Merker, H.-J., Druginduced damage to the embryo or fetus (Molecular and multilateral approach to prenatal toxicology), Curr. Top. Pathol., 69, in press.

Richmond, A., Elmer, W.A., 1980, Purification of a mouse embryo extract component which enhances chondrogenesis in vitro, Develop. Biol., 76, 366 - 383.

Saxén, L., Lehtonen, E., 1978, Transfilter induction of kidney tubules as a function of the extent and duration of intercellular contacts, J. Embryol. exp. Morph., 47, 97 - 109.

Schacter, L.P., 1970, Effect of conditioned media on differentiation in mass cultures of chick limb bud cells, Exp. Cell Res., 63, 19 - 32.

Solursh, M., Ahrens, P.B., Reiter, R.S., 1978, A tissue culture analysis of the steps in limb chondrogenesis, In vitro, 14, 51 - 61.

Solursh, M., Reiter, R., Ahrens, P.B., Pratt, R.M., 1979, Increase in levels of cyclic AMP during avian limb chondrogenesis in vitro, Differentiation, 15, 183.

Summerbell, D., Lewis, J.H., Wolpert, L., 1973, Positional information in chick limb morphogenesis, Nature, 244, 492 - 496.

Thorogood, P.V., Hinchliffe, J.R., 1975, Analysis of condensation process during chondrogenesis in embryonic chick hind limb, J. Embryol. exp. Morph., 33, 581.

Umansky, R., 1966, The effect of cell population density on the developmental fate of reaggregating mouse limb bud mesenchyme, Develop. Biol., 13, 31 - 56.

Wilby, O.K., Ede, D.A., 1975, A model generating the pattern of cartilage skeletal elements in the embryonic chick limb, J. theor. Biol., 24, 199 - 217.

von der Mark, H., von der Mark, K., Gay, S., 1976, Study of differential collagen synthesis during development of the chick embryo by immunofluorescence. I. Preparation of collagen type I and type II specific antibodies and their application to early stages of the chick embryo, Develop. Biol., 48, 237 - 249.

Wolpert, L., 1978, Pattern formation and the development of the chick limb, in: Birth defects, original article series, Vol. XIV, (Bergsma, W. Lenz, eds.), pp. 547 - 559, Alan R. Liss, Inc.

Zimmermann, B., Neubert, D., Bachmann, D., Merker, H.-J., 1975, Induction of skeletal malformations in organ cultures of mouse limb buds, Experientia, 31, 227 - 228.

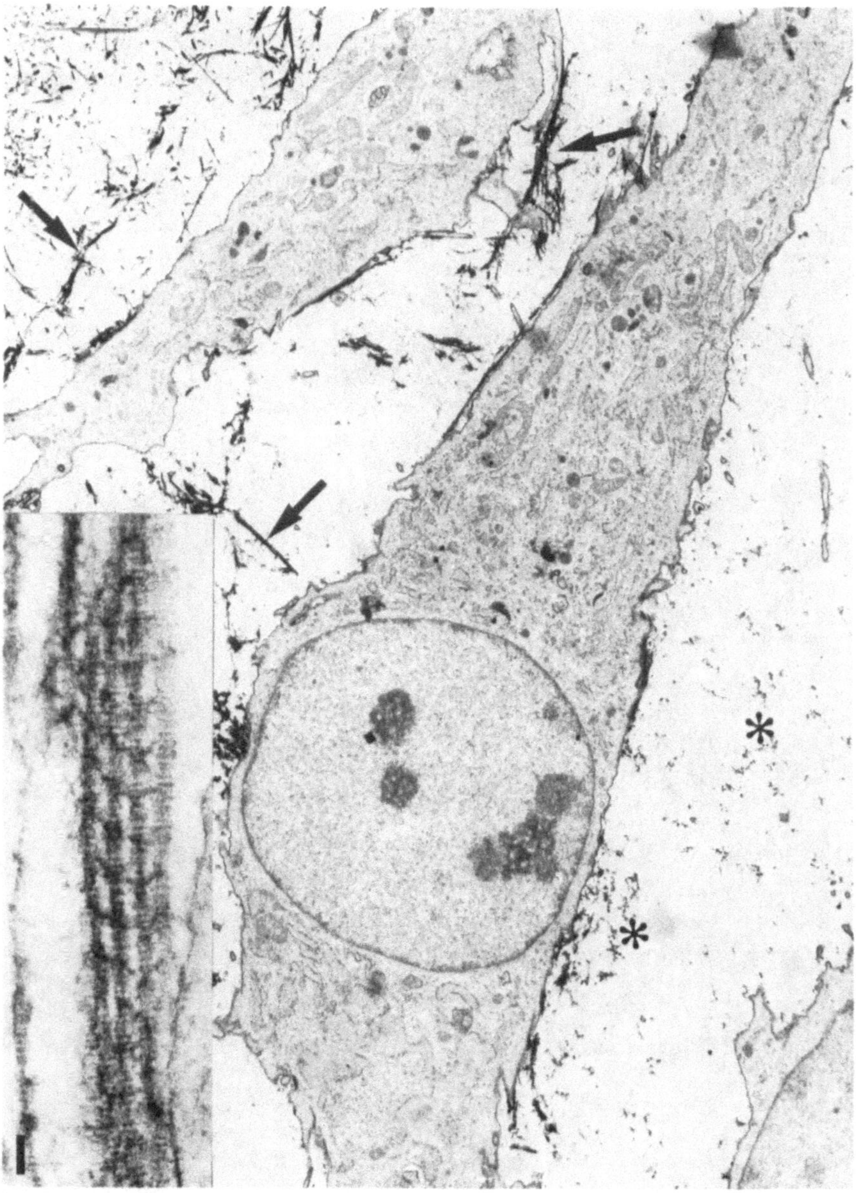

Fig. 1: Isolated blastemal cells from the upper limb buds of 11-day-old mouse embryos after two days in monolayer culture at low cell density. Regularly distributed flat and stretched FLC with numerous organelles. In the intercellular space - tannic-acid-positive granular material (*) and collagen fibrils (↓). x 8 400.
Inset: Higher magnification of a collagenous fibrillar bundle. x 90 000.

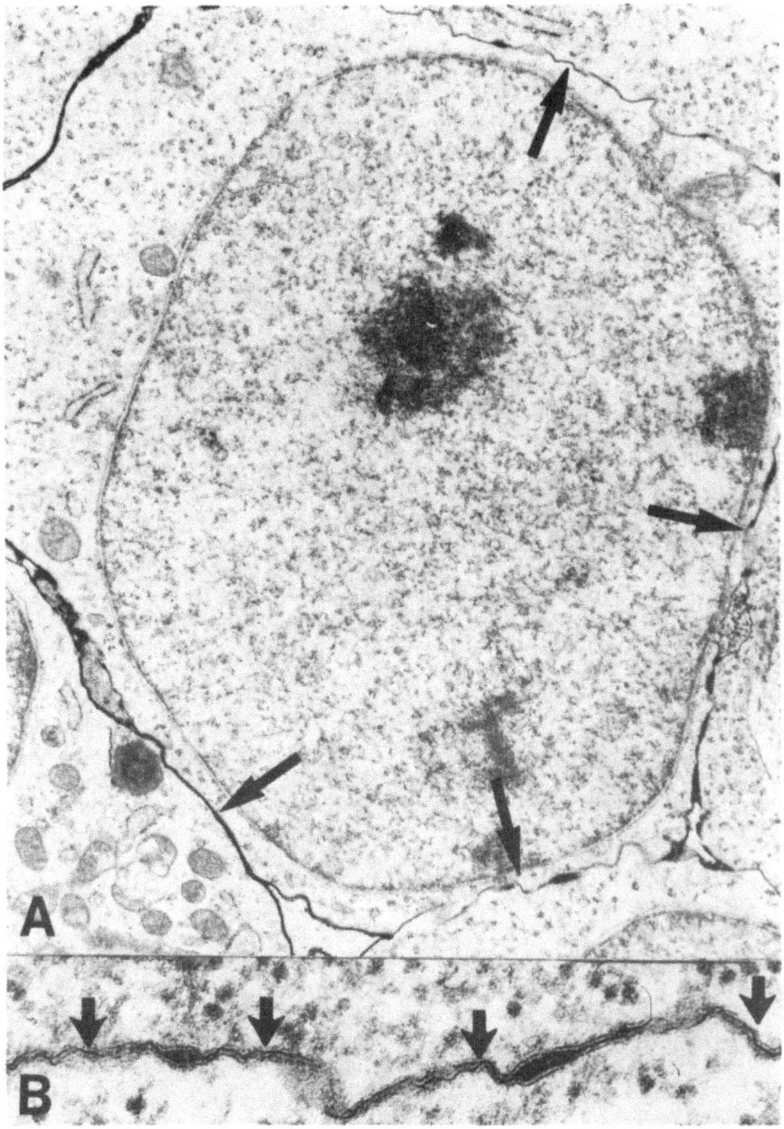

Fig. 2: Isolated blastemal cells from the upper limb buds of 11-day-old mouse embryos after two days in high density culture.

A. Densely packed cells with numerous contacts with neighbouring cells (↓). x 17 500.

B. Higher magnification of a contact zone with gap junctions (↓). x 120 000.

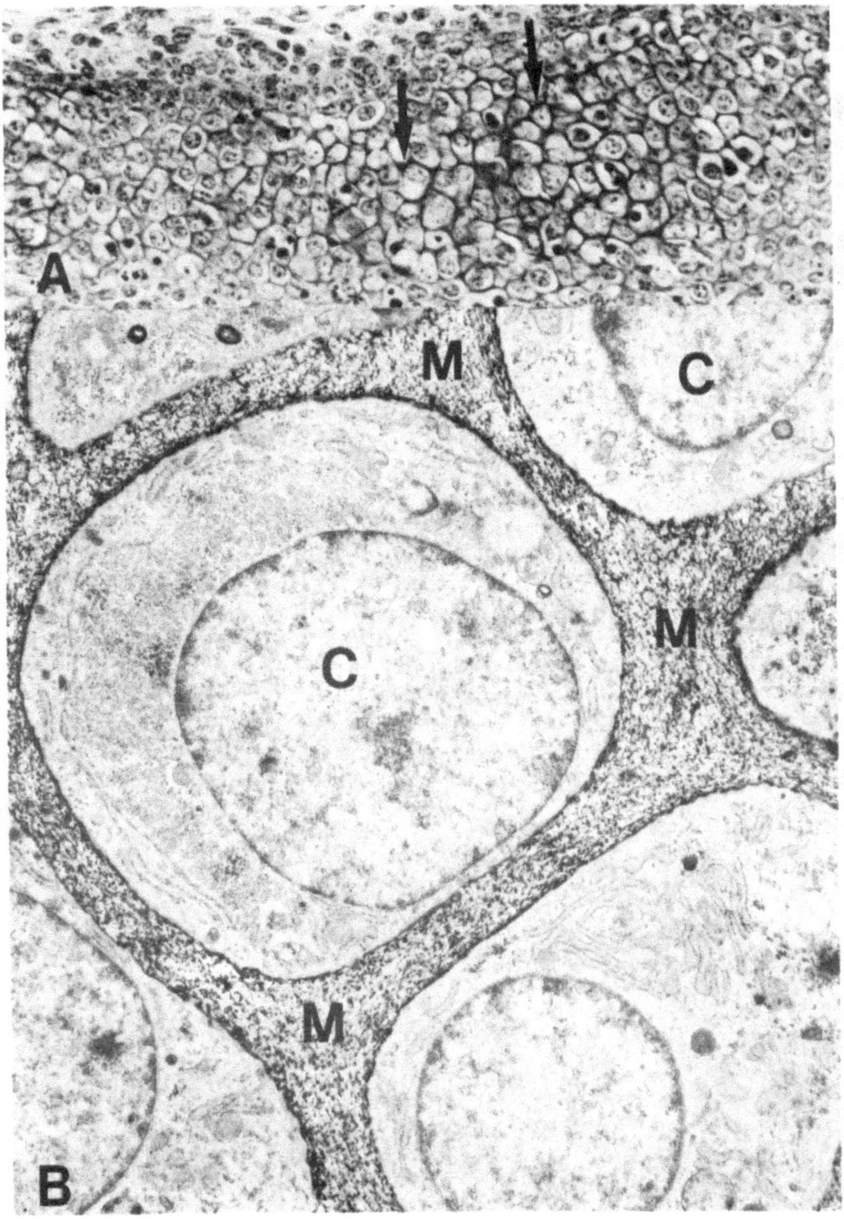

Fig. 3: Isolated blastemal cells from the upper limb buds of 11-day-old mouse embryos after six days in high density culture.

A. Light microscopical picture. The dark areas between the cells (↓) represent metachromatic material.

B. Electron microscopical picture. Typical chondrocytes (C), in between these chondrocytes cartilage matrix (M). x 17 000.

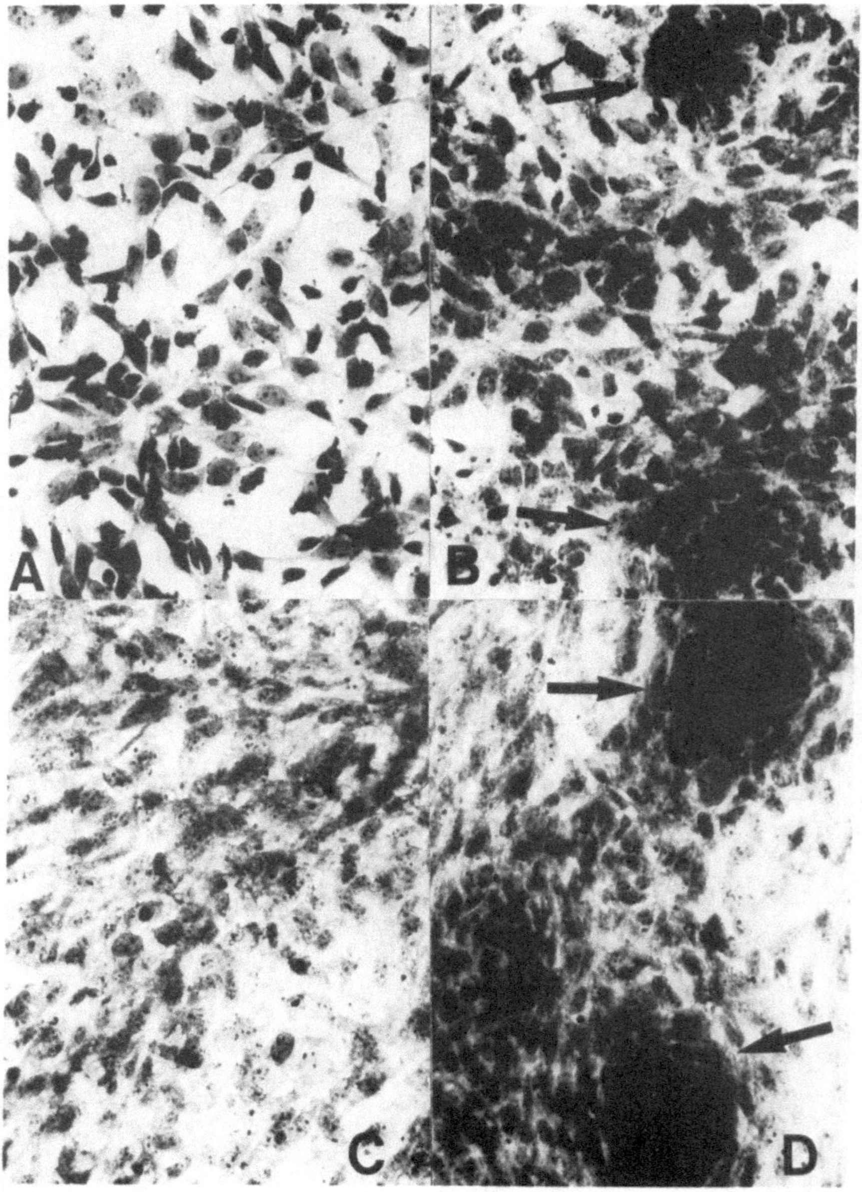

Fig. 4: Isolated blastemal cells from the upper limb buds of 11-day-old mouse embryos grown in monolayer culture at low cell density with and without the addition of isolated membrane fragments.
A. After 24 hours in vitro, without membrane fragments.
B. After 24 hours in vitro, with membrane fragments. Note the densely packed nodules (*).
C. After four days in vitro, without membrane fragments.
D. After four days in vitro, with membrane fragments. Enlargement of nodules (↓).

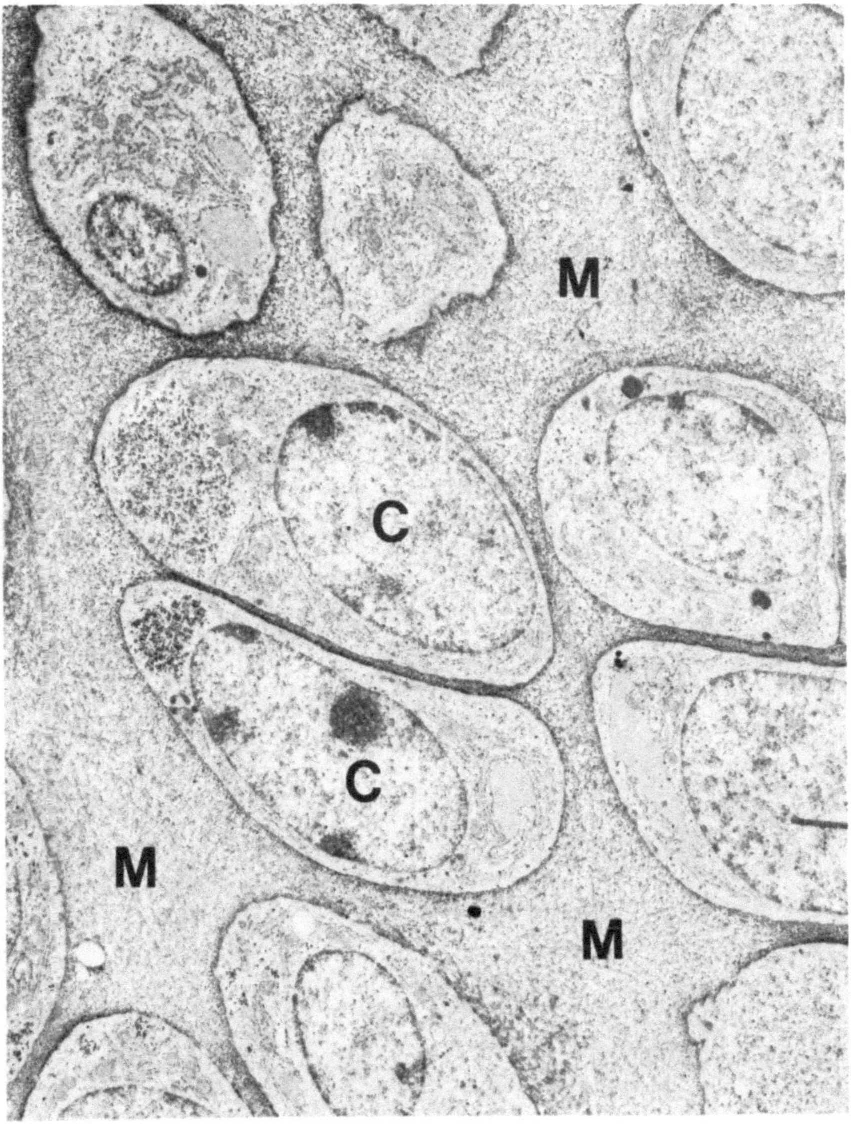

Fig. 5: Isolated blastemal cells from the upper limb buds of 11-day-old mouse embryos, first grown for four days in monolayer culture at low cell density, subsequently re-isolated and grown for six days in high density culture. Characteristic cartilage tissue with chondrocytes (C) and matrix (M). x 7 000.

Effects of Surface Coat Influencing Substances on the Limb Bud Blastema in Vitro

Bernd Zimmermann

Institut für Toxikologie und Embryonal-Pharmakologie, Freie Universität Berlin
Garystraße 9, D-1000 Berlin 33

INTRCDUCTION:

Skelettogenesis is one of the important processes in the development of mammalian limbs. It involves at least three different events:

1. migration of mesenchymal cells,
2. formation of blastema,
3. synthesis of matrix substances.

Blastema formation is a prerequisite for cartilage differentiation. Electron microscopically, the blastema is characterized by pronounced specific cellular contacts between individual cells. These contacts can be considered as gap junctions (GOODENOUGH, 1974; MERKER et al., 1980).

In order to investigate formation and significance of these cellular contacts, we tried to disturb blastema formation in vitro by adding substances which were supposed to have an effect on the cell surface or on cell surface components. Substances were applied only during blastema formation, and subsequent inhibition of chondrogenesis was taken as criterion of action.

METHODS:

Two different methods were applied:

1.) Limb buds of 11-day-old mouse embryos were grown in a modified organ culture according to TROWELL (1959). Limbs were dissected and placed on a membrane filter (SARTORIUS SM 11303) on a stainless steel grid at the medium-air interface. HAM'S F12 medium supplemented with 20% fetal calf serum (SEROMED, München), EAGLE'S amino acid mixture 1%, 75 µg/ml ascorbid acid, 400 mg/l glucose, 50 IU/ml penicillin and 50 µg/ml streptomycin was used as growth medium. During the first three days of culture, blastema formation occurred. Chondrogenesis started at approximately day 4. After six days, most of the cartilage anlagen of the limb were formed. Consequently, the limbs were grown for 6 days, but the substances were added only on the first three days.

2.) In a second culture technique actual contact behaviour of the cells was investigated. The limb buds of mouse embryos of day 11 or 12 were dissociated into single cells (0.2% Trypsin in CMF), which were grown in a micro mass culture. 10 µl of a cell sediment from a filtered (20 µm nylon mesh) cell suspension were placed in holes of 1.5 mm diameter made in a silikon plate of 1 mm thickness lying on a membrane filter in an organ culture. With this technique the cell mass grew at the same medium-air interface as the limbs in the limb bud culture. Here again chondrogenesis occurred after three days in culture and cartilaginous nodules developed after 6 days. Again, the cells were cultured for 6 days, but the substances were added only on the first three days.

Teratology of the Limbs

After the culture period, the limb bud cultures were fixed in 10% formol and stained with methylene blue for detection of cartilage. The micro mass cultures were fixed in BOUIN'S solution, embedded in paraffin, sectioned and stained with HE/alcian blue. Electron microscopical investigations were carried out in routine techniques. For substances and doses see Table 1.

RESULTS:

1. Limb bud cultures:
In our control cultures only proximal parts of the limb (humerus, proximal parts of the radius and ulna) developed in a satisfying manner, whereas the distal parts showed large variations. So we refrained from doing a quantitative evaluation. Consequently, only the occurrence or the absence of cartilage was considered. The results are summarized in Table 1 (file 3).

Neither lectin concanavalin A nor substances, which disturb PG synthesis, such as Bacitracin, xylosides and DON, have any influence on chondrogenesis in limb bud cultures. Hyaluronic acid does not have any influence either. Hyaluronidase, however, clearly inhibits chondrogenesis. Galactosamine, one of the carbohydrates and carbohydrate derivatives tested so far, has a pronounced inhibiting effect. Thiodigalactoside, which inhibits myoblast fusion (GARTNER and PODLESKI, 1975) does not effect blastema formation, whereas vitamin A acid has a marked inhibiting effect.

2. Micro mass culture:
In this special type of culture, densely packed cells show large and pronounced cellular contacts between adjacent cells as early as after 6 hours in culture (Fig. 1). At higher magnification, these contacts are recognizable as typical gap junctions (Fig. 2). Also some necrotic cells occur, and some contacts between healthy and necrotic cells are observed (Fig. 1). After three days in culture, most of the contacts are opened and a small intercellular space occurs (Fig. 3) without considerable amounts of matrix substance. After 6 days, however, cartilage has developed. Electron microscopically, we found typical chondrocytes embedded in a cartilaginous matrix (Fig. 4). In the light microscope staining with alcian blue in combination with HE-stain shows large cartilaginous nodules (Fig. 5). These nodules occur within a densely packed cell mass which does not show any specific signs of differentiation. In the centre of the culture necroses are recognizable. The influence of the different substances on cartilage development is also summarized in Table 1 (file 4). Because of the impossibility to perform exact measurements of histological sections, we renounced quantitative evaluations. Here again the question was whether cartilage was formed or not.

Under the influence of concanavalin A a clear increase in chondrogenesis is seen (Fig. 6). Not only the number of cartilage nodules seems to be increased but also the amount of matrix between the chondrocytes. The proteoglycan inhibiting substances do not show any inhibiting effect on chondrogenesis when given at the beginning of blastema formation. Hyaluronic acid has no influence on chondrogenesis either. But in contrast to the limb bud culture, hyaluronidase does not cause inhibition of chondrogenesis. Inhibition of cartilage only occurs after application of galactosamine or vitamin A acid (Fig. 7). A slight inhibition is also seen after thiodigalactoside.

DISCUSSION:

It has to be kept in mind that the substances in all experiments described here were applied only on the first three days of the culture period, that means in the period of blastema formation and before the onset of matrix production. First, it has to be pointed out that substances, which disturb proteoglycan synthesis, do not have any inhibiting effect on blastema formation. The same holds true for limb bud as well as micro mass cultures. Hence PGs are not necessary either for blastema formation or the genesis of cell contacts. On the other hand, it is well known that DON (LINSENMAYER and KOCHHAR, 1979) as well as xylosides (HJELLE and GIBSON, 1979; LOHMANDER et al., 1979) inhibit chondrogenesis. But these inhibitions occur after blastema formation in the course of matrix synthesis (see ZIMMERMANN, this volume).

Galactosamine in both techniques shows a pronounced inhibition of blastema and contact formation. The hepatitis-inducing effect of galactosamine is well known, the toxic effect this substance has on the liver is interpreted as influence on protein synthesis, as change in membrane surface or as effect on galactosamine receptors. In our cultures this action seems to be rather specific, because none of the galactosamine analogous substances (glucosamine) nor galactosamine derivatives (galactose, galactose-1-phosphate, galactosamine-1-phosphate, N-acetyl-galactosamine) have any inhibiting effect (ZIMMERMANN, unpublished). Also, vitamin A acid inhibits blastema formation in both cultures. Owing to the various effects this substance has on cellular processes and on cellular membrane (LEWIS et al., 1978; FRASER and TRAVILL, 1978) inhibition should be expected.

More interestingly, however, are substances, which show different effects in both techniques. Concanavalin A does not show any effect in limb bud culture, but in micro-mass culture chondrogenesis is increased. It could be shown that concanavalin A leads to an agglutination of cells (WLODARSKI et al., 1974). Furthermore, trypsinization of cells increase the number of concanavalin A receptors on the cell surface (SINGER and MORRISON, 1976; see also BURGER, 1973). In micro-mass culture, an increase in chondrogenesis may be due to enhanced agglutination of the single cell mediated by concanavalin A. This is a strong indication of the importance of cellular contacts for blastema formation and subsequent chondrogenesis. On the other hand, hyaluronidase inhibits chondrogenesis in limb bud culture, not however, in micro-mass culture. This finding indicates that cell migration is of great significance for blastema formation in limb buds. According to TOOLE (TOOLE et al., 1972) a hyaluronic micro milieu is the prerequisite for cell migration and blastema formation. If hyaluronic acid is digested by hyaluronidase, cell migration is inhibited. However, in micro-mass culture cell migration is no longer necessary for blastema formation. Owing to the densely packed cells, an almost spontaneous contact between cells occurs, so that hyaluronidase cannot have any influence on blastema formation in this case.

Thiodigalactoside is reported to inhibit fusion of myoblasts (GARTNER and PODLEWSKI, 1975). This finding stimulated us to study the effect this substance has on contact behaviour and blastema formation. However, only a slight inhibition was seen after application in micro-mass culture. To gain more insight into these problems, further studies are necessary.

In summary, migration followed by contact organization of mesenchymal cells is necessary for blastema formation and subsequent chondrogenesis. While the micro-mass culture seems to be an excellent model for studying contact development, limb bud cultures can be used for investigating both migration as well as contact behaviour.

<u>Fig. 1</u>: Blastemal cells from limb buds of 11-day-old mouse embryos after 6 hours in micro-mass culture. Between adjacent cells many cell contacts are seen (arrows). Contacts are also recognizable between a healthy and a necrotic (N) cell. x 19 000.

<u>Fig. 2</u>: High magnification of cell contacts shows typical gap junctions (arrows) at cross sections. x 128 000.

<u>Fig. 3</u>: Blastemal cells from limb buds of 11-day-old mouse embryos after 3 days in micro-mass culture. Nearly no cell contacts are detectable. A small intercellular space without considerable amounts of matrix substances has developed (arrows). x 19 000.

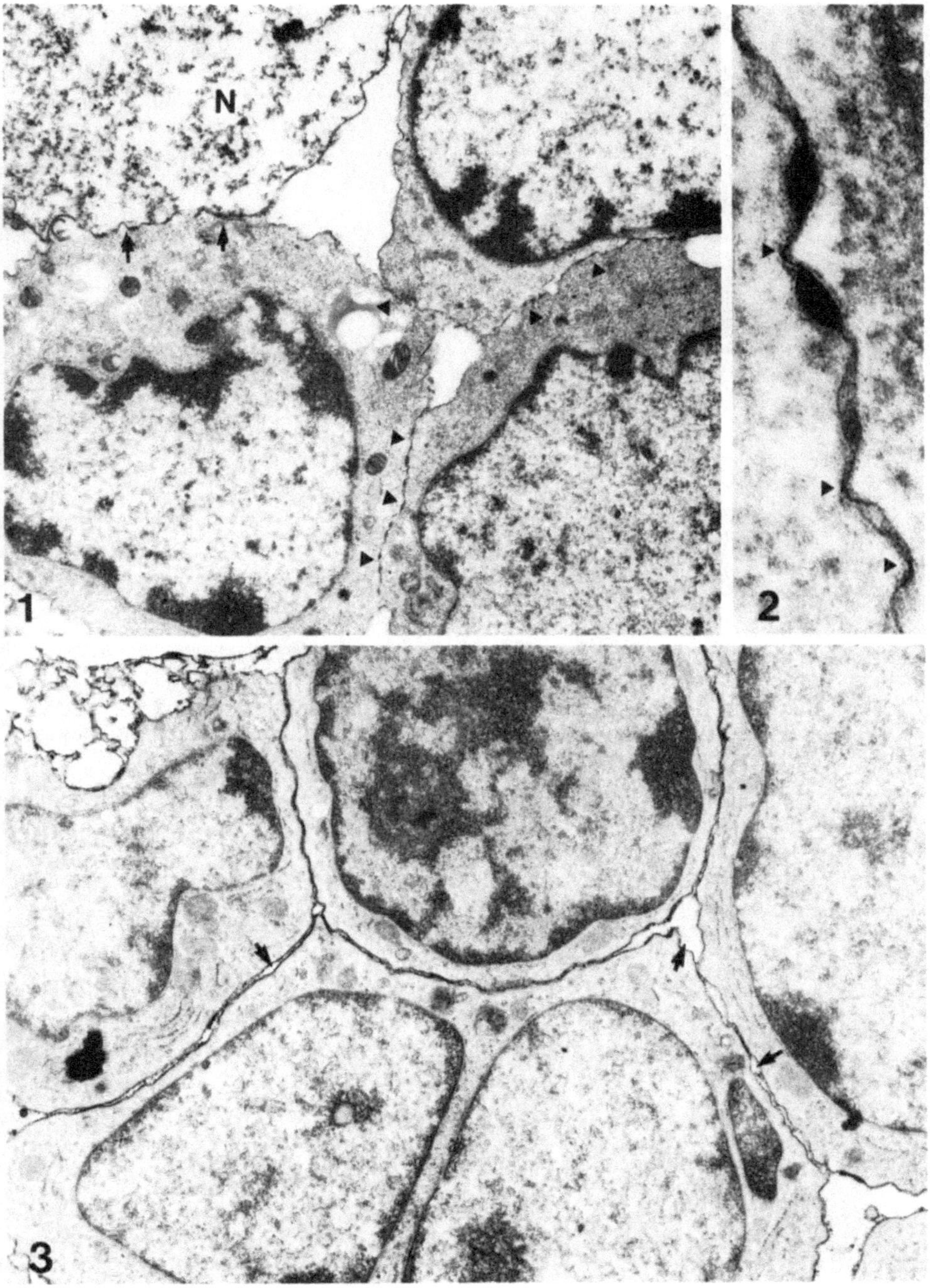
N
1
2
3

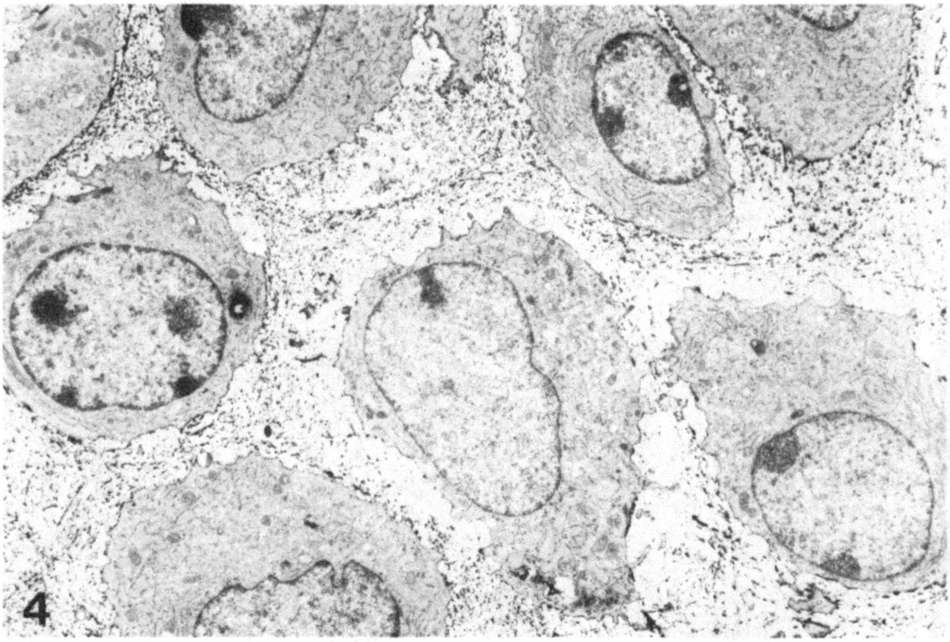

Fig. 4: Electron microscopical picture of a cartilage nodule of a micromass culture after 6 days. Typical cartilage with chondrocytes and an intercellular matrix has developed. x 7 700.

ACKNOWLEDGEMENTS

I wish to thank Mrs. HEIDI SOMOGYI for doing the electron microscopical techniques and Mrs. HELGA STÜRJE for doing the histological techniques. This work was supported by grants of the Deutsche Forschungsgemeinschaft awarded to Sfb 29.

Table 1:

EFFECT OF DIFFERENT SUBSTANCES ON CARTILAGE DEVELOPMENT IN VITRO AFTER APPLICATION AT THE BLASTEMA STAGE ON DAYS 1 TO 3

Culture period: 6 days

	Dose	Limb Bud Culture	Micro Mass Culture
Concanavalin A	200 µg/ml	=	↑
Bacitracin	100 µg/ml	=	=
Nitrophenyl-ß-D-xyloside	1 mM	=	=
6-Diazo-5-oxo-norleucine (DON)	20 µM	=	=
Hyaluronic acid	1 mg/ml	=	=
Hyaluronidase	125 IU/ml	↓↓	=
Glucuronic acid	10 mM	=	=
Galactosamine	10 mM	↓↓	↓
Thiodigalactoside	10 mM	=	(↓)
Vitamin A acid	1 µg/ml	↓↓	↓↓

= : cartilage development as in controls
↓ : strongly reduced
↓↓ : hardly any cartilage
↑ : increased formation of cartilage

Fig. 5: Histological section of a micro-mass culture after 6 days (control). Cartilage nodules (X) are seen within a cell mass without any signs of differentiation (HE-alcian blue staining). x 320.

Fig. 6: Histological section of a micro-mass culture (6 days) after application of 200 µg concanavalin A/ml for the first three days of culture. Compared to the control, cartilage nodules are more prominent with more densely stained matrix (HE-alcian blue staining). x 320.

Fig. 7: Histological section of a micro-mass culture (6 days) after application of 1 µg vitamin A acid/ml for the first three days of culture. Only a small cartilage nodule (arrow) is seen with weakly stained matrix besides many necrotic cells (X), (HE-alcian blue staining). x 320.

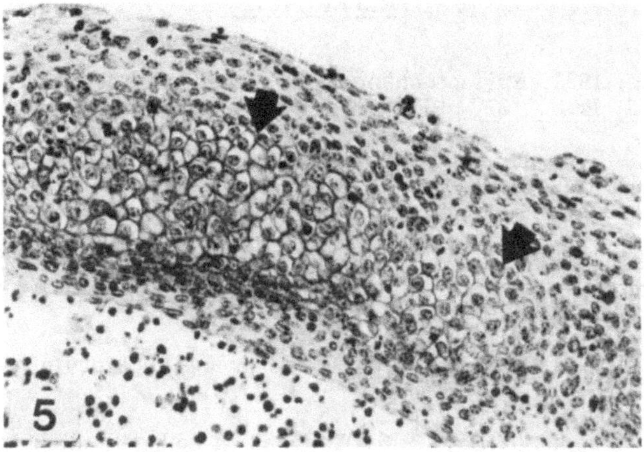
5

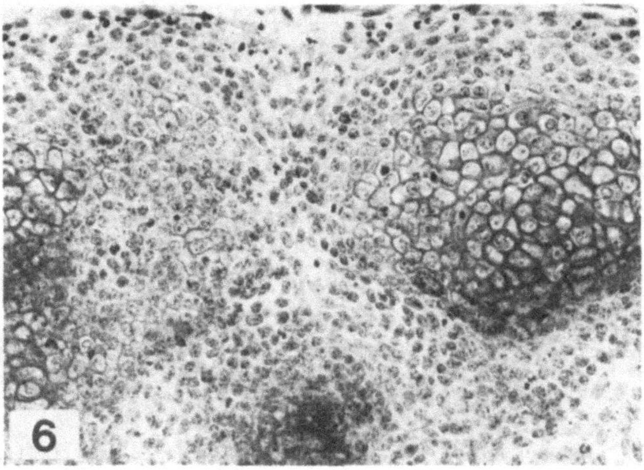
6

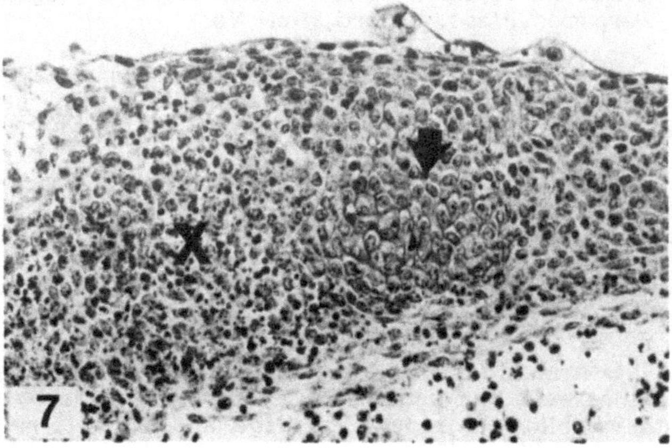
7

REFERENCES

Burger, M.M., 1973, Surface changes in transformed cells detected by lectins, Fed. Proc., 32, 91 - 101.

Fraser, B.A., Travill, A.A., 1978, The effect of retinoic acid on chondrogenesis in the fetal hamster tibia in vivo, J. Embryol. exp. Morph., 48, 23 - 25.

Gartner, T.K., Podleski, T.R., 1975, Evidence that a membrane bound lectin mediates fusion of L6 myoblasts, Biochem. Biophys. Res. Comm., 67, 972 - 978.

Goodenough, D.A., 1974, Bulk isolation of mouse hepatocyte gap junctions, J. Cell Biol., 61, 557 - 563.

Hjelle, J.T., Gibson, K.D., 1979, Changes in collagen ultrastructure, macroscopic properties and chemical composition of chick embryo cartilage induced by administration of a ß-D-xyloside, J. Embryol. exp. Morph., 53, 179.

Lewis, C.A., Pratt, R.M., Pennypacker, J.P., Hassell, J.R., 1978, Inhibition of limb chondrogenesis in vitro by vitamin A: Alterations in cell surface characteristics, Develop. Biol., 64, 31 - 47.

Linsenmayer, T.F., Kochhar, D.M., 1979, In vitro cartilage formation: Effects of 6-diazo-5-oxo-L-norleucine (DON) on glycosaminoglycan and collagen synthesis, Develop. Biol., 69, 517 - 528.

Lohmander, L.S., Hascall, V.C., Caplan, A.I., 1979, Effects of 4-methyl umbelliferyl-ß-D-xylopyranoside on chondrogenesis and proteoglycan synthesis in chick limb bud mesenchymal cell cultures, J. Biol. Chem., 254, 10551.

Merker, H.-J., Zimmermann, B., Grundmann, K., 1980, Differentiation of isolated blastemal cells from limb buds into chondroblasts, in: Tissue culture in medical research, (R.J. Richards, K.T. Rajan, eds.), pp 31 - 39, Pergamon Press, Oxford, New York.

Singer, J.A., Morrison, M., 1976, Effect of metabolic state on agglutination of human erythrocytes by concanavalin A, Biochem. Biophys. Acta, 426, 123 - 131.

Toole, B.P., Jackson, G., Gross, J., 1972, Hyaluronate in morphogenesis: Inhibition of chondrogenesis in vitro, Proc. Nat. Acad. Sci. USA, 69, 1384 - 1386.

Trowell, O.A., 1959, The culture of mature organs in a synthetic medium, Exp. Cell Res., 16, 118 - 147.

Wlodarski, K., Ostrowski, K., Chlopkiewicz, B., Koziorowska, J., 1974, Correlation between the agglutinability of living cells by concanavalin A and their ability to induce cartilage and bone formation, Calcif. Tiss. Res., 16, 251 - 255.

Proliferation Behaviour and Surface Coat in the Limb Bud Blastema of Mouse Embryos. An Autoradiographic Study

R. Herken

Institut für Toxikologie und Embryonal-Pharmakologie, Freie Universität Berlin
Garystraße 9, D-1000 Berlin 33

INTRODUCTION:

The first visible step in limb skelettogenesis is the densification of mesenchymal cells to the blastema. The next step is the differentiation of the mesenchymal cells of the blastema into cartilage cells. At the same time, in the marginal region of the blastema, mesenchymal cells develop to form the perichondrium.

When determining the generation times of cells from the upper limbs of the mouse during chondrogenesis in vitro (HERKEN, 1975), it was striking that addition of ^{3}H-thymidine did not lead to a labelling of blastemal cells. We took this finding as an indication of a difference between the proliferation behaviour of blastemal cells and that of other limb cells. To gain more insight into this problem, we followed the proliferation behaviour of blastemal cells until chondrogenesis. For this purpose, the limb bud culture technique established at our institute (NEUBERT et al., 1974) was applied and the limb buds were labelled with ^{3}H-thymidine. It was the aim of our studies to be able to make statements as to which phases of the skelettogenesis of limbs may be disturbed by drugs interfering with cell proliferation.

Apart from the proliferation behaviour of blastemal cells, we also wanted to investigate to what extent the synthesis of a glycoprotein-containing surface coat plays a role in blastema formation. A striking morphological criterion of blastema formation is the close contact of the cells of this region (MERKER et al., 1980). Since it is known that the surface coat of the cells, which predominantly consists of glycoproteins, is of great importance for specific cellular contacts (Review by MARCHESI et al., 1978), it is feasible that blastema formation is accompanied by a synthesis of glycoproteins of the surface coat. Incorporation studies using labelled fucose (BENNETT, LEBLOND, 1970; BENNET et al., 1974) are especially suitable for the demonstration of glycoprotein synthesis. The specificity of an autoradiographic demonstration is based on the fact that fucose is a carbohydrate which is specifically incorporated into carbohydrate side chains of glycoproteins (COFFEY et al., 1964; BEKESI, WINZLER, 1967); we tried to demonstrate the glycoprotein synthesis of cells involved in chondrogenesis by in vitro labelling of the limb buds with ^{3}H-fucose.

MATERIAL and METHODS:

The investigations were performed on NMRI mice kept at a normal day/night cycle. The animals received Altromin and water ad libitum. The mating period was two hours. The presence of a vaginal plug at 8 a.m. indicated day 0 of gestation.

The embryos were removed on day 11 + 3 hours (42 somites) and the upper limb buds were dissected. The limb buds were grown in a modified

Biggers medium (BIGGERS et al., 1961). Details of the limb bud culture have been described elsewhere (NEUBERT et al., 1974; HERKEN, 1977).

^{3}H-Thymidine labelling

On days 2, 3, and 4 in vitro, the limb buds were placed for 1 hour into a medium containing 2 µCi/ml ^{3}H-thymidine (spec. act. 5 Ci/mmol, Amersham). Subsequently, the preparations were removed and fixed in 3% glutaraldehyde plus 3% paraformaldehyde in cacodylate buffer (pH 7.2). Postfixation was carried out in 1% OsO_4 in cacodylate buffer (pH 7.2). This was followed by embedding in Mikropal (Ferak).

Another group of limb buds was placed into medium on days 1, 2, and 3. This medium also contained 2 µCi/ml ^{3}H-thymidine. Thus, the amount of thymidine added to the medium was far below the dosis which is able to influence cell proliferation in vitro (PAINTER et al., 1964). 24 hours later, i.e. on days 2, 3, or 4 in vitro, the limb buds were removed and prepared further, as described above.

^{3}H-Fucose labelling

On days 2, 3, and 4 in vitro the limb buds were placed in medium for 30 minutes or 4 hours, respectively. This medium contained 25 µCi/ml ^{3}H-fucose (spec. act. 15 Ci/mmol, Amersham). Further preparation of the limb buds was carried out as described above. From the embedded material 1 µ thick serial sections were cut in longitudinal direction and dipped into an Ilford K5 photoemulsion. After exposure at +4° C, the preparations were developed in Amidol, fixed in sodiumthiosulphate, stained with alkaline Giemsa solution and covered in Euparal.

FINDINGS:

^{3}H-Thymidine labelling

After pulse labelling for one hour, none of the blastemal regions showed any cell labelling. This indicates that DNA synthesis does not proceed in these cells of the blastema. It was also striking that we failed to detect mitoses in the blastema. This absence of DNA synthesis and mitoses was not restricted to the blastema of certain limb regions, but was also true of all bone anlagen.

In the regions where differentiation of blastemal cells into cartilage cells had become recognizable, the labelling behaviour did not change after pulse labelling with ^{3}H-thymidine. The marginal region of these blastemata, which was weakly labelled in certain areas, had not yet been transformed into the perichondrium.

It was only at the developmental stage, when blastemal cells had completely differentiated into cartilage cells and the perichondrium had developed in the marginal region, that cartilage and perichondral cells were labelled after pulse labelling with ^{3}H-thymidine. In addition, single mitoses could now be observed in the cartilage.

Even after 24-hour labelling with ^{3}H-thymidine hardly any cell labelling could be detected in the blastemata (Fig. 2). However, in contrast to pulse labelling, pronounced labelling was seen in those areas where chondrogenesis sets in (Fig. 3). But the centre of the blastema, where typical cartilage cells are located, was not labelled; labelling was confined to the marginal regions. In those areas of the limbs, where blastemal cells had differentiated into typical cartilage cells surrounded by a perichondrium, strong labelling of cartilage, but also of perichondral cells, was found.

^{3}H-Fucose labelling

30 minutes after the addition of ^{3}H-fucose, the regions where mesenchymal cells had densified to form the blastema, a clear-cut punctiform labelling was recognized in the cytoplasm of blastemal cells. After a four-hour application of ^{3}H-fucose, the extent of labelling had increased. The major part of labelling was no longer seen in a punctiform fashion in the cytoplasm of blastemal cells, but the labelling formed a kind of fringe around the cells.

In regions of the limb buds, where first indications of differentiation of blastemal into cartilage cells were seen, a relatively weak punctiform labelling was detected after 30-minute labelling with ^{3}H-fucose. Four hours after the addition of ^{3}H-fucose this punctiform labelling was much more pronounced. In addition, a relatively weak labelling was also observed in regions of the cell surface. It can be generally stated that those regions of the blastema where cartilage cells are recognizable, show a weaker labelling than regions where the blastema still consists of densely packed mesenchymal cells.

In regions of the limbs, where blastemal cells had already differentiated into typical cartilage cells and were surrounded by a perichondrium, the labelling of cartilage cells after 30-minute or 4-hour additions of ^{3}H-fucose resembled that described above at the beginning of chondrogenesis (Fig. 4). After a 30-minute addition of ^{3}H-fucose a relatively weak and diffuse labelling in the perichondrium had become more pronounced. Besides a rather diffuse labelling a punctiform labelling was recognizable in cytoplasmic cells.

DISCUSSION:

The present study shows that the proliferation behaviour of blastemal cells clearly differs from that of the neighbouring limb cells. Cell labelling was not detected in our limb bud cultures in the blastemal region either after one hour nor after 24-hour additions of ^{3}H-thymidine. We also failed to observe mitoses in these areas. This indicates that the blastemal cells were neither in the S-phase of the cell cycle, when ^{3}H-thymidine could have been incorporated into DNA, nor in the mitosis phase. It can therefore be assumed that the blastemal cells do not pass the cell cycle but are either arrested in the G_2- or in the G_1-phase. Since the G_2-phase only represents a relatively short transitional phase between the S-phase and mitosis, in which the cell structures necessary for mitosis are synthesized, it seems to be unlikely that the blastemal cells are arrested in this phase of the cell cycle. However, the G_1-phase of the cell cycle is of fundamental importance for processes of cell differentiation, since during this phase proteins specific for each cell are synthesized (GRAHAM, 1973). The more differentiated a cell is, i.e. the more specific proteins have to be synthesized in the cell, the longer takes its G_1-phase compared with the overall length of the cell cycle. We assume that the blastema is differentiated in such a way that the blastemal cells are arrested for a certain period in the G_1-phase of the cell cycle, in order to synthesize the specific proteins which they require for the differentiation into cartilage cells. However, after differentiation of mesenchymal cells of the blastema into cartilage cells, DNA synthesis and thus, further cell proliferations, do not set in immediately. During the phase of development, at which cartilage cells were detected, labelling of these cells with ^{3}H-thymidine had not yet taken place. The first labelled cells were observed when a perichondrium was recognizable. Owing to the temporal dependency of the labelling of cartilage cells on the formation of the perichondrium we assume that the formation of the perichondrium plays a decisive role in the termination of the proliferation stop of the blastema. The significance of the perichondrium for the re-occurrence of cell proliferation in the blastema was also strengthened by the fact that the first labelled cartilage cells were not seen in the centre of the blastema but in the marginal regions, where the perichondrium developed.

The labelling behaviour of the cartilage cells after 24 hours addition of ^{3}H-thymidine corresponded to the picture we had expected. Here it became even more obvious than after pulse labelling that the proliferation of cartilage cells sets in close to the perichondrium.

It was surprising to see that even 24 hour additions of ^{3}H-thymidine did not lead to a labelling of the blastema. If the mesenchymal cells had proliferated until shortly before the formation of the blastema, it could have been expected that within the 24 hours of ^{3}H-thymidine application at least part of the cells had been labelled before the densification of mesenchymal cells to blastemal cells.

During the further course of development, these labelled cells would have been integrated into the blastema so that after 24 hours, labelled cells would have become recognizable in the blastema. Since this was not the case, we assume that the mesenchymal cells of the later blastema had been already arrested in the G_1-phase of the cell cycle for a certain period prior to blastema formation. This would indicate that the densification of blastemal cells is not the triggering factor, which, for example, by way of contact inhibition, leads to proliferation inhibition. It is more likely that the formation of the blastema is a result of proliferation inhibition.

While the stage of blastema formation is characterized by an inhibition of cell proliferation, the findings obtained after the application of ^{3}H-fucose indicate that glycoprotein synthesis proceeds in blastemal cells. Using this method we tried to investigate glycoprotein synthesis and the speed at which this surface coat material is transported to the cell surface. Therefore, ^{3}H-fucose was administered for 30 minutes and four hours, respectively. The synthesis of the carbohydrate side chains of the glycoproteins of the surface coat takes place in the sacculus of the Golgi apparatus of the cell (BENNETT et al., 1974). Thus, after a short labelling period, the major part of the incorporated fucose is to be seen in the cytoplasm, provided that glycoprotein synthesis has taken place in the cell. The glycoprotein-containing surface coat material is then channelled to the cell surface via the turnover of the membrane, so that a labelling of the cell surface would have to be expected. Thus, it follows that besides the occurrence of glycoprotein synthesis also the extent of the membranous turnover of a cell can be deduced from the different labelling situation after 30 minutes and four hours application of ^{3}H-fucose.

After a four hour application of ^{3}H-fucose, part of the labelling was detected on the cell surface of blastemal cells. While at the beginning of the differentiation of the blastema into cartilage cells, a weak labelling was still to be seen in the cell surface after four hours application of ^{3}H-fucose, in the fully differentiated cartilage ^3H-fucose incorporation was only detected in the cytoplasm, even after the same period of drug administration. This suggests that with progressing differentiation of blastemal into cartilage cells, a reduction in the membranous turnover of the cells takes place in addition to a decrease in glycoprotein synthesis. Here blastemal cells exhibit the highest, and cartilage cells the lowest membranous turnover. The labelling behaviour of the perichondrium does not differ essentially from that of the cartilage. The extent of glycoprotein synthesis and membranous turnover in the perichondrium is low, as compared with that of blastemal cells.

On the basis of our findings, the following statements can be made as to the influenceability of the different phases of blastemal differentiation of the limbs by pharmaceutical drugs: the blastemal phase can most likely not be influenced by substances interfering with cell proliferation, since blastemal cells do not reproduce at this stage. Disturbances in cell proliferation can only be triggered when differentiation into cartilage has almost been completed. Our findings however, indicate that the formation of the blastema can possibly be disturbed by drugs interfering with glycoprotein synthesis.

SUMMARY:

Limb buds of 11-day-old mouse embryos (42 somites; strain NMRI) were grown in an organ culture until the formation of blastema and cartilage (day 2 to 4 in vitro). In order to investigate the proliferation behaviour of cells involved in blastema and cartilage formation, the limb buds were labelled in vitro for one hour or 24 hours with ^3H-thymidine. Neither pulse labelling nor long-term labelling with ^3H-thymidine led to any labelling of the blastemal cells. Indications suggesting an arrest of these cells in the G_1-phase of the cell cycle are discussed. It was only after formation of the perichondrium was recognizable in addition to a differentiation of blastemal cells into cartilage cells, that labelling of cartilage cells could be observed.

To investigate glycoprotein synthesis and the extent of the migration of surface coat material to the cell surface of blastemal and cartilage cells, the limb buds were labelled with ^3H-fucose for 30 minutes and four hours on days 2, 3, and 4 in vitro. After 30 minutes application of ^3H-fucose the most pronounced labelling was seen in the region of the blastemal cells. Cartilage and perichondral cells which had already differentiated showed weaker labelling. After four hours application of ^3H-fucose the major part of labelling of blastemal cells was observed on the cell surface, whereas in the fully differentiated cartilage after the same period, labelling was restricted to the cytoplasm of cartilage cells. Thus, it can be concluded that the blastemal cells are characterized by a faster membranous turnover, as compared with typical cartilage cells.

ACKNOWLEDGEMENTS

The expert technical assistance of Mrs. H. STÜRJE and H. WOHLFEIL is gratefully acknowledged.

The work was supported by grants of the DFG awarded to Sfb 29.

REFERENCES

Bekesi, J.G., Winzler, R.J., 1967, The metabolism of plasma glycoproteins. Studies on the incorporation of L-fucose-l-^{14}C into tissue and serum in the normal rat, J. Biol. Chem., 242, 3873 - 3879.

Bennett, G., Leblond, C.P., 1970, Formation of cell coat material for the whole surface of columnar cells in the rat small intestine, as visualised by radioautography with L-fucose-^{3}H, J. Cell Biol., 46, 409 - 416.

Bennett, G., Leblond, C.P., Haddad, A., 1974, Migration of glycoprotein from the Golgi apparatus to the surface of various cell types as shown by radioautography after labelled fucose injection into rats, J. Cell Biol., 60, 258 - 284.

Biggers, J.D., Gwatkin, R.B.L., Heyner, S., 1961, Growth of embryonic avian and mammalian tibiae on a relatively simple chemically defined medium, Exp. Cell Res., 25, 41 - 58.

Coffey, J.W., Miller, O.N., Sellinger, O., 1964, The metabolism of L-fucose in the rat, J. Biol. Chem., 239, 4011 - 4017.

Graham, C.F., 1973, The cell cycle during mammalian development, in: The Cell Cycle in Development and Differentiation (1st Symp. Br. Soc. Develop. Biol.), (M. Balls, F.S. Billet, eds.), pp. 293 - 310, Cambridge University Press, London.

Herken, R., 1975, Autoradiographic investigations with ^{3}H-thymidine in limb bud cultures, in: New Approaches to the Evaluation of Abnormal Embryonic Development (D. Neubert, H.-J. Merker, eds.), pp. 200 - 212, Georg Thieme Publ., Stuttgart.

Herken, R., 1977, The influence of D-penicillamine on the proliferation rate of cells from the upper limb bud of mouse embryos in vitro, Teratology, 15, 159 - 162.

Marchesi, V.T., Ginsburg, V., Robbins, P.W., Fox, C.F., 1978, Cell surface carbohydrates and biological recognition, Progr. Clin. Biol. Res., 23, Alan R. Liss, Inc., New York.

Merker, H.-J., Zimmermann, B., Barrach, H.-J., Grundmann, K., Ebel, H., 1980, Simulation of steps of limb skelettogenesis in vitro, this book.

Neubert, D.H., Merker, H.-J., Tapken, S., 1974, Comparative studies on the prenatal development of mouse extremities in vivo and in organ culture, Naunyn-Schmied. Arch. Pharmacol., 286, 251 - 270.

Painter, R.B., Drew, R.M., Rasmussen, R.E., 1964, Limitations in the use of carbon-labelled and tritium-labelled thymidine in cell culture studies, Radiat. Res., 21, 355 - 366.

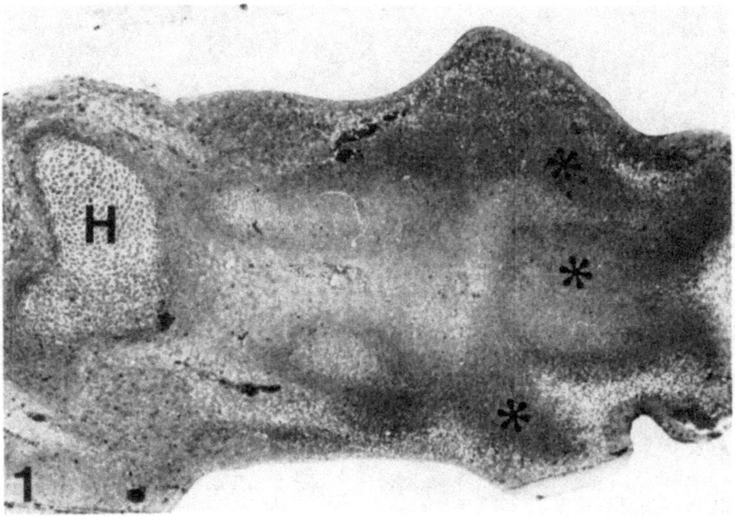

Fig. 1: Longitudinal section of a limb bud on day 3 in vitro. Asterisk: densification of mesenchymal cells in the region of the hand skeleton. H = cartilage of the humerus.
x 64.

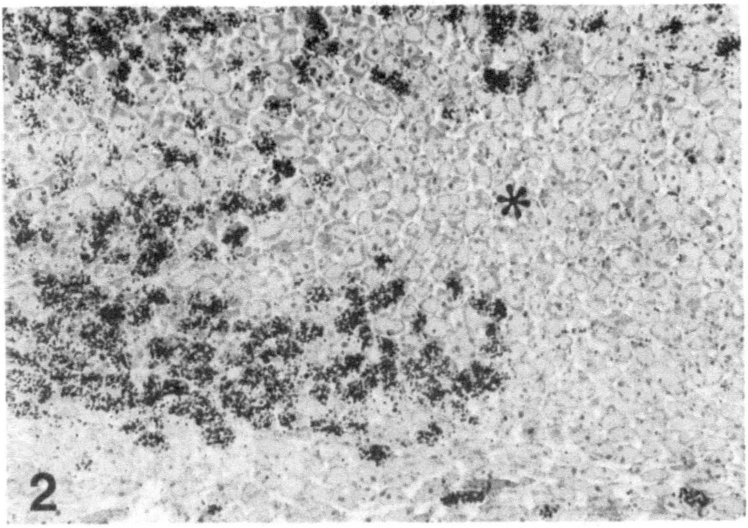

Fig. 2: Blastemal region of a limb bud on day 3 in vitro after 24 hours labelling with ^{3}H-thymidine. Asterisk: unlabelled centre of the blastema.
x 400.

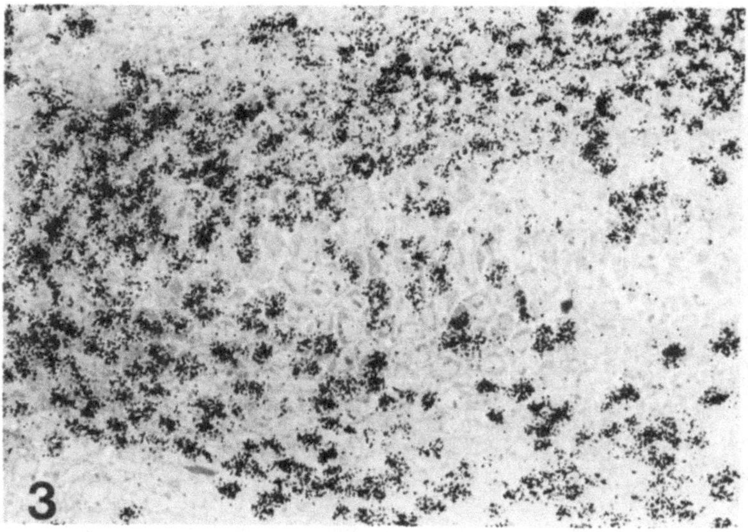

Fig. 3: Beginning differentiation of the blastema of a limb bud into cartilage on day 3 in vitro. 24 hour labelling with ^{3}H-thymidine. x 400.

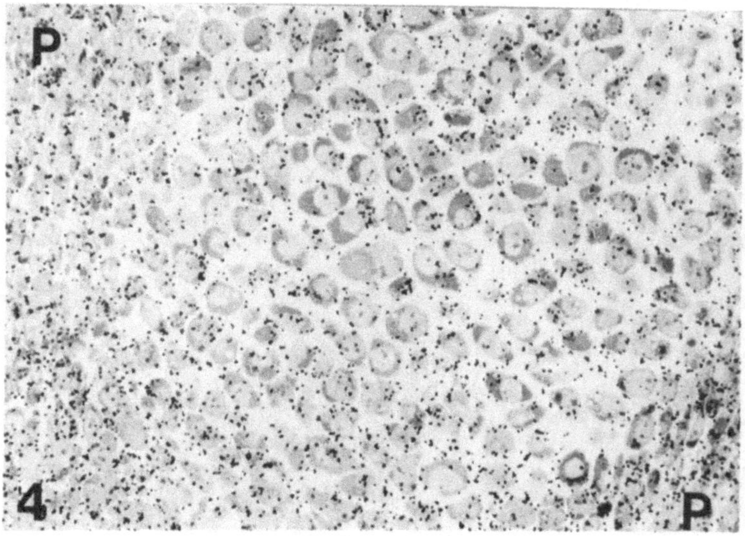

Fig. 4: Cartilage anlage of a humerus on day 3 in vitro after four hour labelling with ^{3}H-fucose. P = region of the perichondrium. x 640.

The Occurrence of Unilateral Abnormality of the Limb Induced by the Teratogen 6-Aminonicotinamide

H.-J. Barrach, I. Dillmann

Institut für Toxikologie und Embryonal-Pharmakologie, Freie Universität Berlin
Garystraße 9, D-1000 Berlin 33

To date, little data has been found in the literature demonstrating evidence of the susceptibility of test animals to a unilateral abnormality induced by a teratogenic agent. To our knowledge, the only well-documented evidence for a teratogenic vulnerability restricted to one of the extremities was published by WILSON et al. (1968). The effect was obtained using carbonic anhydrase inhibitors in rats, and it affected the right front limbs. In this paper, we will present a detailed documentation of a unilateral abnormality which occurred in our laboratory using the teratogen 6-aminonicotinamide (6-AN) with random-bred NMRI mice as experimental animals. Biochemical aspects of this teratogenic effect have been published elsewhere (NEUBERT et al., 1980).

A single dose of 10 or 15 mg/kg 6-AN was given to the mice on day 9 or 10 of pregnancy. At day 18 of gestation, the fetuses were taken, and examination revealed a wide variety of abnormalities of the limbs in addition to other malformations, such as rib or dorsal vertebra anomalies. Most of these very severely malformed limbs were hind limbs. Pictures of those limbs are presented to demonstrate the severity of the anomalies (Figs. 1 - 4).

When the data were examined, it was found that there was a preference for the malformation to occur in the left hind limb more often than in the other limbs. By listing the paw malformations in percent of the malformed animals, distributions were obtained which clearly pictured this phenomenon of limb preference.

In the first experimental series, a dose of 10 mg/kg 6-AN was given subcutaneously (s.c.) on day 9 of pregnancy. Upon examination of 302 fetuses taken from the treated mice, 34 were found to have malformed paws. Figure 5 shows the distribution of malformed paws in each fetus. The most significant finding was that 80% of the fetuses had malformed left hind limbs only. There was no single malformation of the right hind paw or left front paw. One fetus had a malformed right front paw. The second and third most frequent occurrence of malformation was the combination of the left hind paw with the right hind paw, or the left hind paw with the right front paw. The last column of Figure 5 shows the sum of left hind paw malformations occurring singly or in combination with other malformations. The data show that 97% of the affected fetuses had a malformation of the left hind paw.

In another experimental series, the malformation pattern was evaluated using a higher dose of 6-AN. A dose of 15 mg/kg 6-AN given on day 9 of gestation did not change the preferential occurrence of malformation in the left hind paw (Fig. 6). Single malformations of the left hind paw occurred in 60% of the malformed fetuses. The sum of fetuses with left hind paw malformations including the combinations was 89%. An abnormality of the right front paw occurred as a single malformation only in 7% of the fetuses. This is higher than in the other experiments; however, there is no

Teratology of the Limbs

increase in the rate of single right hind paw malformations. Only one fetus had the left front paw malformed in combination with an abnormal right front paw.

It has been found that 6-AN interferes with the regulation of the body temperature in rodents (COPER et al., 1971). The authors used adult rats for their experiments and found a hypothermal effect as a result of the 6-AN treatment. The question therefore arose as to how the hypothermy (35 - 36, ° C) of the mother animals in our experiments might interfere with the embryotoxic action of the dose 10 mg/kg 6-AN s.c. At an ambient temperature of 36°C, the body temperature of the treated mice remained normal (37 - 38 ° C). Under these conditions, the percentage of malformed fetuses was higher than the percentage obtained when the mother animals were kept at a temperature of 23° C, or even when the higher dose of 15 mg/kg 6-AN was administered (Table 3). Again, the highest percentage (over 50%) of single paw malformations occurred in the left hind paw, with the next most frequent occurrence being the combination of left and right hind paws. The sum of left hind paw malformations occurring singly or in combination with other malformations was 95%.

When the mother animals were treated at day 10 of pregnancy, the number of fetuses with malformed paws decreased. Table 4 shows the data obtained when the test animals were kept at room temperature. After treatment with 10 mg/kg 6-AN s.c., only malformations of the hind paws occurred, and single malformations occurred only in the left hind paw. The right hind paw was affected only in combination with the left hind paw.
Table 5 shows the results obtained when the treated animals were kept at 36° C. A malformation occurred in the left hind paw of 71% of the fetuses examined, while the combination of malformed left hind paw and right hind paw accounted for another 21%. One fetus had the left hind paw malformed in combination with the right front paw, and one fetus had malformed hind paws plus a malformed left front paw.

Preliminary studies with other mouse strains suggested that the side specific effect of 6-AN could also be induced in other strains of mice, such as C57 black. The results are summarized in table 6. The mother animals were treated with 15 mg/kg 6-AN at day 9 of pregnancy. Over 40% of the fetuses examined showed a single malformation of the left hind paw, while the total percent of left hind limb malformations occurring singly or in combination with other anomalies was 59%. Although the left hind limb was the most frequent location of malformed paws, there is a slight difference between the NMRI and the C57 strain. In 30% of the C57 strain fetuses which were examined, malformation of the right front limb occurred as the second most frequent event of a single limb abnormality. The left front limb of those examined was always normal in this group of treated mice.

To summarize, in this study using NMRI mice and the teratogen 6-aminonicotinamide, we examined 746 fetuses treated at day 9 of gestation, the most sensitive stage in which limb malformations occur as a result of application of 6-AN. Of those fetuses examined, 252 had developed paw malformations. The left hind paw was affected at a rate of between 89 and 97%, either singly or in combination with other malformations, whereas the left front paw was malformed in only 0 to 6% of the fetuses. Although this effect is really quite pronounced, we have no clue as to the mode of action of this very specific teratogenic effect. It should be mentioned that, when using a variety of other teratogenic agents with the same mouse strain, no such preferential action on one side of the body was observed.

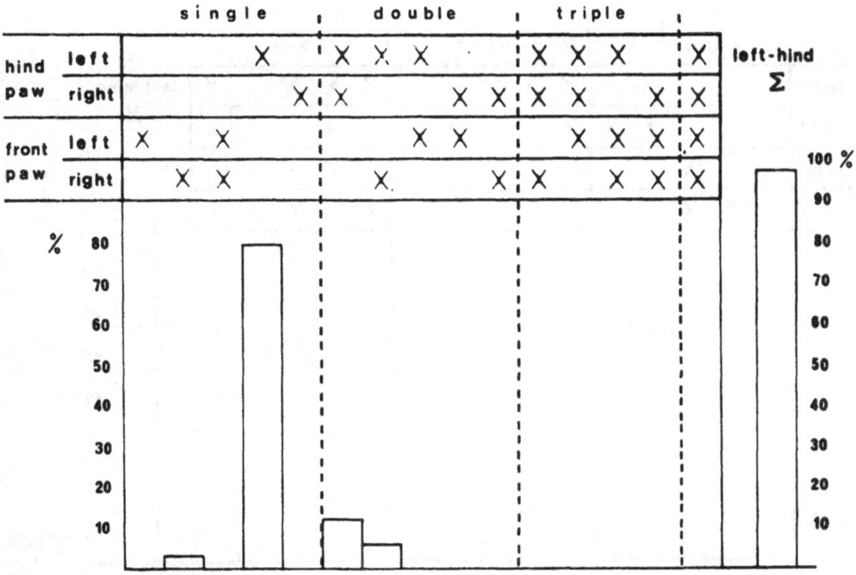

Table 1: NMRI mice were treated on day 3 of gestation with 10 mg/kg 6-AN and kept at 23° C ambient temperature. 302 fetuses were examined of which 34 fetuses had malformed paws.

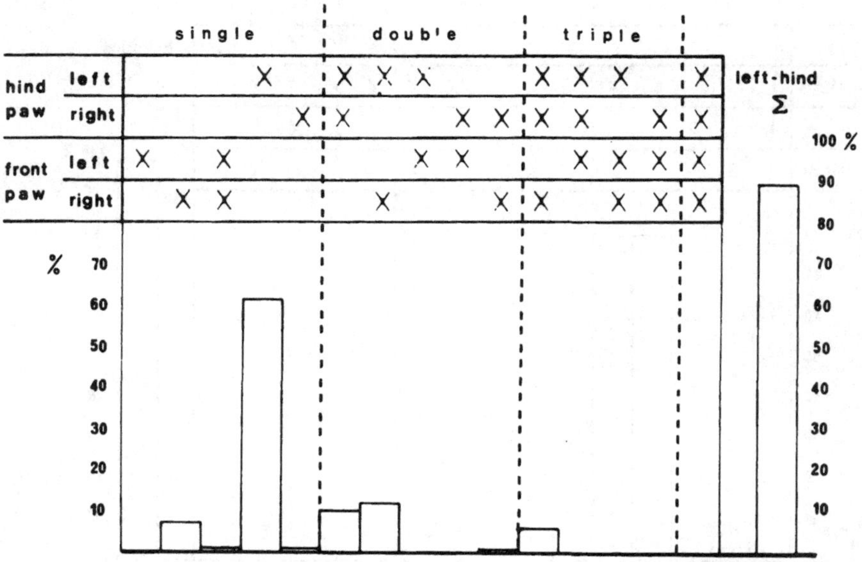

Table 2: Mice (NMRI) were treated on day 3 of gestation with 15 mg/kg 6-AN and kept at 23° C ambient temperature. Of the 167 fetuses examined 63 offspring had malformed paws.

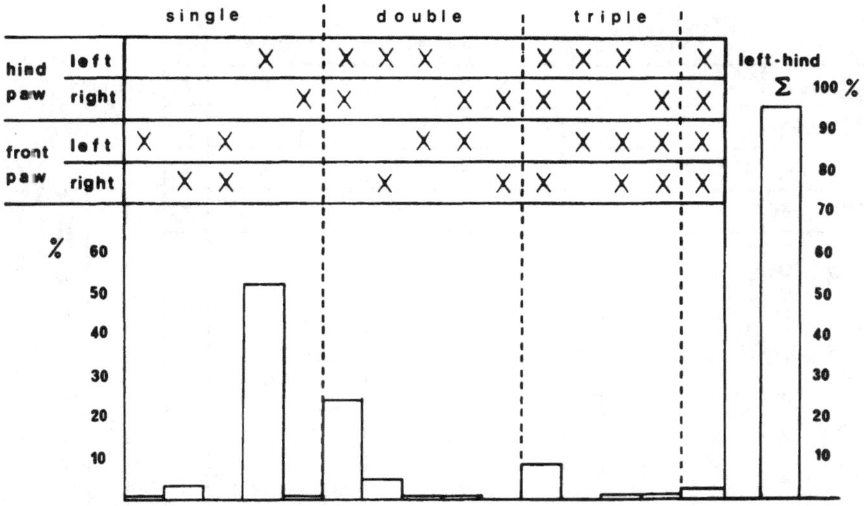

Table 3: The mice (NMRI) were treated on day 9 of gestation with 10 mg/kg 6-AN. The ambient temperature was raised to 36° C for 10 hours starting at the time of treatment with the drug. 277 fetuses were examined, of which 149 fetuses had malformed paws.

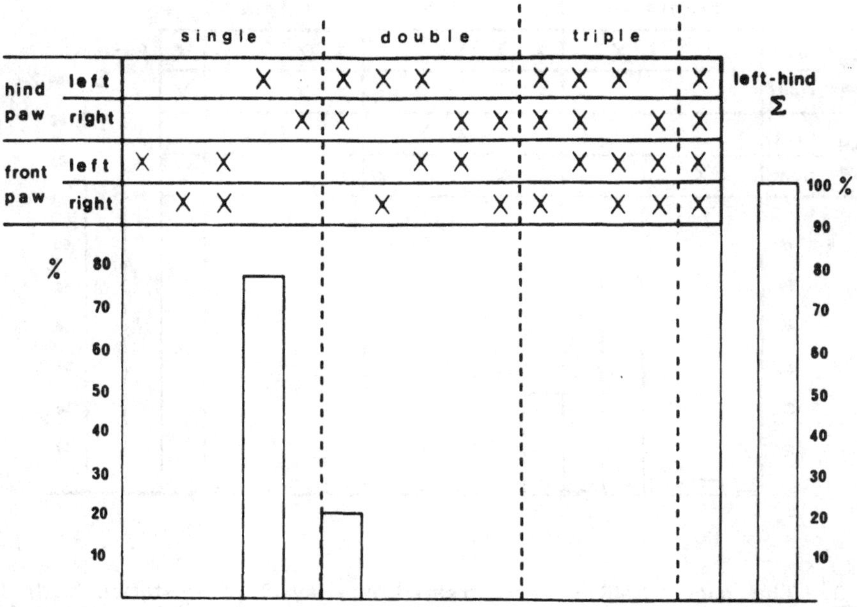

Table 4: NMRI mice were treated on day 10 of pregnancy with 10 mg/kg 6-AN and kept at room temperature. 166 fetuses were examined: 9 fetuses had malformed hind paws only.

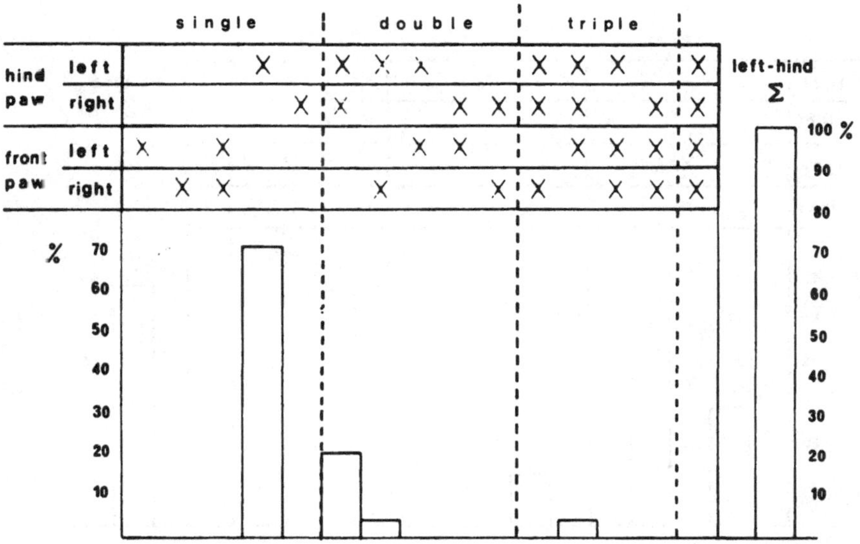

Table 5: When the NMRI mice were treated with 10 mg/kg 6-AN and kept at 36° C ambient temperature, 24 fetuses of the 166 examined had malformed paws.

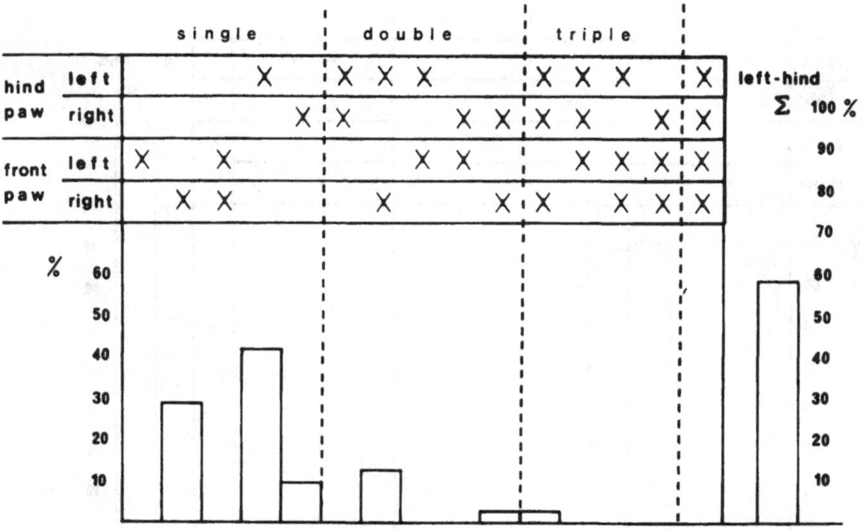

<u>Table 6</u>: Mice of the inbred strain C57 black were treated on day 9.5 with 15 mg/kg 6-AN and kept at room temperature of 23° C. 104 fetuses were examined, of which 31 had paw malformations. Although this mouse strain had a higher incidence of right front paw malformations, the effect on the left hind limb was the more frequent.

REFERENCES

Coper, H., Lison, H., Rommelspacher, H., Schulze, G., Strauss, S., 1971, The influence of adrenergic receptor-blocking agents, amphetamine, and 6-aminonicotinamide on thermoregulation, Naunyn-Schmied. Arch. Pharmak., 270, 378 - 391.

Neubert, D., Barrach, H.-J., Merker, H.-J., 1980, Drug-induced damage to the embryo or fetus (Molecular and multilateral approach to prenatal toxicology), in: Current topics in pathology, (E. Grundmann, ed.), Vol. "Drug-Induced Pathology", Springer, Heidelberg, (in press).

Wilson, J.G., Maren, T.H., Takano, K., Ellison, A., 1968, Teratogenic action of carbonic anhydrase inhibitors in the rat, Teratology, 1, 51 - 60.

Figures 1 - 4: Mouse hind limbs, day 18 of pregnancy.

Fig. 1: This picture shows the control right hind limb.

Fig. 2: This picture shows the hind limbs of a fetus after treatment of the mother animal with 15 mg/kg 6-AN day 3 of gestation. Aplasia of the left hind limb and syndactylism of the right hind limb.

Fig. 3: This is the offspring of a mouse which was treated the same way as in Fig. 2. The picture shows a paw skeleton reduced to one digit in the left hind paw and to two digits in the right hind paw. The right front limb in this case is unaffected.

Fig. 4: This picture shows syndactylism and one digit missing from the left hind limb of a fetus after treatment of the mother with 10 mg/kg 6-AN on day 9 of pregnancy.

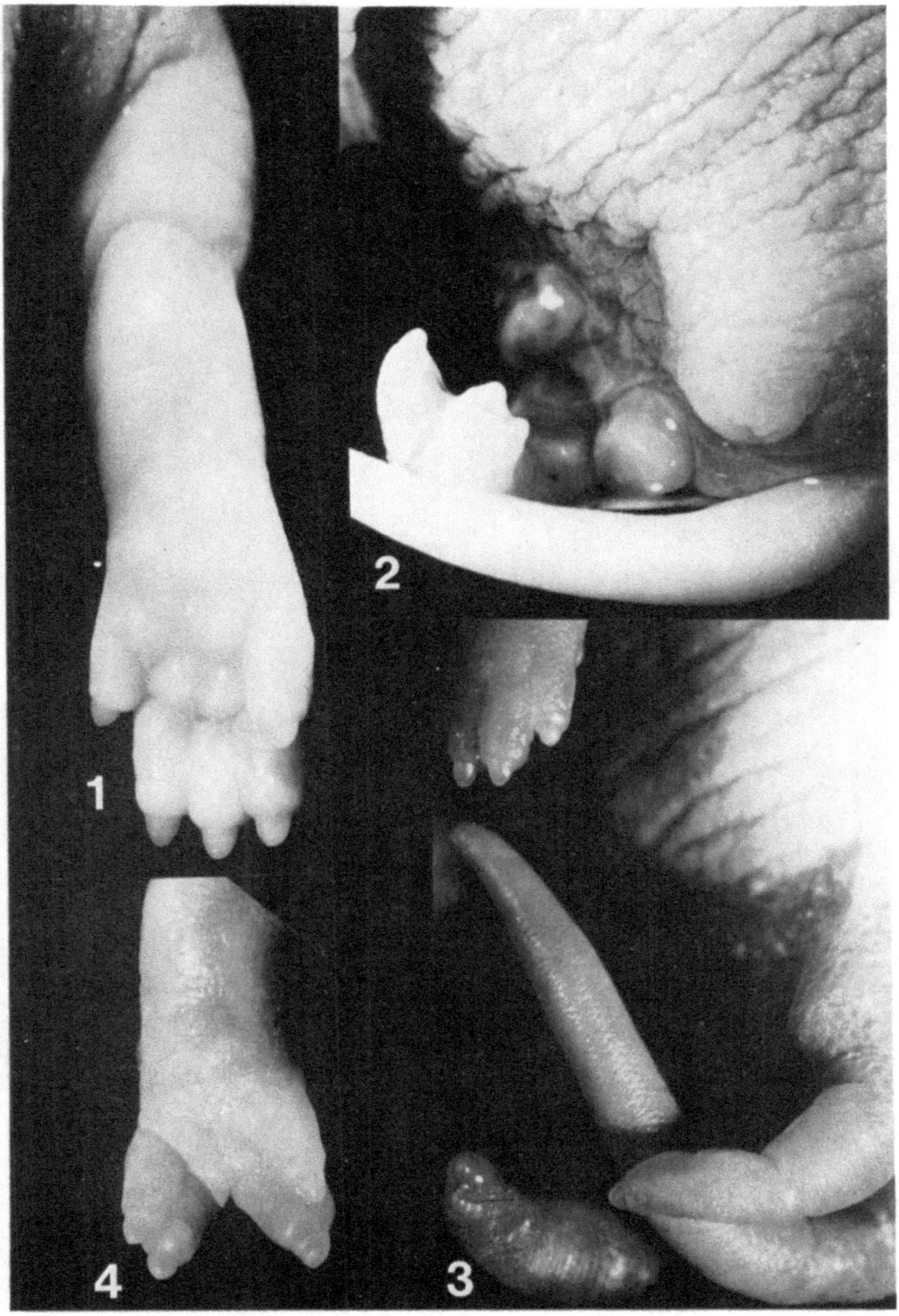
1
2
3
4

Ascorbic Acid Content of Limb Buds at Different Stages of Mammalian Embryonic Development

Gudrun Blankenburg, Margret Rautenberg und Diether Neubert
Institut für Toxikologie und Embryonalpharmakologie, Freie Universität Berlin,
Garystraße 9, D-1000 Berlin 33

Collagen synthesis plays an important rôle during embryonic development and is of great significance particularly to the differentiation of the anlagen of the skeletal system and naturally also to the development of the extremities.

There are a number of factors which are essential for collagen synthesis to proceed. Among these ascorbic acid seems to be of special importance. We studied some characteristics of ascorbic acid metabolism in mammalian embryonic tissues during the stage of limb bud differentiation.

In a rodent species two possibilities of ascorbate supply to the differentiating embryonic tissues may be visualized:

1) Since the enzymes necessary for catalysing the conversion of D-glucurono-γ-lactone into ascorbate are present in some adult tissues it is conceivable that embryonic tissues possess the capacity for synthesizing ascorbate to a certain extent of their own requirements.

2) Since the majority of adult tissues are supplied with ascorbate via the blood stream, ascorbate being synthesized mainly in liver tissues and in some species in the kidneys, the embryo may receive at least part of its essential ascorbate quantity from the maternal compartment via maternal blood.

This paper is intended to contribute to the solution of the following four questions:

A) Are embryonic tissues of rodents capable of synthesizing ascorbate to a certain extent?

B) What is the concentration of ascorbate in embryonic tissues, especially in limb buds?

C) Is it possible to modify the ascorbate concentration in embryos by an increased supply of ascorbate from the maternal compartment?

D) What happens to ascorbate as a component of the medium during the organ culture period of embryonic tissues?

A) Are embryonic tissues of rodents capable of synthesizing ascorbate to a certain extent?

Ascorbate is synthesized in a variety of animal species via a pathway involving D-glucurono-γ-lactone, L-gulono-γ-lactone and 2-keto-L-gulono-γ-lactone (cf. CHATTERJEE, 1970). In primates - including man - and in a

Teratology of the Limbs

few other mammalian and bird species the capacity for synthesizing ascorbate was lost during evolution and hence ascorbate became a vitamin for these species (CHATTERJEE et al., 1961).

When the formation of ascorbate from glucurono-γ-lactone is measured in liver tissues of mice it becomes obvious (Fig. 1) that this capacity is low during the perinatal period and rapidly increases postnatally so that a rate comparable to that of adult liver is reached about four days after birth. This finding corroborates preliminary data obtained in rats by CHATTERJEE et al. (1965). In our studies, the rate of ascorbate formation from measured in homogenates of fetal liver amounts to roughly $^1/_{10}$ of that found in adult liver. However, it is interesting that the enzymic capacity can be detected already at rather early fetal stages and that, based on total cell protein, the capacity of ascorbate formed in livers of 11-day old embryos does not greatly differ from that found in 18-day old fetuses.

We have not been able to detect any conversion of D-glucurono-γ-lactone into ascorbate in homogenates of limb buds of 11- or 12- day old mouse embryos (Tab. 1). But the limit of detection with the method used is 0.2 ng ascorbate formed $\times$ µg $DNA^{-1} \times min^{-1}$. Therefore, we can only state that the enzymic activity in limb buds is at least 2 - 3 times lower than in the liver of the same embryo.

From the data presented it appears feasible that ascorbate is synthesized in embryonic liver already on day 11 of gestation and that this synthesis may be supposed to contribute to the ascorbate content of embryonic tissues.

B) <u>What is the concentration of ascorbate in embryonic tissues, especially in limb buds?</u>

When the ascorbate content is measured in whole mouse embryos our data (Fig. 2) clearly show that the ascorbate concentration is significantly lower at early embryonic stages - for example day 10 - when compared with that of older embryos (12-day old). It seems that the transfer of ascorbate to the embryo varies at different stages of development. Therefore it is conceivable that, at certain stages of development, the embryo has a "physiological deficiency" of ascorbate - also under normal conditions.

We also studied the ascorbate content in limb buds of the mouse during late embryonic and early fetal development. From the data given in Fig. 2 two results are obvious:

1) The ascorbate content in limb buds is lower than that of the whole embryo at all developmental stages studied, and

2) the ascorbate concentration also increases during development (day 10.5 and 13 of gestation) in a similar way as in the whole embryo.

Hence, at the beginning of limb bud formation rather low concentrations are available to the differentiating cells.

C) <u>Is it possible to modify the ascorbate concentration in embryos by an increased supply of ascorbate from the maternal compartment?</u>

We investigated whether it is possible to increase the ascorbate content in embryonic tissues by injecting extremely high doses of ascorbate intravenously into pregnant mice. The data show (Fig. 3) that the maternal serum concentration is raised about 100-fold by this very high dose of ascorbate (2 g/kg bodyweight). These doses are needed to achieve a certain increase of the ascorbate concentration in embryonic tissues (Fig. 2). However, ascorbate is rapidly removed from the serum (Fig. 3) and 8 hours after a single intravenous injection the concentration in the maternal serum is only increased to about 4-fold of control.

Since laboratory animals tolerate these high doses of ascorbate it is possible to increase the ascorbate concentration in the whole embryo as well as in limb buds by about 30 % above the normal level (Fig. 2).

D) <u>What happens to ascorbate as a component of the medium during the culture period of embryonic tissues?</u>

We found that, when limb buds differentiate in organ culture, considerable problems arise with respect to the maintenance of ascorbate - within the tissues as well as in the culture medium (NEUBERT et al, 1978). At a physiological pH ascorbate is extremely unstable.

In a culture medium ascorbate is oxidized within approximately 2 hours to about 50 %. Ascorbate is broken down and completely disappears from the culture medium within 24 hours (Fig. 4 a).

This effect can, to some extent, be prevented by increasing the ascorbate concentration in the medium (Fig. 4 b). But still, the rate of oxidation - organ culture requires aerobic conditions - is considerable and the ratio of reduced ascorbate to oxidized ascorbate is changed drastically in the medium within a few hours.

We also found that at the same time the ascorbate content in the limb buds kept in organ culture is reduced to about $^{1}/_{3}$ of the initial concentration within a few hours (NEUBERT et al., 1978). This reduced concentration seems to remain stable for a couple of days.

We tried a number of ways to stabilize ascorbate in the explants or to re-increase the concentration to that found under in vivo conditions. But so far, we have neither been successful in increasing the ascorbate concentration in the explants under the in vitro conditions nor in stabilizing ascorbate in the medium for a sufficiently long period.

Although it has been known for a long time that ascorbate, at a physiological pH and under aerobic conditions, is very unstable many investigators include ascorbate in a culture medium assuming that this compound will continue to be active over a prolonged incubation period. Owing to the experiences taken in our studies and all our attempts we are rather pessimistic at present that this goal can be achieved by simple means.

SUMMARY

1) Homogenates of embryonic mouse liver on day 11 of gestation and that of fetal livers are capable of converting enzymatically D-glucurono-γ-lactone into ascorbate. But the rate is only about $^{1}/_{10}$ of that found with homogenates of adult livers. Nevertheless, it seems feasible that rodent embryos can meet some of their needs for ascorbate by de-novo synthesis. We have not been able to detect the occurrence of synthesis in the limb buds.

2) The ascorbate concentration in whole embryos is low at early stages of development - for example day 10 of gestation - and significantly increases at later stages of development (day 12 of gestation). The ascorbate concentration in limb buds is lower than that of whole embryos, but the increase of concentration during development corresponds to that of whole embryos.

3) The ascorbate concentration in whole embryos or in limb buds can be increased to about 30 % above normal level by intravenous injections of extremely high doses of ascorbate into the mother animal.

4) The ascorbate concentration of limb buds drastically decreases during the initial stages of organ culture and it has not yet been possible to counterbalance this effect by supplementing the medium with ascorbate.

A possible rôle of ascorbate in abnormal skeletal development has not been considered so far. From our findings it seems likely that changes in ascorbate concentration occurring in embryonic tissues may influence normal or pathological development.

Acknowledgement

The studies presented in this paper were supported by grants given by Deutsche Forschungsgemeinschaft to Freie Universität Berlin (Sonderforschunsbereich 29).

We are indebted to Ruth Kreft for her help in preparing the manuscript and to Ursula Bluth for her technical assistance.

ng ascorbate formed x min^{-1} x µg DNA^{-1}

day of gestation	embryonic liver	limb bud
11	0.4	<0.2
12	0.7	<0.2

Table 1: Ascorbate formation by homogenates of mouse organ anlagen. With the method used, the limit of detection is 0.2 ng ascorbate formed × µg DNA^{-1} × min^{-1}. Ascorbate synthesis in limb buds is significantly lower than in the liver of the same embryo.

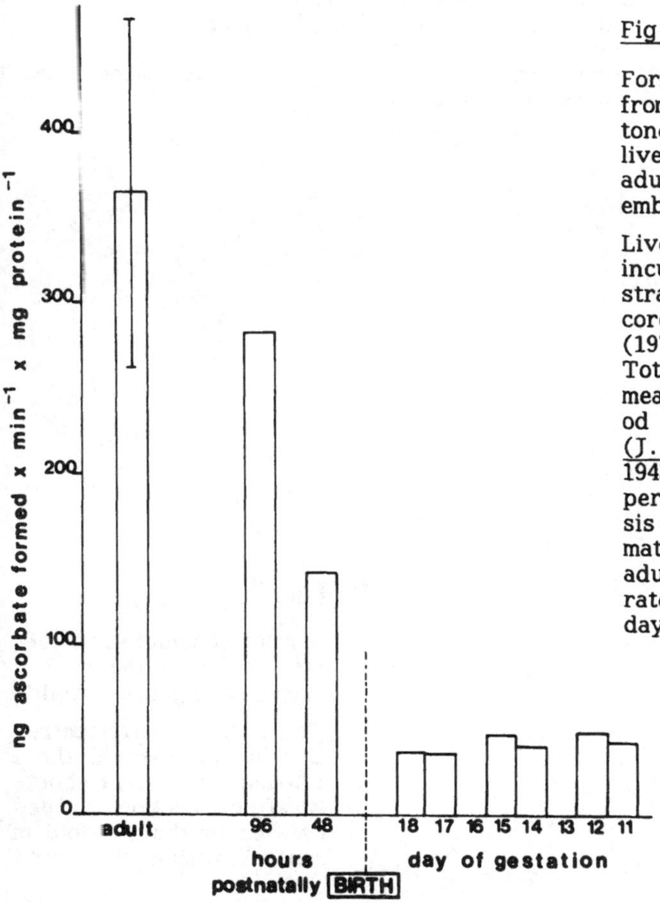

Fig. 1:

Formation of ascorbate from D-glucurono-γ-lactone-semicarbazone by liver homogenates from adult mice and mouse embryos.

Liver homogenates were incubated with the substrate for 1.5 hours according to CHATTERJEE (1970).
Total ascorbate was measured with the method of ROE and KUETHER (J. Biol. Chem. 147, 399, 1943). In the prenatal period ascorbate synthesis amounts to approximately $^{1}/_{10}$ of that in adult liver. The adult rate is reached within 4 days after birth.

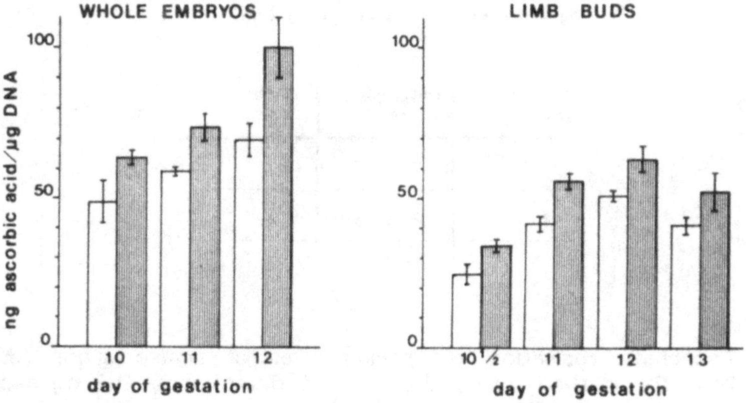

Fig. 2: Ascorbate content in embryonic tissues of mice:
□ - in whole embryos and in limb buds of untreated mice;
▥ - 3 hours after i.v. injection of 2 g ascorbate/kg mouse into the mother animal.
The ascorbate content in whole embryos and in limb buds is raised about 30 % above normal level 3 hours after injection.

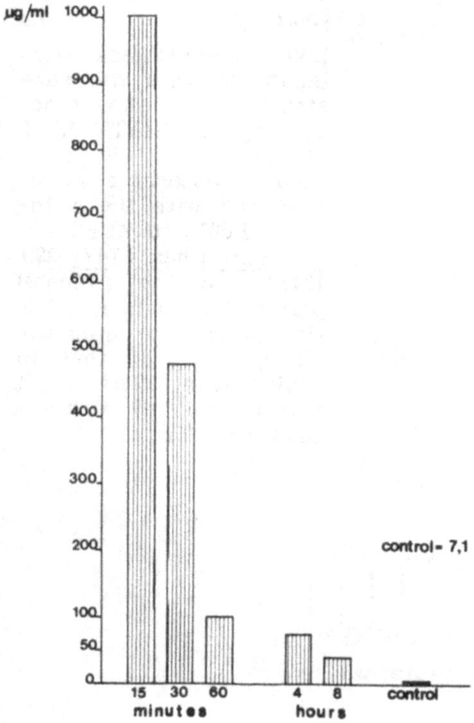

Fig. 3:

Serum concentration after i.v. injection of 2 g ascorbate/kg bodyweight.

The ascorbate concentration is increased to about 100-fold of control shortly after injection. It decreases to about 4-fold of control within 8 hours.

(a)

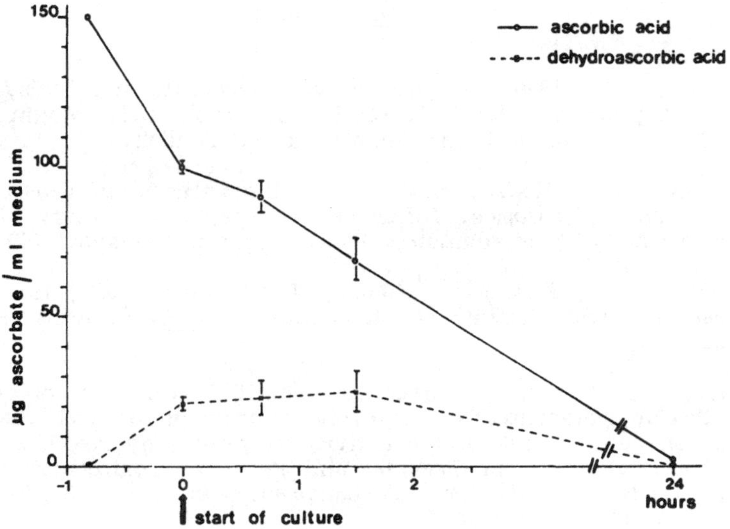

(b)

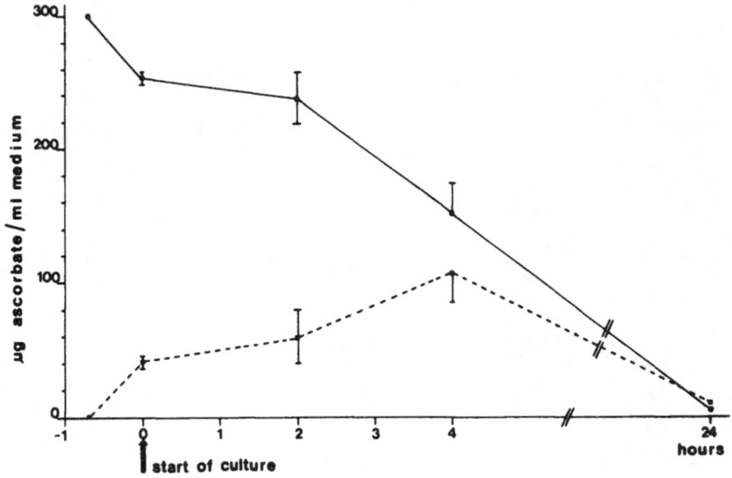

Fig. 4: Ascorbate concentration in culture medium.

Under the conditions of organ culture ascorbic acid is oxidized to about 50 % within a few hours and is decomposed after 24 hours.

The concentration can be raised to some extent by increasing the dose from 150 µg/ml (a) to 300 µg/ml medium (b).

REFERENCES

Chatterjee, I.B., 1970, Biosynthesis of L-ascorbate in animals, in: Methods in Enzymology Vol. XVIII (D.B. McCormick, L.D. Wright, eds.), pp. 28 - 34, Academic Press, New York and London.

Chatterjee, I.B., McKee, R.W., 1965, Biosynthesis of L-ascorbic acid in rat liver microsomes: Influences of age, sex, dietary changes, and whole-body X-irradiation, Arch. Biochem. Biophys. 109, 62 - 67.

Chatterjee, I.B., Kar, N.C., Ghosh, N.C., Guha, B.C., 1961, Aspects of ascorbic acid biosynthesis in animals, Ann. N.Y. Acad. Sci. 92, 36 - 56.

Neubert, D., Tapken, S., Baumann, I., 1978, Influence of potential thalidomide metabolites and hydrolysis products on limb development in organ culture and on the activity of proline hydroxylase, in: Role of Pharmacokinetics in Prenatal and Perinatal Toxicology (D. Neubert, H.-J. Merker, H. Nau, J. Langman, eds.), pp. 359 - 382, Georg Thieme Publ., Stuttgart.

II. Experimental Embryology and Teratology

A. Experimental Embryology

Abnormalities along the Proximo-Distal Axis of the Chick Wing Bud: The Effect of Surgical Intervention

Amata Hornbruch

Department of Biology as Applied to Medicine, The Middlesex Hospital Medical School, Cleveland Street, London W1P 6DB, U.K.

The chick wing bud grows out from the flank between somites 15 - 20, as a slight swelling from stage 17 (HAMBURGER and HAMBURGER, 1951). Outgrowth is rapid and within 48 hours cell differentiation has started at the proximal end. The early bud consists of mesenchyme enclosed by an ectodermal envelope with the characterisitic apical ectodermal ridge (AER) running along the antero-posterior edge. The AER is of great importance in normal development. Loss of the ridge or major parts of the ridge results in loss of distal structures. SAUNDERS (1948) removed the AER from successively older stages and found that the early stages were severely truncated while later stages suffered progressively smaller losses. The ridge in some way maintained the cells of the underlying mesenchyme at the tip. SUMMERBELL, LEWIS and WOLPERT (1973) have proposed the progress zone model in which they attribute to the AER the function of keeping the cells near the tip in a labile state in which their positional value changes autonomously. The cells that have already left the progress zone have their positional value fixed. Thus as the limb grows out, and cells leave the progress zone, the pattern is laid down in a proximo-distal sequence.

Does the chick limb bud regulate when parts are removed or added and if so to what extent? HAMPÉ (1959) and KIENY (1967, 1977) consider that regulation of the proximo-distal axis of the limb takes place when tissue is removed from the bud as well as when extra tissue is added. Conversely, SUMMERBELL and LEWIS (1975) find that the limb is largely of mosaic character along the proximo-distal axis. When they exchange distal tips between embryos of different stages they find deficiencies in one, and extra cartilagenous elements in the other of the pair. The progress zone model itself does not predict regulative or mosaic behaviour. However, it seems reasonable that the labile cells (in the progress zone) are more likely to regulate than those more proximal. Outside the progress zone there is a proximo-distal sequence of positional values. Removal of tissue leads to apposed surfaces with different positional values and the cells are no longer labile. One expects mosaic behaviour. Inside the progress zone it seems likely that cells all have the same positional value. Removal of tissue leads to apposed surfaces with the same positional value and the cells are labile. One expects regulative behaviour. If one of the apposed surfaces comes from inside the progress zone and the other one from outside the progress zone does one expect regulation? The stage of the limb bud and the size of the slice is important, the earlier the stage the better the restoration because the discrepancy of the positional value outside and inside the progress zone is small. The older the stage and the larger the slice removed, the less likely it is for the progress zone to be able to fill in the missing values.

In this paper I describe experiments which deal with removal of tissue from the proximo-distal axis only. I examine the regulation of the skeleton along this axis and the results are based on measurements of the total length of the axis and do not describe changes in the total volume of tissue. However there were no obvious effects on the other two axes.

Teratology of the Limbs

The experiment compares the percentage length of the proximo-distal axis of the bud left after the operation with the percentage length of the wing skeleton at day ten. The percentages are calculated in comparison to the unoperated (control) left bud or wing. (SUMMERBELL and WOLPERT, 1973).

The result is based on the total length (l) of the proximo-distal axis of the skeleton of the wing at ten days.

$$l_{wing} = l_{stylopod} + l_{zeugopod} + l_{autopod}$$

This is then expressed as the percentage (p) of its normal length by comparing it with the unoperated left control wing.

$$P\ observed = \frac{l\ operated}{l\ control}$$

I then compared this with the expected percentage length had the bud not regulated (see Fig. 1).

$$P\ expected = \frac{l\ stump + l\ tip}{l\ total\ bud}$$

(See LEWIS, 1975 and SUMMERBELL, 1977 for a discussion of the relationship between the length of the bud and the length of the wing skeleton).

The same method can be used to determine the level of any deficiencies and which of the elements is effected.

The series of experiments starts at stage 19 when the mesenchyme consists of a homogenous population of cells and follows through all stages up to and including stage 25 when the proximal parts of the limb have already differentiated.

A narrow strip of tissue, including the AER, and about 100 - 150 µm thick, was removed by cutting along the sub-apical sinus. A slice of the proximo-distal axis parallel to the first cut was then excised and dicarded; then, the tip was grafted back onto the stump. Measurements of the total length of the proximo-distal axis of the limb bud before and after the operation were recorded as well as the proximo-distal length of the discarded slice (Fig. 1). The experiment started with a sham control in which no tissue was discarded then continued with progressively larger slices discarded until the base of the limb was reached, and the grafted tip made contact with the flank. All operations were carried out on the chick's right wing bud while the left wing was left intact to serve as a size control. The embryos were sacrificed on the 10th day of incubation. Both wings were fixed, stained and prepared as whole mounts (SUMMERBELL and WOLPERT, 1973) and the skeletal elements measured and analysed.

601 operations were carried out. 145 embryos were dead on day 10 of incubation and could not be analysed. The most common cause of death was post operative haemorrhage particularly where large slices of limb bud were removed and major blood vessels disrupted. There was a dramatic fall in survival rate from stage 23 and older stages over the earlier stages. 26 operations were excluded from the analysis because of trivial problems such as, the tip had fallen off after the operation or a blood clot had formed between the tip and the stump and prevented a normal healing process to take place, or some injury occured to the skeleton of the wing during processing so that measurements could not be made accurately. Finally 430 embryos were examined and both wings measured.

In this short report I will consider only some stages. The missing stages can be assumed to occupy an intermediate position to those on which the extent of the defect is shown.

The maximum proportion of the bud that can be removed at stage 19 is 70%, the other 30% is the tip. This can still result in some cases in a morphologically normal looking wing with all the skeletal elements present as well as elbow joint and wrist being normal. However, the measurements reveal that the zeugopod is proportionately slightly short compared to the stylopod and autopod. On the whole the regulation is very good.

Removal of up to 40% of the bud for stage 21 results in a wing of approximately normal size. Larger deficiencies lead to severe reduction of the zeugopod and removal of 60 - 80% of the bud even reduces the humerus by up to 50% of its normal length. But at the level of the hand the morphology is normal and the size compatible with the control side, the wrist has the normal complement of carpals. Regulation is less good, (Fig. 2).

Stage 23 is difficult because the primary site of deletion is the wrist, which because it is so small the contribution is insignificant to the measurement of length of the wing. Removal of 40% and more of the bud leads to severe dificiencies of the forearm and the wrist, and digit 3 is also shorter, the humerus has normal size. Removing more than 60% bud will also reduce the humerus to 50% of its normal length and the elbow joint is almost always abnormal. In most cases ulna and radius are missing but when they are present they are often fused with the humerus displaying an inverted Y structure.

The autopod suffers the first loss in operations carried out on stage 25 embryos. After excision of only 300 µm of the proximo-distal axis of the bud, which is less than 15%, the metacarpals are proportionately considerably shorter than humerus, ulna and radius, which have normal size. 30 - 60% loss of bud still maintains a normal humerus while ulna and radius are reduced by 50% length. The wrist is missing and digit 3 is just under 40% of the normal length. The metacarpals show greater deficiencies than the phalanges. Taking away more than 60% results in even greater loss of digit 3 and in many cases it is difficult to identify each digit because they are so severly reduced. Ulna and radius have completely disappeared and only a short humerus is left (Fig. 3).

The purpose of the experiment was to see if regulation can be improved by making sure that the region of positional disparity was in or near the progress zone. The early stages of the chick limb bud do not appear to be greatly effected by the removal of large sections of the proximo-distal axis. The skeleton looks normal, the total length of the wing falls just short of the expected 95% obtained for the sham control grafts, and the proportions are normal for stylopod and autopod while zeugopod show small deficiencies which increase with older stages. However later stages, while showing the same regulative tendencies when the slice removed is small, show marked mosaic behaviour when the slice is large.

As the width of the tip is kept constant throughout, the single overriding factor cannot be the presence of the progress zone, unless the width of the progress zone narrows with age. The positional value of cells outside the progress zone at proximal levels of an early bud will still not be very different to those inside the progress zone. The disparity can be overcome by generating new intermediate values. The mechanism could involve short range interaction from cell to cell aided by the presence of the AER. It will need about one extra cell cycle time to substitute for half the ulna and radius, for example.

Later stages show much greater deficiencies caused perhaps by the greater positional disparity or by older cells being very non labile. Stage 23 is of particular interest. So far the hand (digit 3) and the wrist showed very small reductions but stage 23 (and older stages) has no wrist when 40% or more of the proximo-distal axis of the bud is removed. This is the first example that cells from the progress zone may be able to overcome a small disparity in positional value. But once the difference exceeds a certain value or time expressed in age of the cells nearest the cut surface they are unable to bridge the gap, no interaction occurs, and the progress zone is unable to generate new values and the wrist is lost. And stages 24 and 25 show no regulation except for a very narrow region proximal to the sub-apical sinus.

To conclude, when the deficiency lies a long way from the progress zone there is no regulation. When the deficiency is close to the progress zone but at a proximal level there is poor regulation, but when the deficiency lies close to the progress zone and is at a distal level there is a good regulation.

ACKNOWLEDGEMENTS

I wish to thank LEWIS WOLPERT and DENNIS SUMMERBELL for their criticism and advice and SARAH RENDLE for her help during the course of the work.

REFERENCES

Hamburger, V., Hamilton, H.L., 1951, A series of normal stages in the development of the chick embryo, J. Morph., 88, 49 - 92.

Hampé, A., 1959, Contribution a l'étude du développement et de la régulation des déficiences et des excédents dans la patte du l'embryon de poulet, Archs Anat. micros. Morph. exp., 48, 345 - 478.

Kieny, M., 1967, Phénomenes de régulation de l'ébauche de membre chez l'embryon de Poulet, Rev. Anat. Embryol. Cell Biol., 39, 1 - 37.

Kieny, M., 1977, Proximo-distal pattern formation in avian limb development, in: "Vertebrate limb and somite morphogenesis", (D.A. Ede, J.R. Hinchliffe, M. Balls, eds.), pp. 87 - 103, Cambridge Univ. Press, Cambridge.

Lewis, J.H., 1975, Fate maps and the pattern of cell division: a calculation for the chick wing-bud, J. Embryol. exp. Morph., 33, 419 - 434.

Saunders, J.W., Jr., 1948, The proximo-distal sequence of origin of the parts of the chick wing and the role of the ectoderm, J. exp. Zool., 108, 363 - 403.

Summerbell, D., 1977, Regulation of deficiencies along the proximal distal axis of the chick wing-bud: a quantitative analysis, J. Embryol. exp. Morph., 41, 137 - 159.

Summerbell, D., Lewis, J.H., 1975, Time, place and positional value in the chick limb bud, J. Embryol. exp. Morph., 33, 621 - 643.

Summerbell, D., Lewis, J.H., Wolpert, L., 1973, Positional information in chick limb morphogenesis, Nature, (Lond.), 244, 492 - 496.

Summerbell, D., Wolpert, L., 1973, Precision of development in chick wing morphogenesis, Nature, (Lond.), 244, 228 - 230.

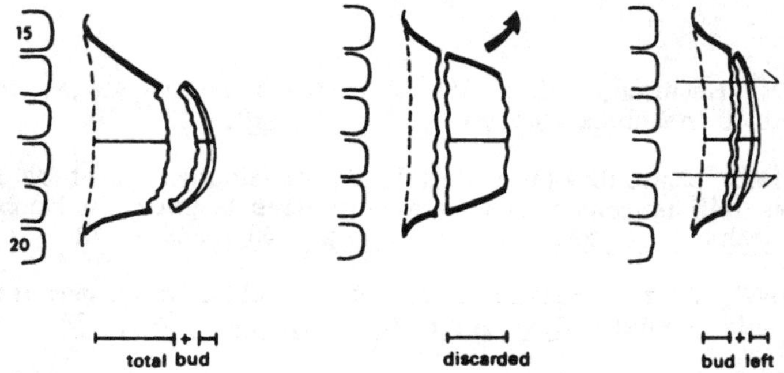

Fig. 1: Schematic drawing of the operation.

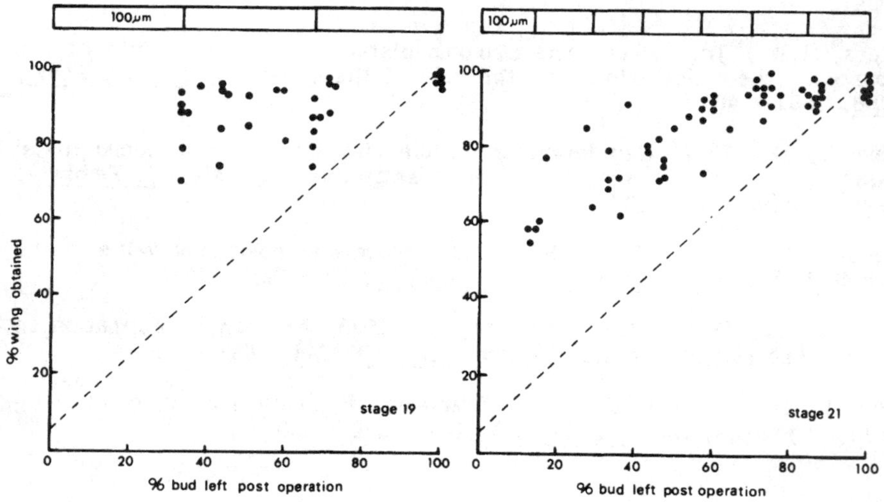

Fig. 2: Scatterplots for stages 19 and 21. The results are plotted comparing the percentage length of the bud left after the operation to the percentage length of the skeleton of the wing at ten days. The broken line is the slope assuming zero regulation (taken from SUMMERBELL, 1977). Above each scatterplot is a scale showing the approximate length of a bud for that stage.

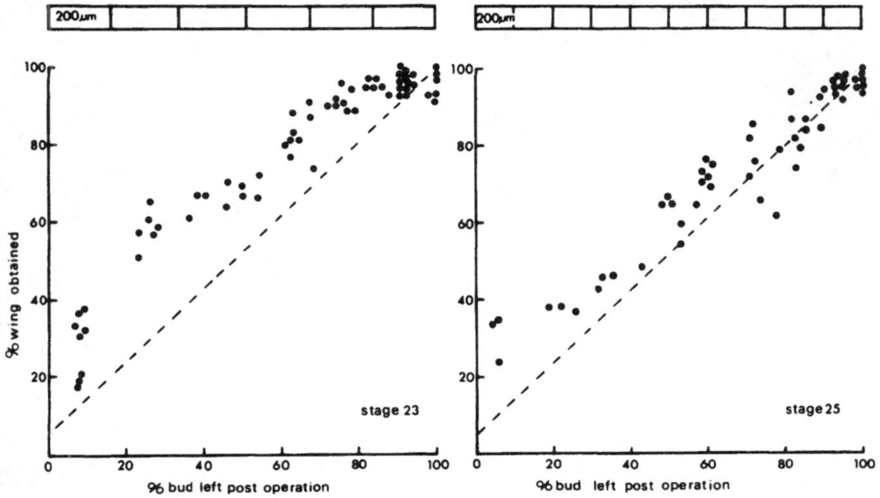

Fig. 3: Scatterplots for stages 23 and 25. The results are plotted comparing the percentage length of the bud left after the operation to the percentage length of the skeleton of the wing at ten days. The broken line is the slope assuming zero regulation (taken from SUMMERBELL, 1977). Above each scatterplot is a scale showing the approximate length of a bud for that stage.

The Effects of X-Irradiation on Limb Development

Dennis Summerbell

Medical Research Council, National Institute for Medical Research,
The Ridgeway, Mill Hill, London NW7 1AA, U.K.

INTRODUCTION:

"The future wing parts are laid down in proximo-distal order and in their definitive spatial pattern" (SAUNDERS, 1948). Here lies the basis of the 'Entwicklungsmechanik' of the limb. The accepted working model envisages a sequence of events, each propagating along the proximo-distal axis so that at successive times successively more distal regions will be passing through the same developmental phase. Thus steps such as specification, determination, chondrogenesis and innervation progress distally along the bud. It comes then as no surprise to discover that X-irradiation of the bud at successive times causes similar types of abnormality at progressively more distal levels (GOFF, 1962). In this paper I re-examine the suggestion of GOFF that it is possible to distinguish more than one such proximo-distal series of malformations, and discuss possible mechanisms.

Chick embryos were staged according to HAMBURGER and HAMILTON (1951), and infertile, dead or abnormal embryos discarded. The remainder were sealed with sellotape and whole eggs irradiated using a MARCONI high voltage X-ray machine at 230 KV with a dose rate of 2.5 $Gy\text{-}min^{-1}$ (1 Gy = 100 rads). The dosage varied from 8 to 20 Gy and the stage of the embryos from 12 to 30. The eggs were returned to the incubator and allowed to develop until day 10 to 12 when the wings of surviving embryos were fixed, stained in Alcian Green then cleared in methyl salicylate (SUMMERBELL and WOLPERT, 1973). Batches of control embryos were incubated with windowing but without X-irradiation.

The wings were examined under a ZEISS stereo IV microscope and the lengths of the humerus, ulna, radius and metacarpal and phalanges of digit 3 measured using a micrometer eyepiece (± 50 µm). In the control population the proportion of the total proximo-distal wing length occupied by each skeletal element is remarkably constant (SUMMERBELL, 1978). The wrist is the only exception. Between days 5 to 11 it is very small and grows hardly at all (SUMMERBELL, 1976), and it has been excluded from this analysis of proportions. The mean proportions are shown in Table 1 together with the standard deviation. Using this control to calculate the range of variations found in a normal population one can estimate accurately small deviations from normal proportions. This gives a sensitive assay for the effect of teratogens.

The irradiated embryos were similarly examined and initially divided into 3 categories: 'dead', those with a clear 'pattern defect' in the skeleton, those in which the skeleton appeared anatomically normal. The lengths of the skeletal elements of the latter group were then measured. Any limbs in which the relative proportions occupied by the skeletal elements differed by more than two standard deviation (95% probability level) from the mean control proportions (see Tab. 1) was categorised as 'malproportioned'. The remaining limbs were categorised as 'normal'. It should be understood that many 'normal' limbs may have been small (but well proportioned) or develop-

Teratology of the Limbs

mentally retarded. The percentage of limbs falling into each category ('dead', 'defective', 'malproportioned' and 'normal') for each dose level can be calculated from Fig. 1. The range of stages (12 - 30) has been subdivided for convenience into sub-groups of consecutive stages that gave similar results.

Pattern defects in the limb rudiment.

GOFF noted two main periods at which X-irradiation caused limb defects: the time of outgrowth of the limb bud, and an earlier period before there is any outward manifestation of the limb. X-irradiation of the limb rudiment (st. 12 - 15) results in a failure to form distal parts. Typically the limb has humerus, radius and digit 2. GOFF explained this as a reduction in the pool of cells available for limb outgrowth so that it became prematurely exhausted before all the distal parts had been formed. I would like to suggest an alternative explanation, that X-irradiation inhibits the normal relationship between the zone of polarising activity (ZPA) and the developing bud. There are three pieces of evidence favouring this idea.

1.) A very similar range of results is produced when a barrier is inserted separating the ZPA from the responding wing tissue (SUMMERBELL, 1979).

2.) When many ZPA cells are grafted to a responding field they produce a full supernumerary limb, as the number of cells is reduced the supernumerary parts formed are reduced in the same order as they are lost following X-irradiation (TICKLE, pers. com.).

3.) Increasing doses of irradiation progressively reduce the ability of a grafted ZPA to produce a supernumerary, again digits fail to form in the appropriate order (SMITH, TICKLE, and WOLPERT, 1978).

Against my suggestion is:

1. The doses that SMITH, TICKLE and WOLPERT used were an order of magnitude higher than those employed by GOFF and by me (but there were important differences in timing).

2. GOFF found a rather inappropriate order of loss of toes in the foot (but abnormal toes are very much more difficult to identify than digits).

Pattern defects in the limb bud.

GOFF described two types of anomaly between stages 18 to 30. 'Reduction', when a skeletal element was thin, distorted, short or missing, and 'fusion', when adjacent elements (antero-posterior or proximo-distal) were joined together. The sequences were best seen in the leg and his evidence was much poorer in the wing. There were no reduction periods for either humerus, ulna or radius, and fusion was widespread. The hand was complex with both reduction and fusion from st. 21 - 29. Despite the wing results the evidence was adequate for GOFF to suggest two successive waves of abnormality progressing down the limb bud. My evidence (see Tab. 2) supports GOFF'S hypothesis. There is a good sequence for fusion, but the sequence for reduction is again less complete with few examples at proximal levels and complicated results in the hand.

WOLPERT, TICKLE and SAMPFORD (1979) have also X-irradiated a range of stages. Their results are compatible with GOFF'S except that at st. 17/18 and 18/19 they obtain fused elbows at low doses (10 Gy). The st. 18/19 results could be a minor difference in staging but those at 17/18 are difficult to understand as GOFF and I both find this stage very resistant to irradiation.

Both GOFF and WOLPERT et al., comment on a peculiarity of elbow fusion. It consisted of a rounded bulge of cartilage projecting posteriorly from the joint. My material shows that its appearance depends on the way in which the three elements in the joint meet. When all 3 epiphyses are lost the shafts fuse to form a characteristic 'Y' shaped element. If the epiphyses of radius and ulna are lost the shafts fuse onto the shaft of the humerus so that the epiphysis of the latter projects posteriorly to form a 'K' shape. When the epiphyses of the humerus and one of the zeugopodal elements are lost the result is an 'L' shape. Examples of each type were found.

Analysis of proportions and growth control.

Variation from normal proportions provides a very sensitive assay for deficiencies. When there is a visible pattern defect the proportions are severely effected (see also WOLPERT et al.), but when the gross pattern appears normal there can still be small, though highly significant, deficiencies in size, (see Tab. 1). In fact while pattern malproportion can be of any magnitude, size malproportion is normally very slight, the limbs clustering close to normal proportions. If one includes size malproportion then there is a clear sequence of reduction deficiencies, (see Tab. 2). At stages 16 to 18 all surviving embryos had normal pattern and proportion but this was followed by a reduction sequence. This again supports GOFF'S idea of a separate proximo-distal sequence of reduction though the phases do not always clearly precede fusion.

One explanation for the disparity between pattern and size malproportion may be a mechanism for growth control, and I have argued elsewhere that such a mechanism must be involved in the control of development across the antero-posterior axis. Provided that all the positional values necessary to the pattern are present, the control acts via a negative feed back loop to maintain the pattern in its appropriate size and proportion. However, one feature of the model is that once disturbed it can never regain perfect size (in a manner analagous to ZENO'S paradox). Thus, assaying some time after irradiation, one would expect to find that all limbs that had complete patterns would have almost, but not quite, perfect proportions. If any of the pattern is lost, the part is obviously unable to regulate its size. An alternative explanation is that the major pattern defects were usually fusion of joints. If this involves destruction of the epiphysis then it seems likely that it could also involve destruction of the adjacent growth plate. This would have a major effect on the growth of the elements involved. When the joint is not affected then one assumes that the adjacent growth plate also survives. There may still be an adverse effect on cells that form the initial diaphysis but once both growth plates start to throw off cells the initial loss rapidly becomes trivial so that the deficiency at day 10 is very small.

The progress zone.

GOFF relied very heavily on differential sensitivity for his explanation of the effects of X-irradiation. Alternative explanations have been proposed by SUMMERBELL (1973) and WOLPERT et al. (1979). Both are based on the progress zone model and both assume that X-irradiation inactivates cells equally throughout the bud. Both models account for a proximo-distal sequence of defects and both make a number of predictions. In SUMMERBELL (1973), the major level specific defect is caused by a reduction in the active population of cells in the progress zone. More proximal cells are then recruited back into the progress zone until it is once more complete. This causes either a loss of positional values or a steepening of the gradient just proximal to the boundary of the progress zone, but distal parts should be of normal size and proportion. WOLPERT et al. (1979) use the same basic mechanism but instead of recruiting proximal cells into the progress zone they allow the surviving cells to gradually return the population to its normal size by cell division. Level specific defects are distal to the boundary of the progress zone and more distal elements are progressively closer to their normal size. Neither model predicts accurately the results obtained by either WOLPERT et al., or myself, but neither model is exclusive of the other and the data suggests that a more accurate fit would lie somewhere in between.

CONCLUSION:

I have tried to show how recent advances in our understanding of normal development can influence our thoughts about teratology. The progress zone model suggests that many teratogens can exert their effect by the same mechanism. Anything that kills cells is likely to cause the same general range of defects and variation will be due to factors such as the number of cells dying and the time course. The primary effect is just general 'nastiness'. You will have noticed that I have avoided throughout the use of specific nomenclature for defects. This is deliberate, the current system emphasises the defects's phenotype and ignores the fundamental mechanisms. I believe this system to be wrong and suggest that an inadequate language hinders our understanding, and the development of the subject.

Table 1: Proportions of skeletal elements.

	Humerus	Ulna	Digit 3 Meta-carpal	Phalanx Proxi-mal	Phalanx Distal
Mean proportion (%)	35.73	29.94	20.11	8.20	4.66
Standard deviation	.74	.64	.54	.42	.55
Mean length (± 50 µm)	4200	3550	2350	950	600
95% probability (±)	±200	±150	±150	±100	±100

Table 2: Stages at which different events effect each proximo-distal level.

	Size reduct.	GOFF'S reduct.	Joint fusion	GOFF'S fusion	AER[1] truncat.	Differ-[2] entiat.
Shoulder			19-22		18	
Humerus	19	22?			18-19	24
Elbow			19-24	19-24	18-19	
Ulna	21-23	22?			19-20	24
Proximal wrist			22-25	(↑)	(↑)	
Carpals	?	?		(24-27)	(21-24)	26
Distal wrist			24-26	(↓)	(↓)	
Metacarpal 3	25-26	?			25-26	27/28
Joint			25-28			
Prox. phal.3	27	(↑)		(↑)	27	29
Joint		(26-29)	27-29	(26-29)		
Dist.phal.3	28 - 29	(↓)		(↓)	28	30

1. Data taken from SUMMERBELL (1974).
2. Data taken from SUMMERBELL (1976).

REFERENCES

Goff, R.A., 1962, The relation of developmental status of limb formation to X-irradiation sensitivity in chick embryos, J. exp. Zool., 151, 177 - 200.

Hamburger, V., Hamilton, H.L., 1951, A series of normal stages in the development of the chick embryo, J. Morph., 88, 49 - 92.

Saunders, J.W., 1948, The proximo-distal sequence of origin of the parts of chick wing and the role of the ectoderm, J. exp. Zool., 108, 363 - 404.

Smith, J.C., Tickle, C., Wolpert, L., 1978, Attenuation of positional signalling in the chick limb by high doses of X-radiation, Nature, (London), 272, 612 - 613.

Summerbell, D., 1973, Growth and regulation in the development of the chick limb, PhD. Thesis, Univ. London, pp. 199 - 200.

Summerbell, D., 1974, A quantitative analysis of the effect of excision of the AER from the chick limb bud, J. Embryol. exp. Morph., 32, 651 - 660.

Summerbell., 1976, A descriptive study of the rate of elongation and differentiation of the skeleton of the developing chick wing, J. Embryol. exp. Morph., 35, 241 - 260.

Summerbell, D., 1978, Normal and experimental variations in proportions of skeleton of chick embryo wing, Nature, (London), 274, 472 - 473.

Summerbell, D., 1979, The zone of polarising activity: evidence for a role in normal chick limb morphogenesis, J. Embryol. exp. Morph., 50, 217 - 233.

Summerbell, D., Wolpert, L., 1973, Precision of development in chick limb morphogenesis, Nature, (London), 244, 228 - 229.

Wolpert, L., Tickle, C., Sampford, M., 1979, The effect of cell killing by X-irradiation on pattern formation in the chick limb, J. Embryol. exp. Morph., 50, 175 - 198.

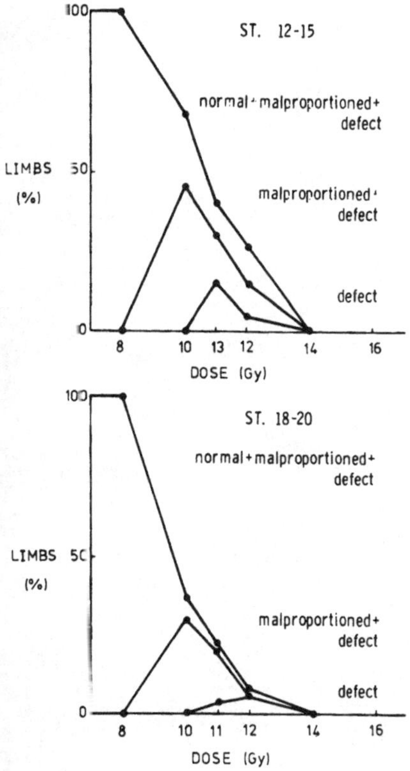

Fig. 1 a, b.

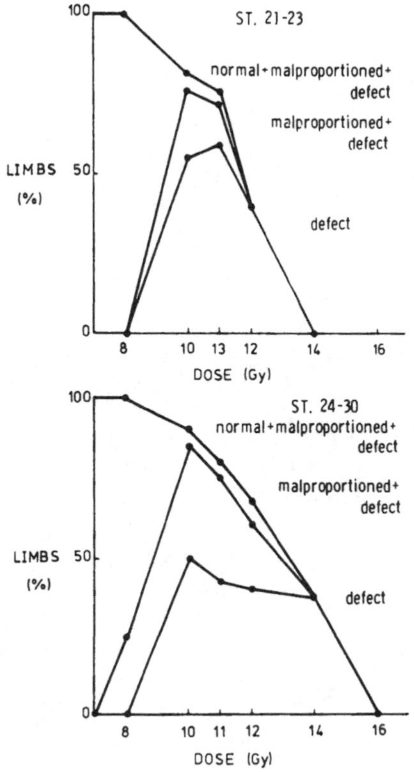

Fig. 1 c, d.

Response at day 10 of embryos at various stages to various doses of X-ray irradiation. See text for description of categories. Normal plus malproportioned plus defect is equal to all surviving limbs.

a.) Stages 12 - 15
b.) Stages 18 - 20
c.) Stages 21 - 23
d.) Stages 24 - 30

Stages 16 - 17 were all either dead or normal:
10 Gy = 46%, 11 Gy = 27% 12 Gy = 13%, 14 Gy = 0% (% survivors).

Effects of Matrix Influencing Substances on Chondrocyte in Monolayer Culture

Bernd Zimmermann

Institut für Toxikologie und Embryonal-Pharmakologie, Freie Universität Berlin,
Garystraße 9, D-1000 Berlin 33

INTRODUCTION:

The development of the limb skeleton of mammalian embryos can be divided into three phases: 1. migration of mesenchymal cells, 2. blastema formation with the development of special cell contacts, and 3. synthesis of cartilaginous intercellular substance.

In order to be able to investigate these different phases of skeletal development separately, we developed in vitro models for the first three developmental steps (MERKER et al., 1980; ZIMMERMANN, 1980). This paper is confined to the experimental investigations of the third step of limb skeletal development, i.e. to matrix sythesis.

MATERIALS and METHODS:

Chondrocytes were obtained from the long bones of fore and hind limbs of day 17 mouse embryos. Epiphyses were dissected from trypsin-cleaned bones and incubated with 0.2% collagenase for chondrocyte isolation. Washed chondrocytes were filtered through a gauze filter and resuspended in medium, which consisted of Ham F12 nutrient mixture supplemented with 15% fetal calf serum, 75 µg ascorbic acid/ml, 50 IU penicillin/ml and 50 µg streptomycin/ml. The initial cell density was adjusted to 1.5 x 10^6 cells/ml and cultivated as monolayers in 35 mm plastic Petri dishes. The culture period was 4 days. For the whole period, some cultures served as controls, others were treated with the following substances: a) chondroitin sulfate, b) hyaluronic acid, c) nitrophenyl-ß-D-xyloside, d) methylumbelliferyl-ß-D-xyloside, e) Arteparon, f) SP54, g) ß-aminopropionitrile, h) D-hydroxyproline and i) poly-L-lysine. After incubation, the cultures were rinsed in HBSS and subsequently fixed in 1% tannic acid plus 1% glutaraldehyde in 0.1 M phosphate buffer. Postfixation with 1% OsO_4 was followed by dehydration in acetone and embedding in Mikropal. Sections were prepared parallel to the direction of cell growth. Electron microscopy utilized a Siemens EM 101.

RESULTS:

In the untreated control cultures, 60 to 80 % of all cells can be considered as typical chondrocytes. They show a round or polygonal shape and are embedded in a metachromatically stained matrix (Fig. 1). Some of these cells are surrounded by a matrix capsule. Staining with FITC-antibodies against different collagen types reveals a reaction only with anti type II collagen (not shown here). Electron microscopically, too, chondrocytes and matrix show the typical and well known morphology (Figs. 2 and 3).

After application of the different substances, characteristic changes in chondrocyte morphology as well as in matrix formation occur. The main results are summarized in Table 1. Treatment with the naturally occurring glycosaminoglycans (GAG's) chondroitin sulfate and hyaluronic acid led to contrary results. After chondroitin sulfate, the amount of matrix increased. Changes in cell morphology or collagen structure were not observed (Figs. 4 and 5). However, hyaluronic acid caused a drastic reduction in the amount of matrix. The thickness of collagen fibrils rose to 40 - 50 nm as compared with the normal thickness of 15 - 25 nm (Figs. 6 and 7).

After treatment with highly sulfated GAG's like Arteparon and SP54, chondrocytes contain vacuoles and enlarged rough endoplasmic reticulum. The matrix has changed strikingly. Dense agglomerations are located around the cells. These agglomerations are collagen complexes of 300 to 500 nm thickness with a typical cross-striation pattern, which is characteristic of segment-long-spacing (SLS) collagen. No typical proteoglycan granules are detectable (Figs. 8 and 9).

Xylosides cause a decrease in the amount of both collagen and proteoglycans. After 0.3 mM, the cells themselves are not yet damaged. In the matrix besides normally thickened filaments, fibrils of 50 to 100 nm thickness occur, which show a distinct cross-striation pattern (Figs. 10 and 11). 1 mM xyloside led to the occurrence of necrotic chondrocytes.

1 mM ß-amonipropionitrile or 1 mg/ml D-hydroxyproline cause similar results. Treatment leads to a decrease in matrix, i.e. both PG's and collagen are reduced and a few necrotic cells occur. Collagen exhibit a very irregular thickness and structure. It seems loosely packed and frayed, only some thicker filaments show indications of cross-striation. The thickness of the filaments varies from 5 nm to 40 nm (Figs. 12 and 13).

Treatment with 0.1 mg/ml of the positively charged polymer poly-L-lysine causes overall necroses of chondrocytes. Interestingly, the fibroblast-like cells remain unchanged (Fig. 14). However, 0.01 mg/ml of the polymer induces hardly any cell lesions, but electron-dense inclusions are seen and the amount of matrix is slightly reduced. Collagen has hardly changed, but a few fibrils of up to 40 nm thickness are detectable. In the matrix large granules are observed, which most likely represent PG precipitations by the polymer (Figs. 15 and 16).

DISCUSSION:

Most of the results shown here are in aggreement with those of other authors, which have, however, been established on different experimental conditions. The effect of chondroitin sulfate to increase the amount of matrix in chondrocyte cultures is considered as a positive feed-back effect between matrix chondroitin sulfate and chondrocytes (NEVO and DORFMAN, 1972; HUANG, 1974; SCHWARTZ and DORFMAN, 1975). The inhibiting action of hyaluronic acid is described by TOOLE and co-workers (TOOLE et al., 1972) and confirmed by others (WIEBKIN and MUIR, 1973; HANDLEY and LOWTHER, 1976). ß-D-xylosides, on the other hand, have mostly been investigated with regard to their effect on GAG synthesis, i.e. on the incorporation of $^{35}SO_4$. In all cases a stimulation of GAG synthesis could be determined besides a dissociation of PG's into single GAG chains and single core proteins (GALLIGANI et al., 1975; HJELLE and GIBSON, 1979). Our findings of a decrease in the amount of PG granules in the matrix is not a contradiction, because in the electron microscope only PG granules are visible and single GAG's are possibly dissolved in the course of fixation and rinsing. In addition, a disturbance of fibrillogenesis is described here (see also HJELLE and GIBSON, 1979). The formation of SLS-collagen after application of highly sulfated GAG's indicate the importance of a certain grade in sulfatation of GAG's for normal fibrillogenesis. In cultures of limb buds these SLS-collagen formations have been described by MERKER et al. (1978). The lathyrogenic substance ß-APN and the unnatural D-form of hydroxyproline yield comparable results. While an increase in the amounts of soluble collagen after application of ß-APN has been reported by ALEO (1969), structural alterations of collagen fibrills as well as a distinct decrease in the amount of matrix PG granules are shown here.

All results indicate a strong interaction between all compartments of the matrix. In fact, it could be assumed from experiments with α,α'-dipyridyl and DON (BHATNAGAR and PROCKOP, 1966; LINSENMAYER and KOCHHAR, 1979) that the synthesis of PG's and collagen are independent, however, HANDLEY et al. (1978) showed, by application of PG extracts a concomitant decrease of collagen and PG synthesis. A strong interaction between matrix and chondrocytes is postulated by many authors (MEIER and HAY, 1974; SOLURSH and KARP, 1975; HOLTZER, 1977) as well as a feed-back regulation of matrix synthesis (HANDLEY, 1978). Our results show that in all cases a disturbance in fibrillogenesis occurs by substances which alter PG formation. On the other hand, a disturbance in collagen synthesis leads to a decrease in the amount of matrix PG's. Hence, cartilage is to be understood as a system of at least three compartments, i.e. chondrocytes, PG's and collagen, which are connected by a strong interaction. Alteration of each of these components results in alteration of the other. Experiments with the positively charged polymer poly-L-lysine show the dependency of the chondrocytes on an intact matrix. Poly-L-lysine leads to an agglutination of the negatively charged PG's, perhaps in concurrence with collagen. PG precipitation by the polymer leads to cell death, but this is a very specific effect on chondrocytes, because fibroblast-like cells remain completely unchanged. It is therfore to be expected that matrix alterations may also affect chondrocytes.

ACKNOWLEDGEMENTS

This work was supported by grants of the Deutsche Forschungsgemeinschaft awared to Sonderforschungsbereich 29 "Embryonale Entwicklung und Differenzierung - Embryonalpharmakologie".

I wish to thank Mrs. HEIDI SOMOGY for her excellent assistance in culture techniques and for doing the electron microscopic preparations.

Fig. 1: Light microscopical picture of a 4 day monolayer culture of day 17 epiphyseal chondrocytes after Giemsa staining. About 70% of all cells can be considered as chondrocytes. They show a round or polygonal shape and are embedded in a metachromatically stained matrix. Some of them are enclosed in a matrix capsule. x 300.

Fig. 2: Electron microscopical picture of a chondrocyte in a 4 day monolayer culture of day 17 mouse embryo epiphyses (untreated control). The cell shows the typical morphology with a nucleus (n), well developed rough endoplasmic reticulum (er) and some mitochondria. The chondrocyte is embedded in a filamentous network of the matrix (m).
x 6 400.

Fig. 3: High power magnification of the matrix of an untreated chondrocyte culture after 4 days shows collagen fibrils of a thickness of 15 - 25 nm, some of them with cross-striation pattern (arrow heads) and proteoglycan (PG) granules. Most of the PG granules are attached to the fibrils (arrows).
x 64 000.

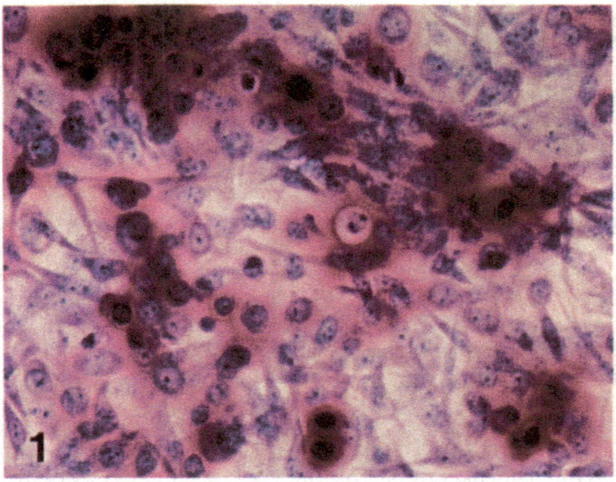
1

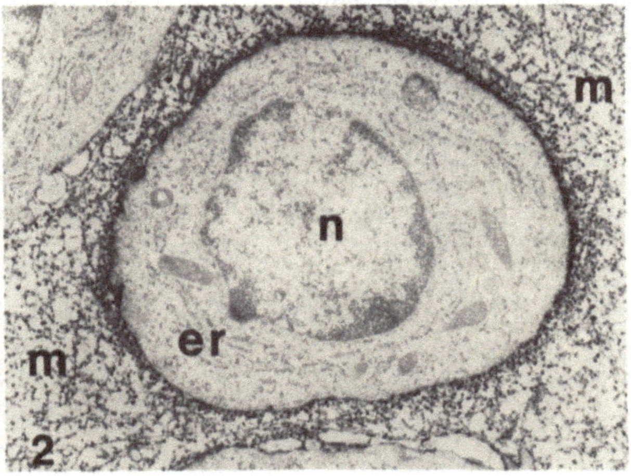
m
n
er
m
2

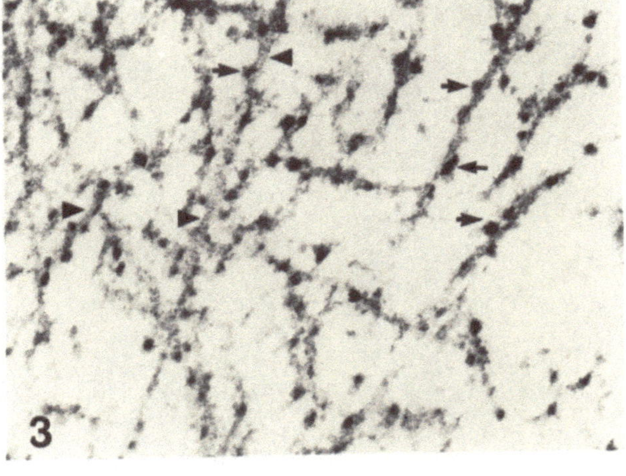
3

Fig. 4: Electron microscopical picture of a chondrocyte of a 4 day culture after treatment with 0.3 mg chondroitin sulfate/ml. The chondrocytes appear in normal morphology with large areas of rough endoplasmic reticulum (er) and some glycogen deposits (g). Large amounts of matrix (m) are recognizable.
x 3 800.

Fig. 5: High power magnification of the matrix of a chondroitin sulfate treated culture shows the normal collagen fibrils of 15 - 25 nm thickness, some of them with cross-striation pattern (arrow heads). The amount of PG granules (arrows) in the matrix is clearly increased, some of them are attached to collagen fibrils. However, some of the granules may represent chondroitin sulfate.
x 64 000.

Fig. 6: Electron microscopical picture of a chondrocyte of a 4 day culture after treatment with 0.3 mg hyaluronic acid/ml. The chondrocyte shows an irregular surface and some vacuoles (v). The rough endoplasmic reticulum (er) seems well developed. n = nucleus. The amount of matrix, however, is drastically reduced.
x 6 400.

Fig. 7: High power magnification of the matrix of a hyaluronic acid treated culture shows besides some normal collagen fibrils with cross-striation pattern (arrow head) also thicker fibrils of up to 40 nm thickness (large arrow). Some PG granules are attached to the collagen fibrils (small arrows).
x 64 000.

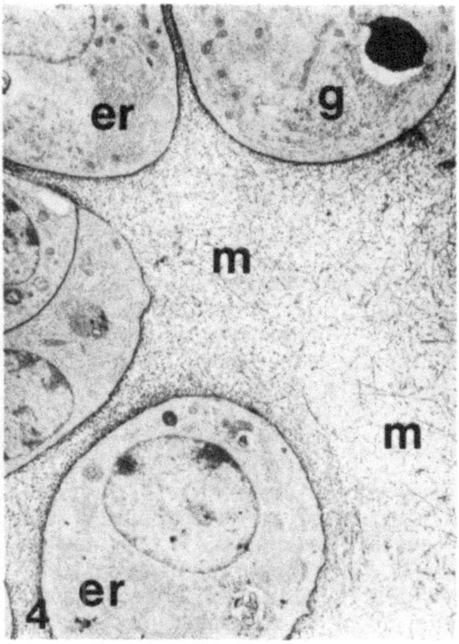
er
g
m
m
er
4

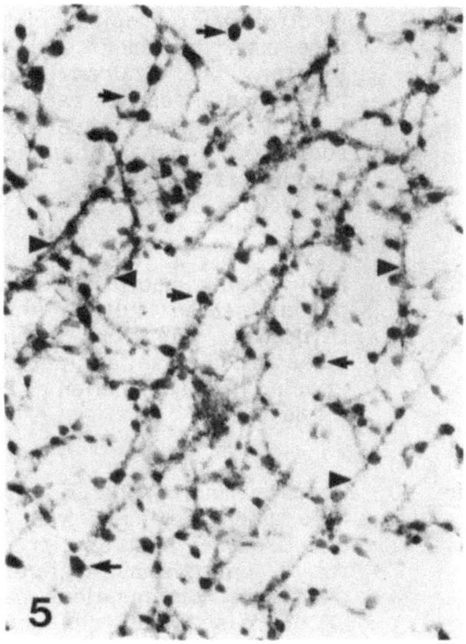
5

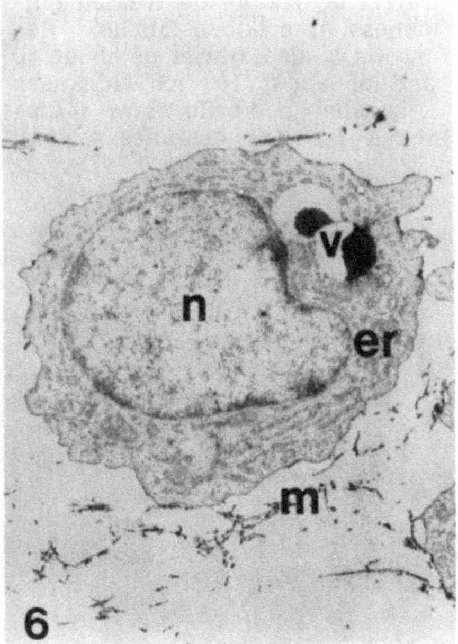
v
n
er
m
6

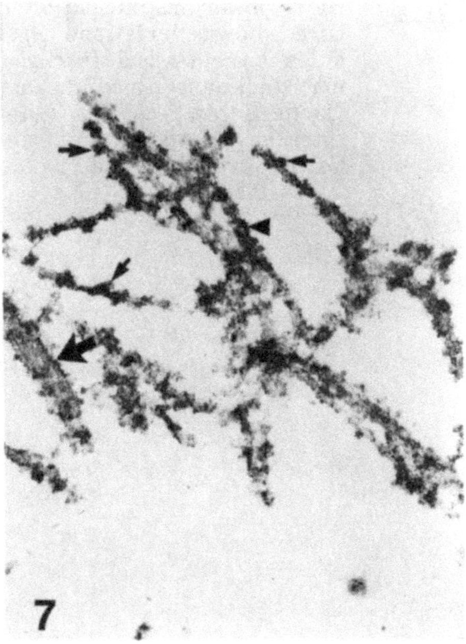
7

Fig. 8: Electron microscopical picture of a chondrocyte of a 4 day culture after treatment with 0.1 mg of the highly sulfated GAG Arteparon. The condrocyte looks quite normal with a well developed rough endoplasmic reticulum (er) and a normal nucleus (n). Some vacuoles (v) are located in the cytoplasm. The matrix around the cell has changed drastically and shows large agglomerations (arrows).
x 6 400.

Fig. 9: High power magnification of a matrix agglomeration of an Arteparon treated culture shows a collagen fibril of about 300 nm thickness. The fibril is characterized by the occurrence of a typical cross-striation pattern as is the case in Segment-Long-Spacing (SLS) collagen. PG granules are absent.
x 64 000.

Fig. 10: Electron microscopical picture of a chondrocyte of a 4 day culture after treatment with 0.3 mM ß-D-nitrophenyl-xyloside. The chondrocyte has an irregular surface and some cisternae of rough endoplasmic reticulum (er). In the nucleus (n) some chromatin condensations can be detected. The amount of matrix is decreased and collagen fibrils seem to be more prominent.
x 6 400.

Fig. 11: High power magnification of the matrix of a xyloside treated culture shows variations in the thickness of collagen fibrils. Besides some normal fibrils (small arrows), also fibrils of about 50 nm thickness (medium arrows) and of about 100 nm thickness (large arrow) can be detected. All collagen fibrils show a distinct cross-striation pattern. Only a few PG granules (arrow heads) are observed.
x 64 000.

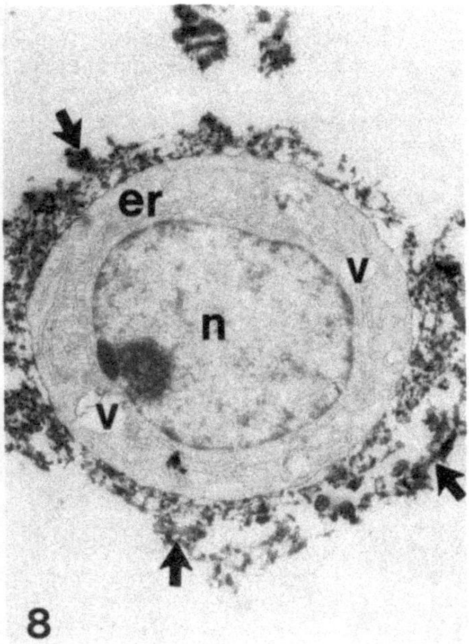
er
v
n
v
8

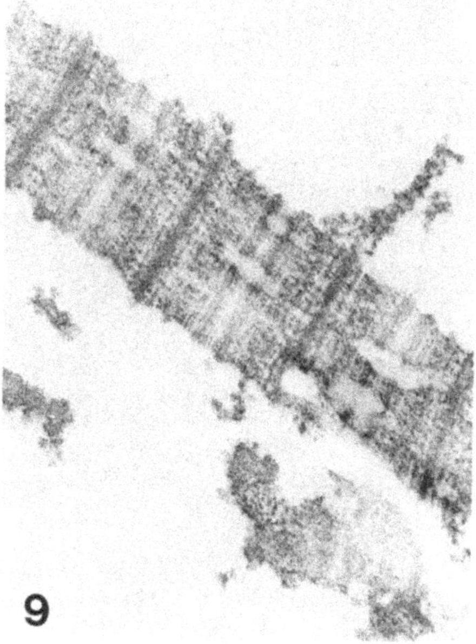
9

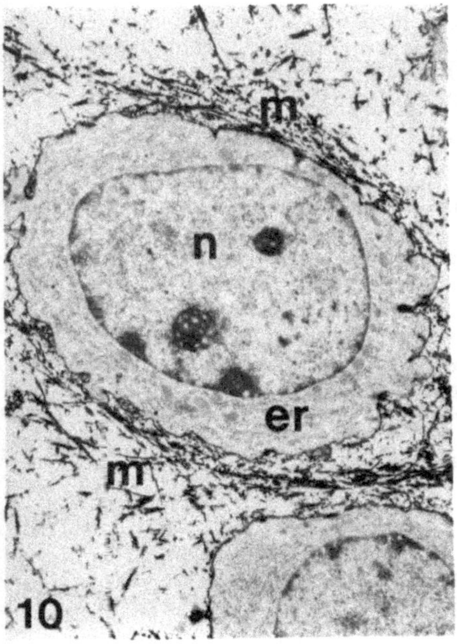
m
n
er
m
10

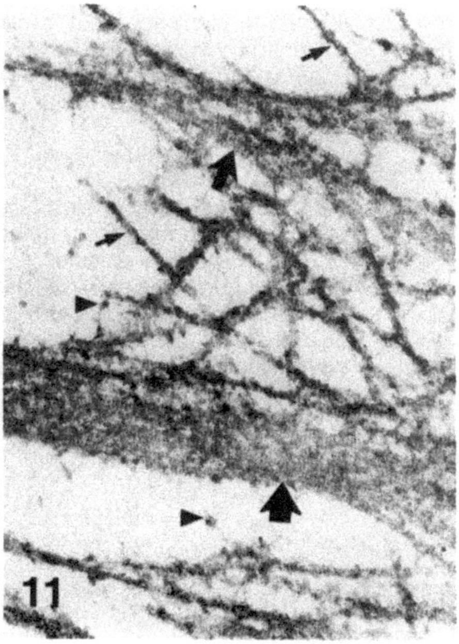
11

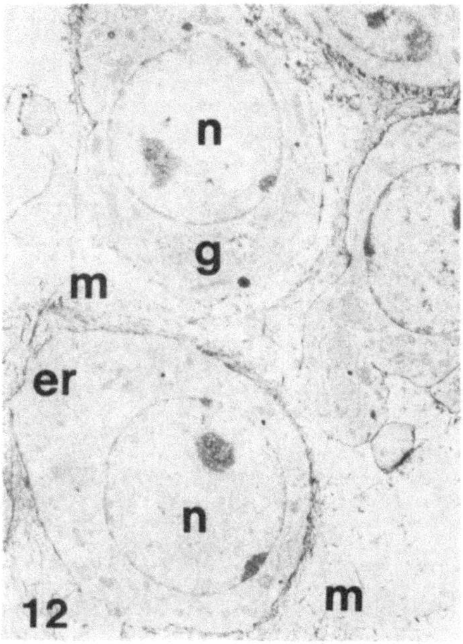

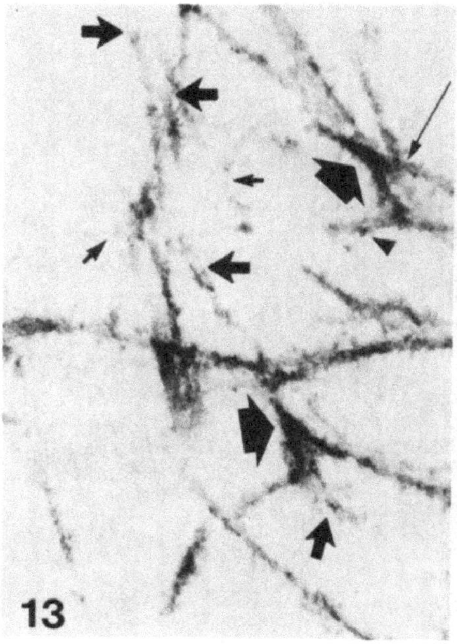

Fig. 12: Electron microscopical picture of chondrocytes of a 4 day culture after treatment with 1 mM ß-aminopropionitrile. The cells show some rough endoplasmic reticulum (er) and glycogen (g). The amount of matrix is clearly reduced (m).
x 3 800.

Fig. 13: High power magnification of the matrix of a ß-aminopropionitrile treated chondrocyte culture. Besides some normal collagen fibrils with cross-striation pattern (long arrow) large variation in fibril thickness can be detected. Thin filaments of about 5 nm thickness (small arrows) are seen as well as much thicker fibrils of up to 40 nm (large arrows). Very often frayed collagen fibrils resembling bunches (medium arrows) are observed. Only very few PG granules are present (arrow head).
x 64 000.

Table 1: Influence of different types of substances on matrix production in chondrocyte monolayer cultures.

Substance	Dose	Matrix changes PG	Matrix changes collagen	Filament thickness* (nm)
Chondroitin sulfate	0.3 mg/ml	↑↑	↑	15 - 25
Hyaluronic acid	0.3 mg/ml	↓↓	↓↓	40 - 50
Xylosides	0.3 mM	↓↓	↓	50 - 100
Highly sulfated GAG's	0.1 mg/ml	↓	↓	300 - 500 (SLS)
ß-Aminopropionitrile	1.0 mM	↓	↓	10 - 40 (frayed)
D-Hydroxyproline	1.0 mg/ml	↓	↓	10 - 40 (frayed)
poly L-lysine	0.01 mg/ml	aggl.	=	15 - 40

* Filament thickness in control cultures: 15 - 25 nm
Changes against controls: ↑ increased; ↑↑ highly increased
↓ decreased; ↓↓ highly decreased
= no change.

Fig. 14: Electron microscopical picture of a 4 day chondrocyte culture after treatment with 0.1 mg poly-L-lysine/ml. All chondrocytes are necrotic (x). However, fibroblast-like cells seem completely unaltered (flc).
x 3 800.

Fig. 15: Electron microscopical picture of a 4 day chondrocyte culture after treatment with 0.01 mg poly-L-lysine/ml. Besides normal appearing chondrocytes (er = rough endoplasmic reticulum), some cells seem to have withdrawn from the surrounding matrix (m). They have an irregular surface and show dark inclusions (arrow) in the cytoplasm. At this magnification, the matrix seems unchanged.
x 6 400.

Fig. 16: High power magnification of the matrix of a 4 day culture after treatment with 0.01 mg poly-L-lysine/ml. Besides normal collagen fibrils with cross-striation pattern (small arrows), fibrils of up to 50 nm thickness are detected (large arrows). No normal sized PG granules are seen. However, large granules (arrow heads) are detectable which may represent PG precipitation by the polymer.
x 64 000.

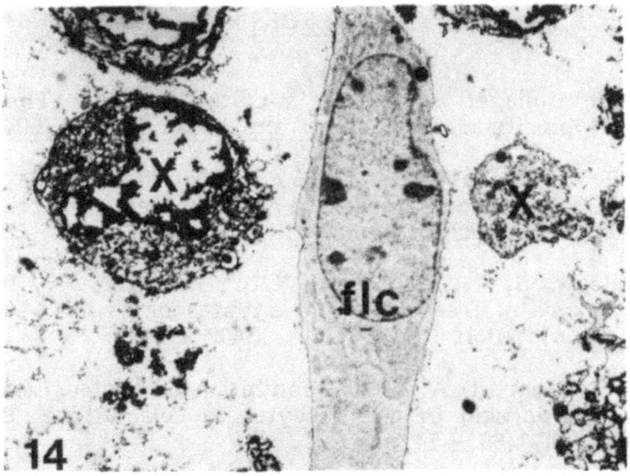
X
X
flc
14

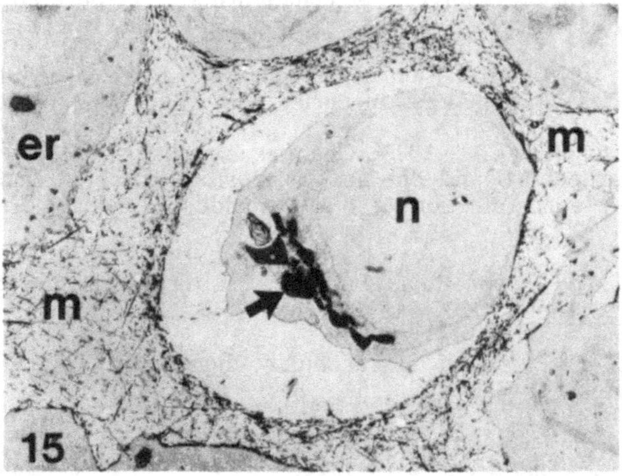
er
m
n
m
15

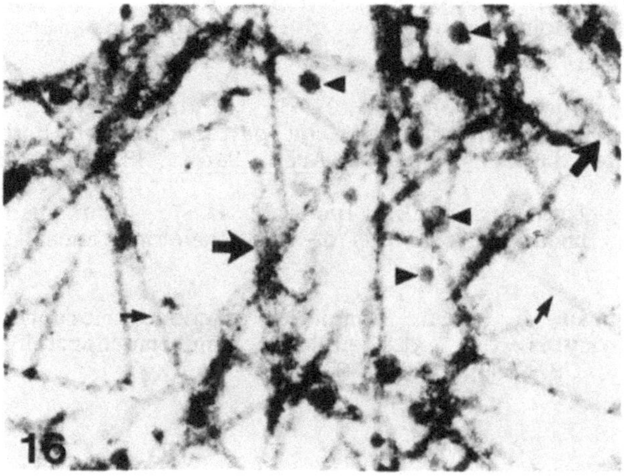
16

REFERENCES

Aleo, J.J., 1969, Collagen synthesis in cultured cells: The influence of beta-aminopropionitrile, Proc. Soc. exp. Biol. Med., 130, 451 - 545.

Bhatnagar, R.S., Prockop, D.J., 1966, Dissoziation of the synthesis of sulphated mucopolysaccharides and its synthesis of collagen in embryonic cartilage, Biochem. Biophys. Acta, 130, 383 - 392.

Galligani, L., Hopwood, J., Schwartz, N.B., Dorfman, A., 1975, Stimulation of synthesis of free cohdroitin sulfate chains by ß-D-xylosides in cultured cells, J. Biol. Chem., 250, 5400 - 5406.

Handley, C.J., Lowther, D.A., 1976, Inhibition of proteoglycan biosynthesis by hyaluronic acid in chondrocytes in cell culture, Biochem. Biophys. Acta, 444, 69 - 74.

Handley, C.J., Brooks, P.R., Lowther, D.A., 1978, Extra-cellular matrix metabolism by chondrocytes. VI. Concomitant depression by exogenous levels of proteoglycan of collagen and proteoglycan synthesis by chondrocytes, Biochem. Biophys. Acta, 544, 441 - 444.

Handley, C.J., 1978, Regulation of biosynthesis of extra-cellular matrix by chondrocytes, Proc. Aust. Biochem. Soc., 11, 40 (abstract).

Hjelle, J.T., Gibson, K.D., 1979, Changes in collagen ultrastructure, macroscopic properties and chemical composition of chick embryo cartilage induced by administration of ß-D-xyloside, J. Embryol. exp. Morph., 53, 179 - 190.

Holtzer, H., 1977, Extracellular matrix-cell interactions and chondrogenesis, Clin. Orthop., 123, 169.

Huang, D., 1974, Effect of extracellular chondroitin sulfate on cultured chondrocytes, J. Cell Biol., 62, 881 - 886.

Linsenmayer, T.F., Kochhar, D.M., 1979, In vitro cartilage formation: Effects of 6-diazo-5-oxo-L-norleucine (DON) on glycosaminoglycan and collagen synthesis, Develop. Biol., 69, 517 - 528.

Meier, S., Hay, E.D., 1974, Stimulation of extracellular matrix synthesis in the developing cornea by glycosaminoglycans, Proc. Nat. Acad. Sci., USA, 71, 2310 - 2313.

Merker, H.-J., Lilja, S., Barrach, H.-J., Günter, T., 1978, Formation of an atypical collagen and cartilage pattern in limb bud cultures by highly sulfated GAG, Virchow's Arch. Path., 380, 11 - 30.

Merker, H.-J., Zimmermann, B., Barrach, H.-J., Grundmann, K., Ebel, H., 1980, Simulation of steps of limb skeleton genesis in vitro, this book.

Nevo, Z., Dorfman, A., 1972, Stimulation of chondromucoprotein synthesis in chondrocytes by extracellular chondromucoprotein, Proc. Nat. Acad. Sci., USA, 69, 2069 - 2072.

Schwartz, N.B., Dorfman, A., 1975, Stimulation of chondroitin sulfate proteoglycan production by chondrocytes in monolayer, Connect. Tiss. Res., 3, 11 - 122.

Solursh, M., Karp, G.C., 1975, An effect of accumulated matrix on sulfation among cells in a cartilage colony: A autoradiographic study, J. Exp. Zool., 191, 73 - 84.

Toole, B.P., Jackson, G., Gross, J., 1972, Hyaluronate in morphogenesis: Inhibition of chondrogenesis in vitro, Proc. Nat. Acad. Sci., USA, 69, 1384 - 1386.

Wiebkin, O.W., Muir, H., 1973, The inhibition of sulphate incorporation in isolated adult chondrocytes by hyaluronic acid, FEBS Letters, 37, 42 - 46.

Zimmermann, B., 1980, Effects on surface coat influencing substances on the limb bud blastema in vitro, this book.

The Influence of Nerve Supply in Limb Development

W. G. McBride, P. A. Stokes, P. H. Vardy
Foundation 41, The Women's Hospital
Crown Street, Sydney 2010, Australia

The factors controlling limb development are still subject to speculation. From his transplant experiments HAMBURGER (1939) concluded that morphogenesis is independent of innervation, and that atypical or completely abnormal morphogenetic development in a large percentage of transplants cannot be attributed to deficient nerve supply. SAUNDERS (1948) showed the importance of the apical ectodermal ridge in the proximodistal sequence of origin or parts of the chick wing. WOLPERT (1971) has emphasised the zone of polarising activity although this concept has recently been criticised by SAUNDERS (1977).

KIENY and FOUVET (1974) found that excision of a portion of the spinal chord in 2-day chick embryos, although made rostral to the prospective leg level, produces a high frequency of proximal hemimelia and a lower proportion of post-axial amelia, and concluded that the question of the influence of the nervous system in limb development is open for further investigation. Excision of part of the brachial section of the neural tube at stages 13 - 15 of development was found to produce deformity of the wing (CIHÁK et al., 1978). Similarly ipsilateral leg deformities were produced by excision of portion of the lumbar neural tube at stages 13 - 16 (McBRIDE, 1979). SINGER (1974) has shown the importance of nerve supply in the regeneration of the forelimb of the adult triturus although YNTEMA (1959) was able to obtain the growth of the limb in aneurogenic amphibia.

As operative interference with the nerve supply to the developing limb results in limb deformities. A study was made of the effects of interference with the function of muscarinic receptors of the cholinergic nerves in the developing chick embryo using the anticholinergics. The drugs used were atropine sulphate 300 µg and 600 µg, hyoscine hydrobromide 200 mg and 400 mg and isotonic saline 400 µl. The eggs used were from a flock of White Leghorns (Inghams Poultry Farms). A total of 500 eggs were incubated at 38 ± 0.1°C and 70 - 80% RH in Qualtex Commercial Incubator. The atropine sulphate and hyoscine hydrobromide were prepared so that 1h of sterile isotonic saline contained 1 g of test drug. In each group 100 eggs were injected with the test drug, atropine sulphate 300 µg, atropine sulphate 600 µg, hyoscine hydrobromide 200 µg and 400 µg, control 400 µl isotonic saline using 1 ml tuberculin syringe after 96 h incubation. The injection sites were sealed with wax. The eggs were opened on the 12th day of incubation. The results of the experiment are summarized in Table 1. It was found that both atropine and hyoscine will produce gastroschisis (Fig. 1) exencephaly (Fig. 2) and reduction deformities of the limbs (Fig. 3). ZACKS (1954) demonstrated the presence of cholinesterase in the embryonic chick from 0 - 96 hour stages. NACHMANSOHN (1939) determined cholinesterase activity in chick nerve and muscle at 6 or 9 days of age. He followed the increasing levels of activity in this enzyme to about the 15th day and showed a higher rate of increase until hatching. It has been found that the cholinesterase inhibitor physostigmine will produce skeletal and limb deformities (BUEKER and PLATNER, 1956). Also the cholinomimetic drugs will produce a consistent syndrome of development defects brevi-

Teratology of the Limbs

collis and muscular hypoplasia of the legs (LANDAUER, 1977). It is thought that in the case of the latter drugs their effects are produced in the first instance by the inactivation of acetylcholinesterase. It can be concluded that interference with the function of the cholinergic nerves will produce deformities in the chick embryo.

As a result of studies of the reduction in number of the neurons in the dorsal root ganglia in rabbit fetuses exposed to thalidomide in utero (McBRIDE, 1974) and the degenerative changes found in the neurons and axons of dorsal root ganglia in day-13 experimental embryos (McBRIDE, 1976), i.e. at least 16 h before the earliest signs of thalidomide dysmelia have been reported in rabbits (VICKERS, 1967) it was claimed that it was the damage to the embryonic neurons that resulted in the peripheral deformities.

In order to study thalidomide distribution within embryonic tissues to determine whether the drug or its metabolites are concentrated at particular sites in the developing embryo. ^{3}H-thalidomide (specific activity 300 µCi-/mg) was prepared by heterogenous platinum-catalysed exchange with ^3H_2O and analysed by thin layer chromatography (radiochemical purity >96%). The radioactive material was added to unlabelled thalidomide prior to suspension in an aqueous solution of 0.5% carboxymethylcellulose and 5% glucose, and was administered by gavage to pregnant New Zealand White Rabbits (3 - 4 kg body weight) at ten days (240 hours) gestation. Blood samples were taken at intervals following treatment and serum was obtained following clot retraction and centrifugation at 1500 r.p.m. for five minutes. The radioactivity present was measured by liquid scintillation counting and the results are shown in the figure. The does were sacrificed by the intravenous injection of sodium pentobarbital at 24, 48, 72 and 96 hours after treatment. The embryos were removed, weighed and digested with N.C.S. solubiliser at 60°C overnight. The levels of radioactivity present were measured by liquid scintillation counting and are shown in Table 2.

Thirteen- and fourteen-day old embryos were frozen in liquid nitrogen and at a later date dissection was performed under a binocular dissecting microscope. For each embryo in turn, the four limb buds, spinal cord region, head and the remaining body wall and contents were divided and placed in separate scintillation vials, weighed, solubilised and measured by liquid scintillation counting. Statistical analysis of the results (Table 2) indicated no significant difference in the levels of radioactivity in each region. Unfortunately, because of the small size of the embryos we were unable to perform a similar study at the earlier developmental stages (eleven and twelve days gestation).

It can be seen from studying Table 2 in conjunction with the figure that there are comparable levels of radioactivity in the maternal serum and the embryo. The rates of decline are parallel suggesting no effective barrier to the exchange of thalidomide and/or its metabolites between mother and embryo. The results in Table 3 demonstrate the complete absence of any specific binding of thalidomide and/or its metabolites to embryonic structures at 72 and 96 hours following administration.

A study was made of the uptake of triated thymidine in the neural tube and limb buds of 10 and 10 3/4 day rabbit embryos some of which were exposed to thalidomide by treating pregnant does with 600 mg/kg from 8 - 10 days; then removed from the uterus and grown in whole embryo culture.

Method of Preparation of Embryos

At 10 or 10 3/4 days of gestation, each pregnant New Zealand White Rabbit was lightly anaesthetised with sodium pentobarbital. Under aseptic conditions, the abdomen was opened and the uterus transferred to either physiological saline or Hartmanns compound sodium lactate solution at 38°C; after dissecting away fat and extraneous tissue, the uterus was transected immediately proximal to each implantation site. It is extremely difficult to peel or cut away the uterine muscle without bursting the amniotic sac. The embryo was revealed lying within the amnion or top of the placenta. The uterine muscle was then trimmed from around and deep to the placenta; great care was taken to maintain the patency of large circular vitelline blood vessels overlying the perimeter of the placenta. Embryos with attached yolk-sacs and placentas were placed in sterile 120 ml bottles containing 10 mls of culture medium at 37°C. The culture medium was made from New Zealand White Rabbit serum which was heat inactivated at 58°C for 40 minutes then stored at -4°C for 1 - 2 weeks before use. Immediately before use 50 µg/ml of streptomycin and 30 µg/ml of penicillin were added. ^{3}H-thymidine (the Radiochemical Centre, Amersham 24 Ci/mmol) was added to the sera (2 µCi/ml serum). The air within the culture bottles was displaced with 100% O_2 and capped with sterile rubber stoppers. The bottles were then rotated 60° from vertical at 35 r.p.m. in an incubator at 37 ± 0.5°C.

During culture, embryos were periodically examined and embryonic status assessed according to the following criteria:

A. Excellent yolk sac circulation
heart rate (H.R.) > 120/min.

B. Fair-good yolk sac circulation
H.R. 60 - 120/min.

C. Poor yolk sac circulation
H.R. 60/min.

D. H.R. absent

After 4 hours in culture intraembryonic distribution of radioactivity was determined autoradiographically. Embryos were fixed in either Carnoys Bouins or formal saline solution, dehydrated, cleaned and embedded in wax. Five micron serial sections were then cut, dewaxed, hydrated and washed for several hours in distilled water. Slides were then dipped in Ilford K2 nuclear research emulsion diluted 1:1 with distilled water at 38°C. Autoradiographs were exposed at 4°C in vertical staining racks in light proof, air tight boxes containing silica gel. Test slides were removed at varying intervals during processing to determine the degree of exposure. Development occurred in Kodak 19 for 7 1/2 minutes at 17°C after lightly staining with H and E.

Counts were made of the silver granules in the cells of the neural tube and limb buds using a Zeiss Microvideomat II linked with a Hewlett Packard computer. The computerized Grain Density Index of the treated and control embryos showed:

1. The treated embryos have less labelling overall than the control embryos. This is confirmed by liquid scintillation counting.

2. The ventro-lateral quadrants of the neural tube of the treated embryos show less signal than the control.

3. The Dorsal Root Ganglia of the treated embryos have low readings of grain density.

4. The distal parts of the limb buds in treated embryos show less signal than the control.

From the experiments carried out in this laboratory it has been shown that surgical excision or chemical destruction of the neurons of the spinal cord will result in reduction deformities of the limbs. It has also been established that interference with the function of muscarinic receptors of the cholinergic nerves of the embryo will produce reduction deformities. The pattern of deformities differs in the two groups. One group being produced by an effect on the neuron and the other by an effect on the peripheral receptors.

Table 1:

The Effect of the Injection of Anticholinergic Drugs into White Leghorn Eggs at 96h Incubation.

Drugs used	No. of Eggs Injected	Living at 12th Day	Total No. Deformed (Rate)	Gastro-schisis (Rate)	Exencephaly (Rate)	Reduction Deformity Legs (Rate)	Wing Deformities (Rate)	Other Deformities
Atropine 300 µg	100	44	14 32%	14 32%	-	-	-	-
Atropine 600 µg	100	25	12 48%	10 40%	2 8%	1 associated with exen-cephaly	-	1 anophthalmia associated with exencephaly
Hyoscine 200 µg	100	46	36 78%	36 78%	-	2 4%	4 9%	-
Hyoscine 400 µg	100	30	6 20%	2 6%	1 3%	2 6%	1 3%	1 cleft palate associated with gastroschisis
Isotonic Saline 400 µl	100	91	-	-	-	-	-	-

Table 2:

Total ^{3}H-radioactivity in rabbit embryos.

Time after treatment (h)	Weight of embryos (mg)	Radioactivity (dpm/g tissue wet wt.)
24	31 ± 6	27001 ± 3015
48	59 ± 10	21409 ± 2473
72	125 ± 18	13708 ± 2240
96	233 ± 28	9945 ± 1009

Dosage administered was as shown in Fig. 4. Each value is the mean of eight embryos, four from each doe (means ± SD).

Table 3:

Distribution of ^3H-radioactivity within rabbit embryos.

	Radioactivity (dpm/g tissue wet wt.)	%	Weight %
13 day embryos			
Limb buds	10349 ± 1384	10	6
Spinal cord	10123 ± 1081	25	24
Head	8932 ± 721	40	44
Remainder	9715 ± 290	25	26
14 day embryos			
Limb buds	8655 ± 668	9	7
Spinal cord	8675 ± 2871	22	18
Head	7475 ± 1082	42	40
Remainder	7076 ± 705	27	35

Dosage administered was as shown in Fig. 4. Each value is the mean of six embryos, three from each doe (means ± SD (%)).

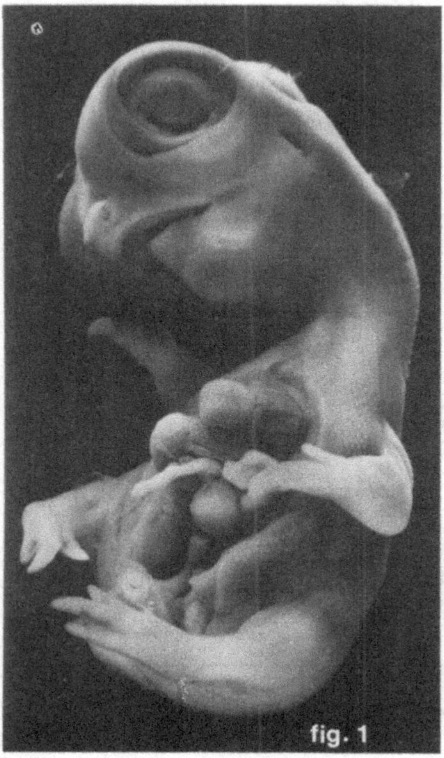

Fig. 1: Chick embryo showing gastroschisis.

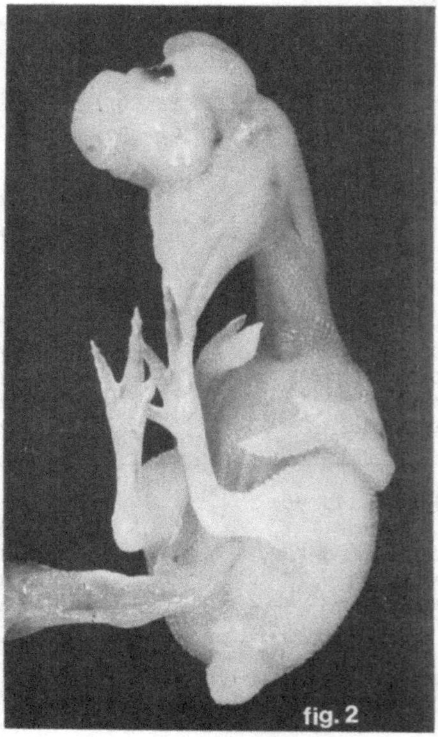

Fig. 2: Chick embryo showing exencephaly and anophthalmia.

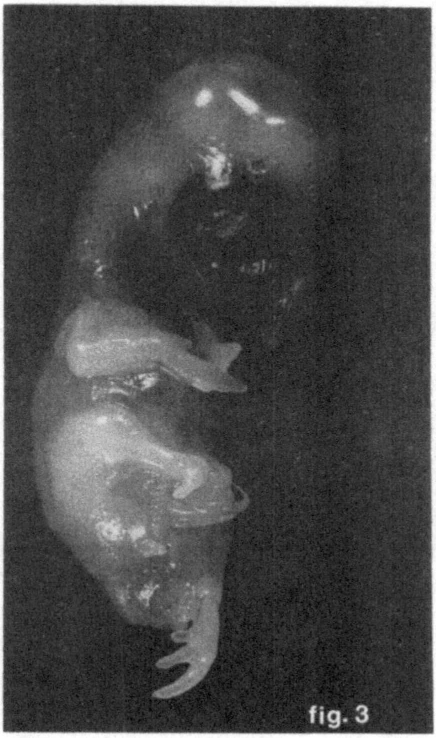

Fig. 3: Chick embryo showing reduction deformity of right leg.

fig. 4

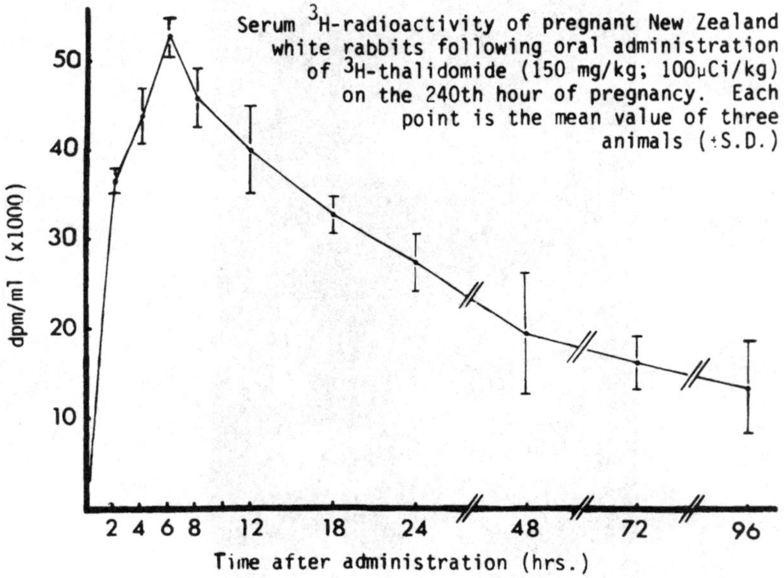

Fig. 4: Serum ^{3}H-radioactivity of pregnant New Zealand White Rabbits following oral administration of ^{3}H-thalidomide (150 mg/kg; 100 µCi/kg) on the 240th hour of pregnancy.

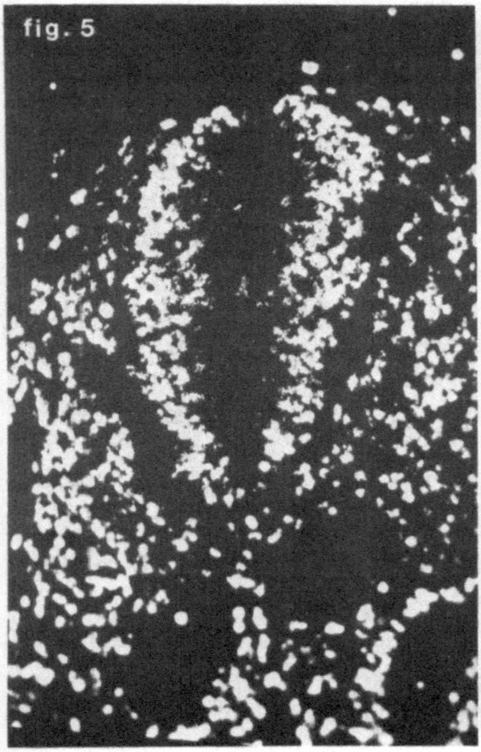

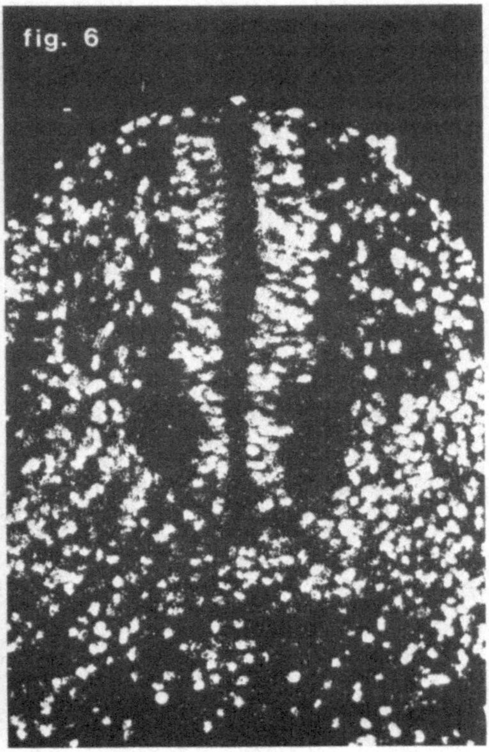

Fig. 5: Autoradiograph of brachial region of neural tube of a control 10 day rabbit embryo grown in culture medium with tritiated thymidine. x 280

Fig. 6: Autoradiograph of the brachial region of the neural tube of a 10 day rabbit embryo exposed to thalidomide in utero for 48 hours prior to culture medium with tritiated thymidine.

REFERENCES

Bueker, E.D., Platner, W.S., 1956, Effect of cholinergic drugs on development of chick embryo, Proc. Soc. Exp. Biol. Med. 91, 539 - 543.

Cihák, R., Doskocil, M., Seichert, V., 1978, Some morphogenetic aspects of the aneurogenic and explanted limb primordia, in: "XIXth Morphological Congress Symposia", pp. 119 - 125, Charles Univ., Prague.

Hamburger, V., 1939, The development and innervation of transplanted limb primordia of chick embryos, J. Exp. Zoo., 80, 347 - 389.

Kieny, M., Fouvet, B., 1974, Innervation et morphogenese de la patte chez l'embryon de poulet, Arch. Anat. Microsc. Morphol. Exp., 63, 281 - 297.

Landauer, W., 1977, Cholinomimetic teratogens. V. The effect of oximes and related cholimesterase reactivators, Teratology, 15, 33 - 42.

McBride, W.G., 1974, Fetal nerve cell degeneration produced by thalidomide in rabbits, Teratology, 10, 283 - 291.

McBride, W.G., 1976, Studies of the etiology of thalidomide dysmorphogenesis, Teratology, 14, 71 - 88.

McBride, W.G., 1979, The inductive influence of neural tissue in limb development in the chick, Aust. J. Zool., 27, 673 - 679.

Nachmansohn, D.J., 1939, Choline esterase involuntary muscle, J. Physiol., 95, 29 - 35.

Saunders, J.W., Jr., 1948, The proximodistal sequence of origin of parts of the chick wing and the role of ectoderm, J. Exp. Zool., 108, 363 - 404.

Saunders, J.W., Jr., 1977, The experimental analysis of chick limb bud development, in: "Vertebrate Limb and Somite Morphogenesis", (D.A. Ede, J.R. Hinchliffe, M. Balls, eds.) pp. 1 - 24, Cambridge University Press.

Singer, M., 1943, The nervous system and regeneration of the forelimb of adult triturus, J. Exp. Zool., 92, 297 - 315.

Vickers, T.H., 1967, Concerning the morphogenesis of the thalidomide dysmelia in rabbits, Br. J. Exp. Pathol., 48, 579 - 591.

Wolpert, L., 1971, Positional information and pattern formation, Curr. Topics Develop. Biol., 6, 183 - 224.

Yntema, C.L., 1959, Regeneration and sparsely innervated and aneurogenic forelimbs of amblystoma larvae, J. Exp. Zool., 140, 101 - 123.

Zacks, S.I., 1954, Esterases in the early chick embryo, Anat. Rec., 118, 509 - 537

Defective Innervation and Defective Limbs: Causes and Effects in the Developing Chick Wing

Julian Lewis

Department of Anatomy, King's College
London WC2R 2LS, U.K.

How is the outgrowth of nerve fibres controlled? How are the paths of outgrowth specified? Why do some of the axons take one route and others another? What decides whether an axon will advance, halt, retreat or die? These problems can be very conveniently studied in the developing limbs of a chick embryo (for review see LANDMESSER, 1980). The spinal cord, the sensory ganglia and the limbs themselves can all be independently perturbed, and the effects on the patterns of nerve outgrowth can be easily assessed by the old techniques of silver-staining (TELLO, 1917; HAMBURGER, 1958), or by the newer methods for tracing connections, such as the retrograde transport of horseradish peroxidase (LANDMESSER, 1978; LANCE-JONES and LANDMESSER, 1980). The data to be presented here as to the factors that define nerve pathways have mostly been gathered with the help of a whole-mount silver-stain which reveals the 3-dimensional system of innervation without the need for sectioning (LEWIS, 1978).

The limb can be considered as a testing-ground on which to examine the behaviour of nerve fibres. This approach rests on a tacit assumption that the developmental interaction between the limb and its nerves is largely one-way: that whereas the tissues of the limb may cause nerve fibres to grow along certain routes and halt at certain targets, the pattern of differentiation and growth of the limb itself is practically unaffected by the presence of the nerve fibres. The conventional view that the pattern of the limb is independent of innervation (HAMBURGER, 1939; KIENY and FOUVET, 1974) has, however, been disputed recently (McBRIDE, 1979; McCREDIE et al., 1978). I shall therefore return to this question at the end of the paper, and present some new data which tend to confirm the old judgment that the limb develops its normal intrinsic pattern even in the absence of nerves.

If we compare the patterns of innervation of the right and left wings of a chick embryo, we find a remarkable symmetry: for example, the same set of nerve branches to each of the twenty-five muscles distal to the shoulder can be seen in precisely corresponding positions. The same pattern, furthermore, is reproduced in other chicks. To understand the genesis of this pattern it is important to know how far it is determined by the specific character of the neurons that innervate the limb, and how far by the intrinsic structure of the limb itself. The question can be answered by grafting an early, uninnervated limb bud to a strange site, such as the head or neck, where it becomes innervated by nerves normally foreign to it. These foreign nerves are found to follow almost exactly the same paths that the normal limb nerves would have taken (HAMBURGER, 1939; LEWIS, unpublished). The paths of nerve outgrowth are thus evidently defined by the intrinsic structure of the limb. They can be regarded as 'public highways', along which axons from any source may advance. The problem is to understand how those highways are specified.

The limb is still quite immature when the nerves first grow into it: muscle and cartilage have just begun to differentiate, but the boundaries between

Teratology of the Limbs

one type of tissue and another are still generally hazy. In the absence of sharply defined landmarks in the intrinsic pattern of the limb, it may seem puzzling that the nerve highways should be so precisely laid out. The tendency of nerves to fasciculate provides an explanation. If one examines the growing end of a nerve - the interosseous, for example, as it advances along the embryonic forearm towards the wrist - one finds that it has a 'frayed' appearance: The individual pioneer axons in this region are taking somewhat erratic and divergent routes. More proximally, however, the axons are not separate, but are bound together in a single fascicle. The axons behind the growing tip evidently cohere to form a nerve whose course represents a compromise choice: its direction of growth is an average or resultant of the divergent tendencies of the individual pioneer growth cones. In this way, through the forces of fasciculation, the vagaries of pathway selection by an isolated axon may be smoothed out. It is not necessary to suppose that the highways for nerve outgrowth are laid out initially as tracks which, though invisible, have the same sharpness that we see in the mature pattern of nerves.

Even though the tracks may be hazy, however, they must in some sense exist. What then are they made of? One approach to this question is to study more closely the pioneer growth cones, to see what might be guiding them. Might they be advancing, for example, by contact guidance along fibrillar material of the extracellular matrix? Electron-microscope studies by LULWAH AL-GHAITH indicate that this is not the case. Instead, the pioneer growth cones appear to be in close contact, over practically the whole of their surfaces, with the membranes of surrounding mesenchymal cells (AL-GHAITH and LEWIS, to be published). This suggests that the pioneer growth cones are guided in their choice of path by the surface properties of the cells of the limb.

Given that the limb is a composite of several different types of cell, what parts do these severally play in guiding nerve outgrowth? Recent discoveries have made it possible to give an answer with regard to muscle cells at least. It has been shown that the myoblasts derive from the somitic mesoderm, and so have a separate origin from the other cells of the limb (CHRIST et al., 1977; CHEVALLIER et al., 1977). Thus by destroying the somitic mesoderm at an early stage it is possible to make limbs that are devoid of muscle cells. The connective tissues of such limbs develop with an astonishing degree of autonomy, as though nothing was amiss, forming a pattern which is normal in almost every way except for the absence of muscle (KIENY and CHEVALLIER, 1979). In collaboration with Drs. MADELEINE KIENY and ALAIN CHEVALLIER, we have studied the innervation of these limbs (KIENY, CHEVALLIER, LEWIS and WOLPERT, to be published). The procedure was to direct a large dose of X-rays onto the somites at the brachial level on one side of the embryo at two days of incubation, and to fix the resultant muscleless wings at various different times, from three days up to eight days thereafter, examining the developing pattern of innervation by means of the whole-mount silver stain.

In a normal wing, the first nerves to appear are the main mixed trunks. The side branches to individual muscles do not become visible until slightly later, at about the time when the first myotubes are forming. The muscle nerve branches originate as short unfasciculated tufts of axons turning aside from the main trunks where they pass close to the rudimentary muscle masses. As the limb grows, the muscles become separated from the main nerve trunks, and the muscle nerve branches are drawn out into the mature, well-fasciculated configuration. In the muscleless wings we found that the main mixed trunks and all their cutaneous branches developed more or less normally, but that practically no muscle nerve branches formed. In almost all those exceptional cases where muscle nerve branches were visible, we were able to show that some residual muscle was present despite the X-irradiation. We checked, by grafting early limb buds reciprocally between normal and irradiated embryos, that the presence or absence of muscle nerve branches did indeed depend on the presence or absence of muscle in the limb, and was not to be explained in terms of accidental damage to the neural tube by misdirected X-rays. The muscle nerve branches were missing from muscleless limbs at all stages: they did not even put in a transient appearance, as far as we could tell. Thus it seems that different parts of the pattern of nerve pathways in a limb are controlled by different classes of limb cell. Muscle cells are necessary to cause axons to turn aside towards the sites of muscles, but the other types of connective tissue cell serve to guide axons along the routes of the main mixed nerve trunks and into the branches that innervate the skin.

In the muscleless wing, do the motor axons initially grow out in company with the sensory axons, and if so, how far do they travel before withdrawing or dying? The answer is obscure because our techniques do not let us distinguish the motor axons from the sensory. One way to find out would be by destroying the sensory neuroblasts as well as the somitic mesoderm, so that any nerve fibre seen subsequently in the muscleless limb could be assumed to be motor. As a first step in this direction, I have attempted to eliminate the sensory component of the wing innervation by destroying the neural crest in the two-day embryo with a focussed beam of ultraviolet light. It turns out to be easy to adjust the dose and the direction of the UV so that all the sensory neurons are eliminated, and easy to adjust it so that all the motor neurons survive; but hard to meet both these requirements at the same time. Fig. 1 shows one of the more successful efforts. Almost all the cutaneous nerve branches in this wing (which has a normal musculature) are missing, and almost all of the muscle nerve branches are present and in the normal locations. This result does at least indicate that motor axons do not depend on sensory axons or on Schwann cells to guide them along the usual paths to their targets (see also HAMBURGER et al., 1966).

It goes without saying that failures were more numerous than successes, and the dose of UV was often excessive, so that the wings were often completely or almost completely deprived of innervation. Such nerveless wings did, however, provide an occasion to check whether wing development is truly independent of innervation. My specimens had the virtue that they had been deprived of their innervation by a method which caused relatively little other disruption, as compared with surgical excision of the neural tube, for example. There were altogether 26 embryos, fixed at 7 - 8 days of incubation, with wings that were completely nerveless or had at most a few thin wisps of nerve extending no further than the elbow. Every one of these wings had a normal-looking skeleton, including humerus, radius, ulna and three digits (Fig. 2, 3). To study the question more systematically, however, I irradiated a total of 31 two-day embryos with the express purpose of destroying the sources of wing innervation totally.

As a source of UV, a 250W high-pressure mercury lamp was used, with an adjustable slit in front of it. An image of the slit was focussed onto the embryo by means of a concave mirror together with a small plane mirror, as in a Newtonian reflecting telescope. The image (in all but three cases) measured 200 μm x 2 500 μm, and this was directed vertically onto the neural tube, so as to destroy it over a length of 2 500 μm posterior to the twelfth somite. The embryo was exposed to the UV for 30 seconds, this being about three times the minimum dose required to create nerveless wings. Of the 31 embryos irradiated, 24 survived to fixation. Of these, 14 were fixed at 8 days of incubation and silver-stained to check that nerves were truly absent from the wings; 6 were fixed at 10 days and stained with alcian green to display the skeleton (SUMMERBELL, 1976), and another 4 were fixed at 16 days, and stained likewise with alcian green. Out of 25 successfully silver-stained wings, 19 appeared entirely nerveless (though nerves were clearly visible elsewhere in the body), and the remaining 6 had no more than thin wisps of nerve, extending no further than the elbow. The skeletons of all the nerveless and quasi-nerveless wings appeared to be complete and normal in their proportions. The cartilage elements can be seen in the silver-stained specimens, but their outlines are not defined clearly enough for accurate measurement. For that purpose I turned to the alcian green specimens (Fig. 4), which could be safely assumed to be nerveless or nearly so. The lengths of the humerus (H), of the ulna (U), and of the middle digit (D) were measured and compared with the data of SUMMERBELL (1976) for the 10 day wings, and with a set of three normal contemporaneous control embryos for the 16 day wings. The uncertainties of staging make the absolute values of the lengths difficult to compare with the standards; but they appeared to lie within the normal range for embryos of their age. For the 8 nerveless wings fixed at 16 days, the mean total length H + U + D was 25.8 mm, with a standard deviation of ± 1.3 mm, as compared with 27.0 ± 1.8 mm for the controls. Fortunately, however, as SUMMERBELL (1976) has shown, the ratios of the lengths H, U and D change very little during the growth of a normal wing. Thus it is possible to check accurately whether the proportions of an experimental wing are normal. For the 12 nerveless wings fixed at 10 days, the average value of U/H was 0.88 with a standard deviation of ± 0.02; and that of D/H was 1.01 ± 0.04. These values are remarkably close to the values of 0.84 ± 0.03 and 0.92 ± 0.05, respectively, read off from SUMMERBELL'S graphs. The 8 nerveless wings fixed at 16 days had U/H = 0.87 ± 0.03 and D/H = 1.02 ± 0.04, as compared with 0.83 ± 0.02 and 1.04 ± 0.02 respectively for the 6 control wings.

I also examined the cleared nerveless wings between crossed polaroid filters to see what muscle was present. As expected from the detailed studies of STRAZNICKY (1967), of SHELLSWELL (1977), and of Dr. EVELYN JAROS (personal communication), I found that an essentially normal pattern of muscles was visible in the nerveless wings fixed at 8 days, but that these muscles gradually atrophied, being distinctly reduced by 10 days of incubation. By that stage the experimental wings were not only less fleshy than normals, but also had their elbows more sharply flexed.

These observations tend to confirm the old view that the development of the limb skeleton is independent of innervation. The finding of a certain proportion of deformities in other studies of nerveless limbs is probably to be explained along the lines suggested by KIENY and FOUVET (1974), as a consequence of other kinds of disturbance incidental to the surgical operations used, affecting circumstances of limb development other than the innervation; for in my series of embryos, in which the innervation was abolished by a method which caused rather less incidental damage and certainly less mortality, the incidence of skeletal deformities was practically zero. Admittedly, the present experiments were done on the wing of the chick, and the legs of chicks and the limbs of mammals might develop according to different principles; but this seems a rather unlikely interpretation of the observations.

ACKNOWLEDGEMENT

I thank the Medical Research Council for support.

REFERENCES

Chevallier, A., Kieny, M., Mauger, A., 1977, Limb-somite relationship: origin of the limb musculature. J. Embryol. exp. Morph., 41, 245 - 258.

Christ, B., Jacob, H. J., Jacob, M., 1977, Experimental analysis of the origin of the wing musculature in avian embryos. Anat. Embryol., 150, 171 - 186.

Hamburger, V., 1939, The development and innervation of transplanted limb primordia of chick embryos. J. Exp. Zool., 80, 347 - 389.

Hamburger, V., 1958, Regression versus peripheral control of differentiation in motor hypoplasia, Am. J. Anat., 102, 365 - 410.

Hamburger, V., Wenger, E., Oppenheim, R., 1966, Motility in the chick embryo in the absence of sensory input, J. Exp. Zool., 162, 133 - 160.

Kieny, M., Chevallier, A., 1979, Autonomy of tendon development in the embryonic chick wing, J. Embryol. exp. Morph., 49, 153 - 165.

Kieny, M., Fouvet, B., 1974, Innervation et morphogenèse de la patte chez l'embryon de poulet, II. Anomalies consécutives à l'excision d'un troncon de tube neural à deux jours d'incubation, Arch. Anat. micr. Morph. exp., 63, 281 - 298.

Lance-Jones, C., Landmesser L., 1980, Motoneurone patterns in embryonic chick limbs following partial deletions of the spinal cord, J. Physiol., 302, 559 - 580.

Landmesser, L., 1978, The development of motor projection patterns in the chick hindlimb, J. Physiol., 284, 391 - 414.

Landmesser, L.T., 1980, The generation of neuromuscular specificity, Ann. Rev. Neurosci., 3, 279 - 302.

Lewis, J., 1978, Pathways of axons in the developing chick wing: evidence against chemo-specific guidance, Zöon., 6, 175 - 179.

McBride, W.G., 1979, The inductive influence of neural tissue in limb development in the chick, Aust. J. Zool., 27, 673 - 679.

McCredie, J., Cameron, J., Shoobridge, R., 1978, Congenital malformations and the neural crest, Lancet, 2, (8093), 761 - 763.

Shellswell, G.B., 1977, The formation of discrete muscles from the chick wing dorsal and ventral muscle masses in the absence of nerves, J. Embryol. exp. Morph., 41, 269 - 277.

Straznicky, K., 1967, The development of the innervation and the musculature of wings innervated by thoracic nerves, Acta Biol. Hung., 18, 437 - 448.

Summerbell, D., 1976, A descriptive study of the rate of elongation and differentiation of the skeleton of the developing chick wing, J. Embryol. exp. Morph., 35, 241 - 260.

Tello, J.F., 1917, Génesis de las terminaciones nerviosas motrices y sensitivas. I. En el sistema locomotor de los vertebrados superiores. Histogénesis muscular, Trab. Lab. Invest. Biol., Univ. Madrid, 15, 101 - 199.

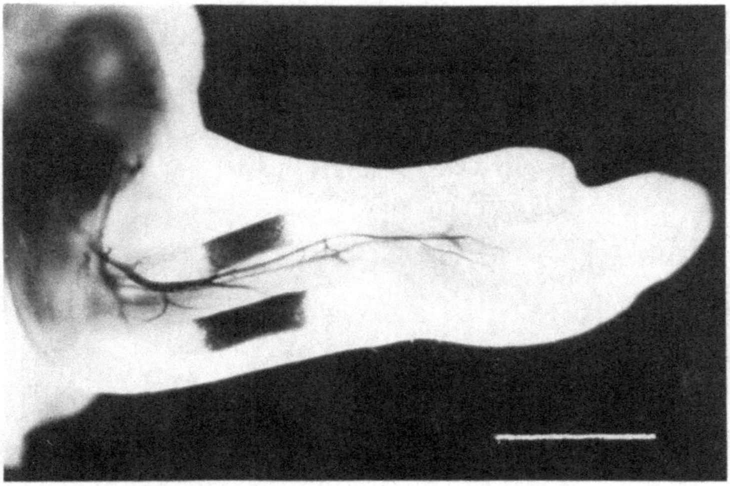

Fig. 1: A silver-stained wing fixed at 8 days of incubation, after UV-irradiation of the neural crest at 2 days of incubation. Dark-ground illumination, dorsal view. Almost all the usual muscle nerve branches are present, and almost all the usual cutaneous nerve branches are absent. Scale bar = 1 mm.

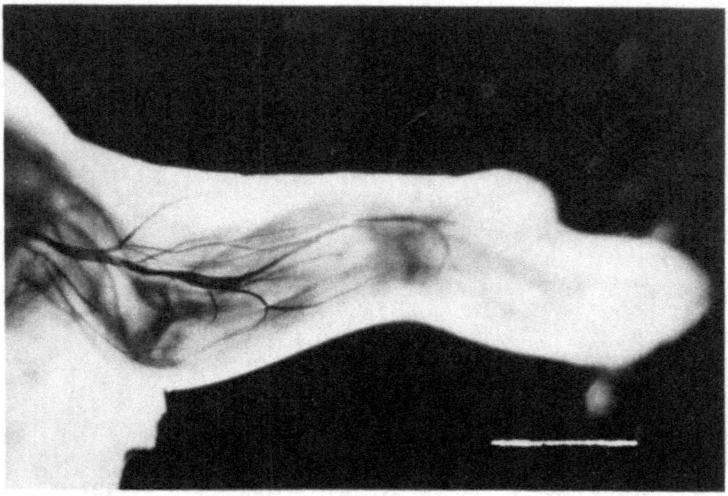

Fig. 2: A silver-stained normal control wing, fixed at 8 days of incubation. Dark-ground illumination, showing the pattern of innervation on the dorsal side. Scale bar = 1 mm.

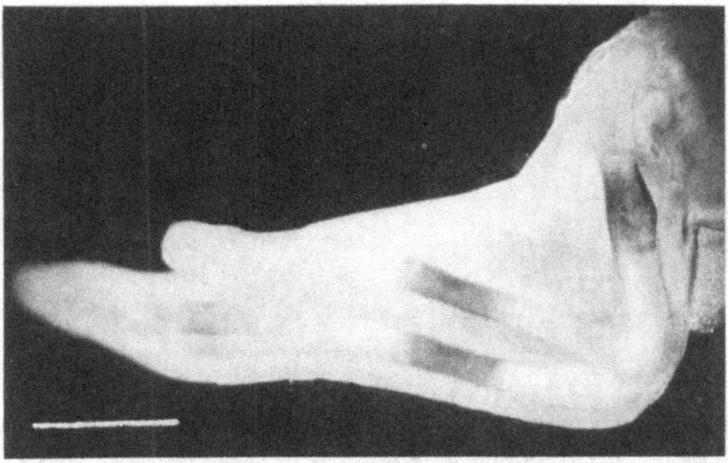

Fig. 3: A silver-stained nerveless wing fixed at 8 days of incubation, from an embryo whose neural tube had been irradiated with UV at 2 days of incubation. Dark-ground illumination, dorsal view. Scale bar = 1 mm.

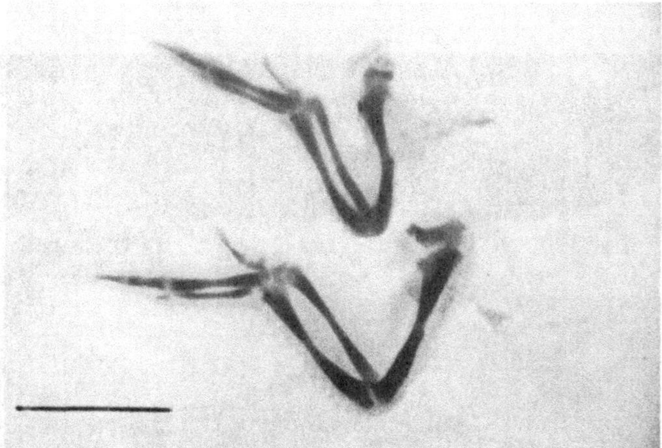

Fig. 4: A nerveless wing (above) and a normal control wing (below), both fixed at 10 days of incubation and stained with alcian green. Scale bar = 2 mm.

B. General Aspects of Teratology

On the Problem of Phase Specificity in Limb Teratogenesis

Diether Neubert and Imke Dillmann

Institut für Toxikologie und Embryopharmakologie, Freie Universität Berlin,
Garystraße 9, D-1000 Berlin 33

INTRODUCTION

When teratogenicity is studied thoroughly or on a larger scale it becomes evident that the induction of a teratogenic effect is a rather specific event. Far from every toxic effect is capable of triggering a malformation; in fact, only few out of hundreds or thousands of agents are "teratogenic". The complex malformation pattern orginating from the action of a given teratogenic agent is determined by a variety of modifying factors. Among these may be included pharmacokinetic and pharmacodynamic parameters of the agent as well as special embryological situations or peculiarities of the developing organism. Understanding the mode of a teratogenic action will only be achieved if the embryological event proceeding during the developmental stage in question has been studied in detail. Vice versa a teratogenic agent may help to elucidate basic steps of embryonic differentiations by modifying or blocking it. A joint approach of embryologists and teratologists to solving questions of normal and pathological experimental embryology therefore seems to be highly desirable.

In this paper will be discussed observations obtained in teratological studies illustrating the complexity of the induction of structural abnormalities and, to some extent, also our present inability to piece together from the toxicological and embryological data available a complete and detailed image of the mode of a teratogenic action. Special emphasis is laid on the occurrence of abnormalities of the extremities - in accordance with the subject of this symposium.

The phenomenon of "phase specificity"

It is a well-established and well-accepted principle that teratogenic effects can only be induced during a defined - and for each type of abnormality rather typical - stage of embryonic development. We may call this prerequisite for the induction of a teratogenic effect "phase specificity". In general, the phase especially susceptible to the interference by a teratogenic agent is the organogenesis period of the particular anlage. Although this principle has been recognized long ago and confirmed in many teratological studies it has predominantly been considered as a "phenomenon" - easily understandable and explainable from the basic embryological events. Little attempt has been made up to now to analyse this phenomenon more closely on a biochemical or toxicological basis.

"Universal" and "specific" teratogenic actions

When the teratogenic action of a variety of agents is elucidated two situations can be identified representing the two extremes of a "scale" of teratogenic effects: There is a certain type of teratogenic agent which, when applied during different stages of development, induces the lesion charac-

Teratology of the Limbs

teristic for the particular stage - and different types of abnormalities when given at various stages of development. X-rays belong to this class of agents, but also chemicals drastically interfering with differentiation and proliferation processes in general, such as alkylating agents, some antimetabolites etc. We suggested to call this class of teratogenic agents: "universal teratogens".

But it becomes quite obvious to an investigator studying the action of many agents with a teratogenic potential that not all chemical agents behave like universal teratogens. With many agents possessing a teratogenic potential only one defect, or a few abnormalities, out of a large variety of defects which can principally be induced at that particular gestational stage will be induced. When applied during other stages of embryonic development such agents may be completely inactive - although the developmental stage, in principle, is susceptible to a teratogenic interference. We suggested to call this class of teratogenic agents: "specific teratogens" (cf. NEUBERT et al., 1980). In praxi, there are few specific teratogens which are only capable of inducing a single defect. The number of different teratogenic manifestations produced also depends on the applied dose. If higher doses are administered it is not only the frequency of a particular abnormality which is increased but other types of defects often occur additionally.

The phenomenon of "drug specificity"

The classification of teratogenic effects in universal and specific teratogenic actions may be considered one aspect of a phenomenon which may be called: "drug specificity".

Two aspects of drug specificity may be discussed: specificity with respect to the gestational phase and specificity with respect to the pattern of induced abnormalities.

Drug specificity with respect to the susceptible period

When a variety of teratogens able to induce an identical abnormality is studied it is found that these teratogenic agents often do not act at the same gestational stage. This has been shown for the induction of cleft palate (cf. NEUBERT et al., 1973) and can also be demonstrated for the induction of abnormalities of the extremities. This aspect is illustrated in Tab. 3. From this schematic presentation it can be seen that of the 4 teratogens studied azathioprine and 6-aminonicotinamide induced limb abnormalities predominantly when applied on day 9 of pregnancy. Cytosine arabinoside, on the other hand, exerts its maximum teratogenic effect when given on day 10 of pregnancy and vitamin A reaches its most pronounced teratogenic effect when given on day 11 of pregnancy. These findings suggest that the abnormality of the extremities caused by the four teratogenic agents is induced via different mechanisms of action. Therefore, it may be supposed that an interference with various developmental differentiations can lead to the same final result, i.e. an identical type of structural abnormality.

Drug specificity with respect to the abnormality pattern

Various teratogenic agents, even when applied during the same stage of pregnancy, in general do not induce the same pattern of abnormalities. Generally, the action of an agent only results in producing a selection of defects, out of a variety of abnormalities which can in principle be triggered at this stage of organogenesis. On the biochemical level this organotropic effect can only be explained as a more or less specific action of the teratogenic agent on several more or less well defined reactions essential for the corresponding normal developmental event.

We wondered whether this phenomenon of drug specificity may be so pronounced that it obscures the phenomenon of phase specificity. Some data on the induction of limb abnormalities are given in the following.

Since in the majority of animal species the forelimb buds develop prior to the hindlimb buds it is conceivable that one and the same teratogenic agent, when applied at different gestational stages, may sequentially induce first malformations of the forelimbs and later on those of the hindlimbs. This would be in agreement with the classical concept of embryology.

When studying the teratogenic effect of α,α-dipyridyl in rats the data obtained (cf. Tab. 4) suggest that there does not exist any such clear-cut sequence. When applied to rats on day 11.5 of pregnancy this teratogen induces abnormalities of the fore- as well as the hindlimbs at about the same frequency. But when given 12 hours later (day 12 of pregnancy) abnormalities of the forelimbs predominate as it is the case when the compound is administered on day 12.5 of pregnancy. No clear-cut preference for upper or lower extremities is found when α,α-dipyridyl is given to rats on days 13, 13.5 or 14.5 of pregnancy. The interpretation of the data, in this case, is complicated since a high percentage of fetuses show abnormalities at both, fore- and hindlimbs, at the same time. However, the data clearly show that abnormalities of the forelimbs as well as those of hindlimbs may be induced by this agent from day 11.5 to 13.5 of pregnancy, with no clear-cut preference for upper or lower extremities.

When using mice as experimental animals, results can be obtained in teratological studies which seem to contradict the laws of phase specificity. Using azathioprine (Tab. 5) it can be seen that on day 9 of pregnancy hindlimb abnormalities are induced exclusively. When the same dose is applied one day later (day 10 of pregnancy) fore- and hindlimb abnormalities can be induced at about the same percentage. The data do not give any indication that forelimb abnormalities are induced at an earlier stage than hindlimb abnormalities. The interpretation of the data is again complicated by the fact that the frequency of fetuses showing abnormalities at fore- as well as hindlimbs is high.

The data obtained using cytosine arabinoside and mice as experimental animals (Tab. 6) are more conclusive. It can be seen that on day 9 of pregnancy predominantly abnormalities of the hindlimbs are induced. Again, no forelimb abnormalities are observed even if the drug is given at an earlier stage. Since hindlimb abnormalities are also the prevailing defects produced on day 10 of pregnancy the data suggest that under the experimental conditions chosen cytosine arabinoside predominantly affects the hindlimbs, with very little effect on the forelimbs. This effect is only slightly modified by varying the dose and time of application of the drug.

Similar results are obtained with the teratogenic compound 6-aminonicotinamide (6-AN) and mice as experimental animals (Tab. 7). Again, the induction of hindlimb abnormalities predominates - being independent of the day of application - and no period of application could be found where a determined dose of the drug resulted in forelimb abnormalities only.

SUMMARY and CONCLUSIONS

The main principle of teratology (phase specificity) stating that a certain type of gross structural abnormality (malformation) can only be induced during a defined gestational period is basically still valid. But the information collected in teratological research within the last decade clearly indicates that teratogenic effects frequently are much more confined to a few organ anlagen and that, in the majority of cases, a typical abnormality pattern is obtained. This "drug specificity" often is so pronounced that it seems to obscure the rules of phase specificity. In its extreme form drug specificity may manifest itself as a teratogenic effect which is confined to one side of the body, i.e. uni-lateral abnormalities. (cf. BARRACH et al., this symposium).

Two points are obvious:

1) We have to realize that teratogenic effects very often are much more specific than had been expected years ago.

2) Several outcomes of teratogenic actions can hardly be explained yet on the basis of our present knowledge in embryology, e.g. teratogenic effects almost exclusively confined to one side of the body.

Much more cooperation of scientists working in basic embryology and toxicologists is needed in order to reach an understanding of the mechanisms involved in normal and pathological mammalian embryonic development.

Experimental procedures

The data presented in this paper were obtained using Wistar rats (Wistar TNO W/74, Versuchstierfarm Winkelmann, Paderborn/FRG) and NMRI mice (Han: NMRI, Zentralinstitut für Versuchstiere, Hannover/FRG) as experimental animals. The animals were mated for two hours (7^{oo} to 9^{oo} a.m.) and if sperms or vaginal plug were found the 24-hour period following mating was considered day 0 of pregnancy. All teratogens studied were applied at single doses. The animals were sacrificed on day 18 (mice) or 21 (rats) of pregnancy and skeletal defects were evaluated after "clearing" and staining of the bones with alizarin red.

For the sake of simplicity the different types of abnormalities of the extremities are not specified in this paper although we realize that a detailed description of the results is essential for a teratological evaluation. The majority of abnormalities mentioned in this paper are defects of the paw skeleton.

ACKNOWLEDGEMENT

The original work presented in this paper was supported by grants by the Deutsche Forschungsgemeinschaft awarded to Sonderforschungsbereich 29 (Embryonale Entwicklung und Differenzierung - Embryopharmakologie) at Freie Universität Berlin.

We are indebted to Ruth Kreft for her help in preparing the manuscript.

REFERENCES

Barrach, H.-J., Dillmann, I., 1980, The occurrence of unilateral abnormality of the limb induced by the teratogen 6-aminonicotinamide, in: This Symposium.

Neubert, D., Barrach, H.-J., Merker, H.-J., 1980, Drug-induced damage to the embryo or fetus (Molecular and multilateral approach to prenatal toxicology), in: Current Topics in Pathology, Vol. "Drug-Induced Pathology" (E. Grundmann, ed.), Springer Verlag, Heidelberg.

Neubert, D., Zens, P., Rothenwallner, A., Merker, H.-J., 1973, A survey of the embryotoxic effects of TCDD in mammalian species, Environment. Health Perspect. 5, 67 - 79.

Table 1:

The abnormality pattern induced by a teratogenic agent can be visualized to depend on three characteristic factors:

1) "Phase specificity"

2) "Drug specificity" (organotropic effect)

3) "Dose specificity"

Table 2:

Two main types of teratogenic agents may be discriminated:

1) "Universal" Teratogens

— agents which can induce various types of abnormalities at different stages of development

2) "Specific" Teratogens

— agents which can induce only one or a few abnormalities at defined stages of development.

Table 3:

Susceptibility of Developing Limbs to Some Teratogenic Agents at Different Developmental Periods

day of pregnancy (mouse)	cytosine-arabinoside	azathioprine	6-AN	Vit. A
8	(+)	+	+	
9	+	+++	+++	
10	++++	++	+	(+)
11	++	+	(+)	++++

(+) : < 10 %)
\+ : 10 - 25 %)
++ : 26 - 50 %) abnormal fetuses
+++ : 51 - 75 %)
++++: 76 - 100 %)

Table 4:

Localization of Malformations at the Extremities

Rat - α,α-dipyridyl - i.p.

day of pregnancy	dose (mg/kg)	fetuses with malformations at: fore-limbs (%)	hind-limbs (%)	fore- + hind-limbs (%)	malformed fetuses* / survivors
11.5	60	29	29	43	7/46 ≙ 15 %
12	60	69	0	31	13/44 ≙ 30 %
12.5	60	52	1	47	79/100 ≙ 79 %
13	60	7	0	93	74/75 ≙ 99 %
13.5	60	5	11	84	19/40 ≙ 48 %
14.5	60	2	1	0	3/93 ≙ 3 %

*Limb abnornalities were considered only.

Table 5:

Localization of Malformations at the Extremities

Mouse - azathioprine - s.c.

day of pregnancy	dose (mg/kg)	fetuses with malformations at: fore-limbs (%)	hind-limbs (%)	fore- + hind-limbs (%)	malformed fetuses* / survivors
9	25	0	100	0	31/47 ≙ 66 %
10	25	33	42	25	106/296 ≙ 36 %
10	50	0	17	83	114/123 ≙ 93 %
11	50	0	71	29	28/83 ≙ 34 %

*Limb abnornalities were considered only.

Table 6:

Localization of Malformations at the Extremities

Mouse - cytosine-arabinoside - i.v.

day of pregnancy	dose (mg/kg)	fetuses with malformations at fore- limbs (%)	hind- limbs (%)	fore- + hind- limbs (%)	malformed fetuses* / survivors
9	10	6	84	10	50/85 ≙ 59 %
9	5	0	100	0	6/41 ≙ 15 %
10	5	8	83	9	77/94 ≙ 82 %

*Limb abnornalities were considered only.

Table 7:

Localization of Malformations at the Extremities

Mouse - 6-AN - s.c. - 36° C

day of pregnancy	dose (mg/kg)	fetuses with malformations at fore-limbs (%)	hind-limbs (%)	fore- + hind-limbs (%)	malformed fetuses* / survivors
8	10	15	62	23	13/78 ≙ 17 %
9	10	4	78	18	149/277 ≙ 66 %
10	10	0	93	8	24/166 ≙ 14 %

*Limb abnornalities were considered only.

The Problem of Growth Retardation

Vincenzo G. Leone
Istituto di Zoologia, Università di Milano
Via Celoria 10, Milano 20133, Italy

Growth retardation is a result repeatedly mentioned as an effect of interferences on normal development. This phenomenon is worthy of consideration in two perspectives. First it has to be considered as a developmental defect, i.e. an alteration of the coded growth chronology of a given limb or body segment, which will be regulated later on, generally after birth. In this perspective it appears as a minor defect in an individual. On the other hand, if this finding becomes statistically significant in a colony or in a situation involving many subjects - it acquires the significance of an alarm signal, which is not to be underestimated when evaluating the teratogenic risk of being exposed to a particular agent or situation. It is even more alarming if the effect is due to low doses of that agent, since this fact could be a warning that the border line to teratogenesis has very nearly been trespassed.

Growth retardation is, actually, a special problem for the embryologist in many respects. First, the understanding of the mechanisms of growth retardation may allow the possiblity of elucidating the mechanisms of normal growth and other developmental problems. For instance, the interrelations between genotype and environmental influences can be evaluated, i.e. epigenetic expressions, and to a certain extent, some mechanisms of the evolutionary pathways may be better understood. Secondly, growth retardation reveals that a moderately deviated developmental process is occurring, and the causes of such deviations have to be investigated.
Thirdly, there are practical implications to growth retardation ranging from human health to poultry and live-stock quality. The acceptance and registration of new drugs and other chemical products which induce retardation should be questioned by governmental agencies.
A fourth problem, derived from the last one, is the necessity of finding standard methods to qualify and evaluate the degree and the risk of the retardation. This paper is mainly aimed for the consideration of this problem. In the majority of cases in which growth retardation is mentioned, authors are referring to skeletal development, particularly of the limbs, in terms of length of skeleton pieces or of the stage of maturity reached by the ossification process.
The bone formation and ossification represent, in fact, a very complex developmental process, exposed to several influences that may interfere with its manifold components. As we have seen from other contributions, these components are represented by mesodermal "anlage" from which the piece of skeleton originates, by the cartilage and matrix that have been formed, by the osteoblast's activity and their enzymatic loading; there are, in addition, the nutritional supply to the individual, in regard to quantity and quality of dietary constituents; the circulating hormones and growth factors; nerve supply and other physiological conditions of the subject - and of the mother when speaking of mammals. Delayed development could be the consequence of defective or lacking synchronization between the developmental stage of the embryo and the physiological condition of the uterus. We must not forget the hereditary make-up, conditioning the chronological and dimensional features of the individual growth, together with

Teratology of the Limbs

the susceptibility and reactivity of the "substratum" to the epigenetic factors, already mentioned. The alteration of a single factor or of many factors of the developmental process give different morphological results, even in quantitative expression.
At this point I hope it can be agreed upon that it is impossible - and useless - even to try and summarize the enormous literature pertinent to the causes, the mechanisms and the correlations implied in growth retardation; most of the participants in this Symposium are credited with contributions on this subject. I would like particularly, however, to report the results achieved by RINALDI et al. (1980, in press) on the effect of thermal stress on the evolution of skeletal development in three groups of Long Evans rats, reared at 23° - 24° C (controls), 27° - 29° C (the 'warm' group), respectively. The young were killed at different ages. Developmental modifications were noticed in both groups kept under stress. In the 'warm' group, development was delayed and irregular, that is not uniform, while in the 'cool' group it was homogeneous and further advanced than the controls. In the animals of the 'cool' group, however, the development of the epiphyseal nuclei of the radius and ulna were retarded by about two days as were the distal epiphysis of both femur and tarsus. Generally speaking, the ossification of the diaphyseal shaft of the long bones was more advanced than that of their epiphyseal nuclei.

The study of the extent of fetal ossification seems in fact to be the most accurate and reliable criterion in evaluating adverse developmental conditions and teratogenic risk, particularly in the case of limbs. In estimating intrauterine growth retardation, the consideration of the fetal weight or the body dimensions does certainly have useful implications, in clinical pediatrics. Teratologists, however, have to bear in mind the findings of FRITZ (1975) and LANSDOW et al. (1976): fetuses of treated females may often weigh less than those of the controls without showing signs of retarded ossification, while, to the contrary, delayed bone differentiation may be found in fetuses with normal weight. The relationship between body weight and ossification of the coccygeal vertebrae in mouse and rat fetuses have been examined by ARIYUKI, HIGAKI, and YASUDA (1980) in order to evaluate fetal growth retardation in teratologic tests. These authors suggest that the correlation coefficients between these two characteristics of the developing subjects should be compared. They also discuss the statistical treatments performed on the relative differences between treated and control groups. In the literature, however, the descriptions of cases with bone growth retardation are generally based on subjective evaluation of the stage and degree of ossification and not on objective parameters such as the number and the extent of the ossification centres, and are not studied in a population large enough to allow statistical evaluation. In addition to the quoted research of RINALDI et al. (1980), the paper by ALIVERTI et al. (1979), provides a reliable quantitative method by which the index of bone growth can be established. This method has been worked out on skeletons of newborn Wistar rat fetuses, delivered by Caesarean section on the 19th, 20th, and 21st day of gestation, respectively. Day 0 of gestation is considered the day when spermatozoa were found in the vaginal smears of the mated females.

The fetuses were cleared and stained with Alizarin red S, according to STAPLES and SCHNELL (1964). The material under consideration consisted of a total of 650 untreated fetuses, of which 84 were delivered from 9 females at day 19; 494 from 50 females at day 20; and 72 from 9 females at day 21. The following skeletal districts were observed with the stereomicroscope: metacarpus, metatarsus, sternum, cervical and caudal vertebrae, proximal phalanges of forelimbs and of the hindlimbs.

The number of ossification centres were correlated with the number of fetuses in which the centres were correlated with the number of fetuses in which the centers were found in each of the three days of gestation considered. The statistical significance of the differences between the discordant groups was analysed by the McNEMAR test (SIEGEL, 1956).

This analysis showed that the ossification develops independently in the different skeletal districts, except for the metacarpal and metatarsal ones, where it runs parallel. Significant differences were found between the subjects of the 19th day and the 20th day, but generally the degree of ossification was sufficiently advanced. On day 21 the results were homogeneous and uniform in all of the skeletal districts examined (Fig. 1). The conclusions that can be drawn from these data are that the skeleton in the rat reaches a definitive stage of development on day 21 and therefore the fetuses of this age are best suited to judge the extent of ossification when utilizing this information as a criterion in assessing the teratogenic risk in a given situation.

In order to evaluate the thalidomide activity interfering with histogenic processes other than embryonic differentiation and growth, a phenomenon which further illustrates growth retardation, LEONE and RINALDI (1969) used as a test the endosteal ossification taking place in the limb bones of adult pigeons at the time of ovulation. This process, induced experimentally by injecting follicular hormone into the birds, makes possible the storage of a large quantity of calcium in the new bone. The calcium can then be easily mobilized to build up the eggshell. Thalidomide did interfere with this osteogenetic process (Fig. 2) and also with the evolution of the callus, the system for repairing broken bones (Fig. 3).

ARIAS and ZAVANELLA (1979), in order to study the teratogenic effects of manganese-ethylenebisdithiocarbamate (MANEB), utilized the regenerating forelimb of the adult newt (Triturus cristatus carnifex) as a test and found malformation of regeneration as well as retardation in reaching the developmental (regenerative) stage in comparison to the controls.

MACI and LEONE (1976), studying the effects of thiamphenicol (TAF) on the chick embryo, found a reduction of the blood islets and, as a consequence, growth retardation. In addition to lowering the blood supply, the TAF inhibits the protein synthesis, particularly that of mitochondrial proteins; the consequence is an inhibition of differentiation and growth of musculature.

I have reported recent studies to show that besides contributions to research on embryonic development, which is our major focus, alternative practical methods have resulted for testing dismorphogenetic potential. These other methods can give complementary information on fundamental phenomena of biological relevance such as growth retardation.

REFERENCES

Aliverti, V., Bonanomi, L., Giavini, E., Leone, V.G., Mariani, L., 1979, The extent of the fetal ossification as an index of delayed development in teratogenic studies on the rat, Teratology, 20, 237 - 242.

Arias, E., Zavanella, T., 1979, Teratogenic effects of manganese ethylenebisdithiocarbamate (MANEB) on forelimb regeneration in the adult newt, Triturus cristatus carnifex, Bull. Environ. Contam. Toxicol., 22, 297 - 304.

Ariyuki, F., Higaki, K., Yasuda, M., 1980, A study of fetal growth retardation in teratological tests: An examination of the relationship between body weight and ossification of coccygeal vertebrae in mouse and rat fetuses, Teratology, 22, 43 - 49.

Fritz, H., 1975, Prenatal ossification in rabbits as indicative of fetal maturity, Teratology, 11, 313 - 320.

Lansdow, A.B.G., Pope, W.D.B., Halsey, M.J., Bateman, P.E., 1976, Analysis of fetal development in rats following maternal exposure to subanestetic concentrations of Halotane, Teratology, 13, 299 - 304.

Lanzani Maci, R., Leone, V.G., 1976, Effetti del tiamfenicolo sullo sviluppo embrionale del pollo, Acc. Naz. Lincei, (Rend. Cl. Sci.) LXV, 641 - 644.

Leone, V.G., Rinaldi, L., 1969, A test for the study of teratogenic-like activities of drugs, in: "Teratology" (Proc. of a Symp.), (A. Bertelli, ed.) pp. 23 - 33, Excerpta Medica Found., Amsterdam.

Rinaldi, L., Cinquetti, R., 1980, Adattamento termico nel ratto. Influenza sulla riproduttività e sullo sviluppo perinatale, Boll. Soc. It. Biol. Sperim., in press.

Siegel, S., 1956, Non parametric statistics for beavioral science, pp. 23 - 33, McGraw Hill Book Co. Inc., New York.

Staples, R.E., Schnell, V.L., 1964, Refinements in rapid clearing technic in the KOH Alizarin Red S method for fetal bone, Stain Tech., 39, 61 - 63.

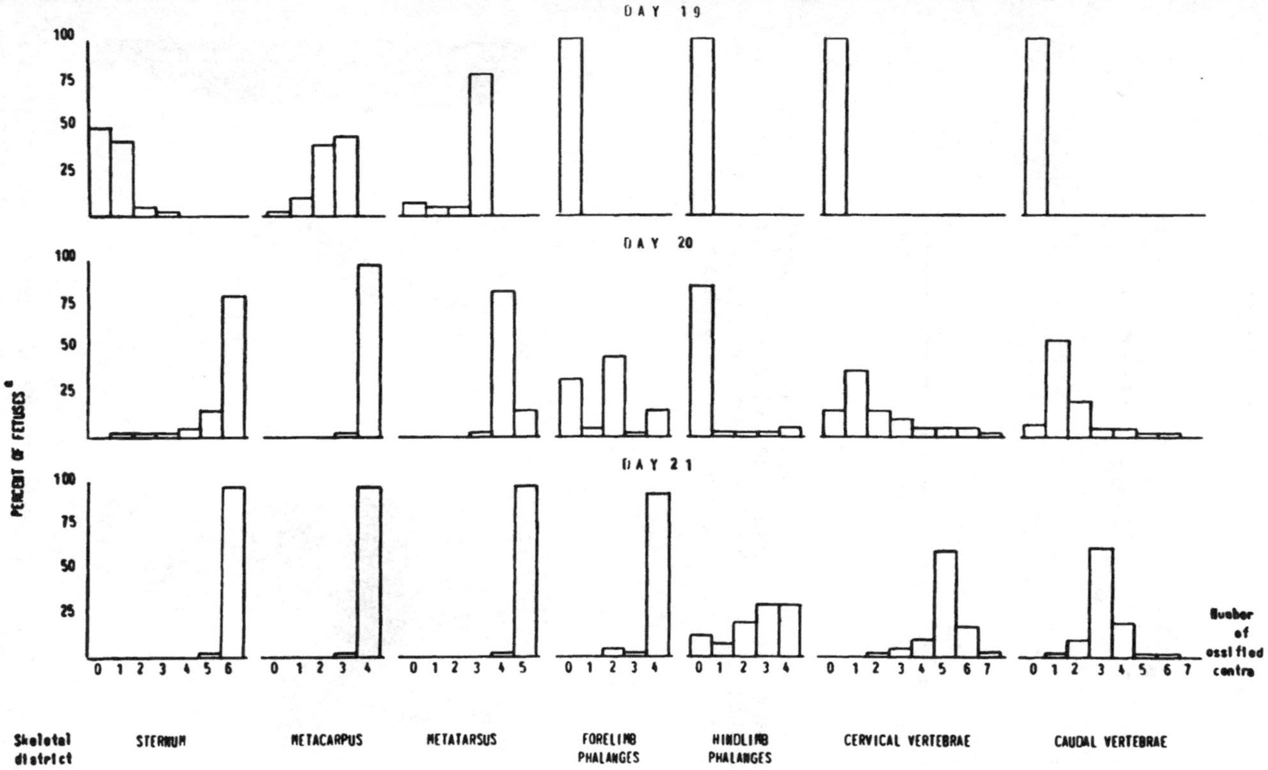

Fig. 1: Histograms of the degree of ossification (number of centres) in the rat fetuses on the last three days before birth.

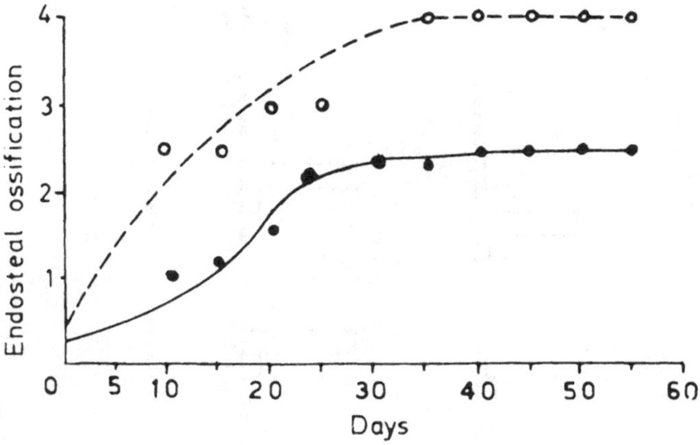

Fig. 2: The extent of endosteal bone formation calculated by evaluation of the ratio between penetration of newly formed trabeculae and mean radius of the long bone shaft in pigeons treated with estrogen (0 - - 0) and with estrogen + thalidomide (0 - 0).

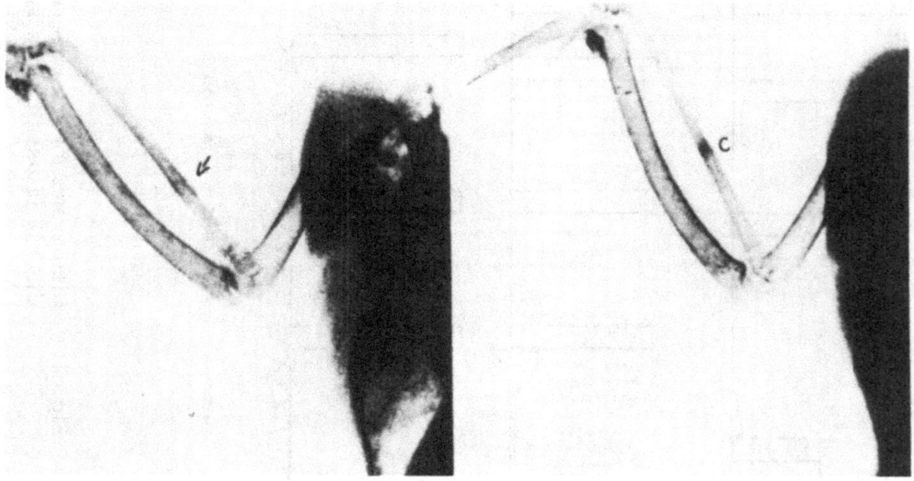

Fig. 3: Radiographs of adult pigeons on day 35 after fracture of the radius. Left: control; the arrow shows the site of complete repair. Right: thalidomide treated pigeon; the callus (C) is still present.

Bilaterally Symmetric and Asymmetric Realization of Limb Malformations

W. Kocher and U. Kocher-Becker

Institut für Toxikologie und Embryonal-Pharmakologie, Freie Universität Berlin, Garystraße 9, D-1000 Berlin 33

Limb malformations in mammals are often observed in only three, two or one of the limbs or the expressivity of malformations found in four limbs varies. With regard to the external bilateral symmetry of the vertebrate body the following distribution patterns of the malformation may occur (Fig. 1):

I. Fore and/or hind limbs are malformed in the same way and to the same degree on both sides of the body (strict bilateral symmetry, mirror image of malformation).

II. The occurrence and/or degree of malformation in the four limbs varies. A side preference of the malformation in fore and/or hind limbs can, however, not be established statistically.

III. The occurrence and/or degree of the malformations present in fore and/or hind limbs show a more or less pronounced side preference (expressed in percent of malformed individuals whose limbs show the side preference in question).

IV. The side preference of the malformation in the fore limbs is contralateral to that of the hind limbs ("crossed asymmetry").

In the present study examples of these various possibilities are presented. They were observed in various related experiments and investigations. The limb malformations investigated either were caused by drugs, caused by a mutant gene effect, occurred spontaneously in the respective +/+ animals or in heterozygotes of the recessive mutant, or were realized by a combined effect of a drug and genes. With regard to the mode of formation, the types of malformation and their symmetry, the following examples shall be given.

Strict symmetry

Strict bilateral symmetry of limb malformations was observed in chick embryos which had been treated with the alkylating substance triethylenemelamine (TEM) during different phases of organogenesis (KOCHER, 1969, 1970). All affected cases showed the same treatment-phase-specific limb malformations in a mirror image fashion on both sides of the body: deficiencies of (or in) skeletal elements, reductions, fusions, and bendings of skeletal elements occurred.

The same kind of mirror image similarity was also observed in terminal limb reductions, which occurred in the chick after treatment with the pentosanpolysulfoester SP54 during later phases of organogenesis (KOCHER-BECKER et al., 1978).

Teratology of the Limbs

Side preference, crossed asymmetry

Homozygotes of the recessive mouse mutant polydactyly (py) exhibit preaxial polydactylism, the expressivity of which varies considerably, depending on the genetic background (KOCHER, 1967, 1977). In cases of low expressivity (presence of a single small preaxial extra element or a diphalangous extra ray) polydactylism was restricted to one of the hind limbs. Here a marked side preference was observed: in approximately 90% of the cases with unilateral manifestation, polydactylism occurred on the right side. During selection breeding towards highest expressivity (+ selection) first both hind limbs, then one and later on both fore limbs were affected. Cases with unilateral polydactylism of the fore limbs showed a preference of the left side which was even more pronounced (98 to 99% of all cases) than that of the contralateral side of the hind limbs.

At a high level of expressivity all 4 limbs could have up to 2 or 3 additional toes or fingers; occasionally the 2nd ray was duplicated (Fig. 2). In these cases the regular first ray was often triphalangous. It could, however, also be reduced. With a further increase in expressivity secondary reductions affected the preaxial element of the zeugopod of the fore limbs: the radius showed distal hypoplasia (Fig. 3) or even aplasia. The number of preaxial extra elements was also reduced secondarily. The reduction of the radius was first observed mostly on one side and with a strong side preference: in 79 of 82 cases it occurred on the left side, in only 2 cases on the right side and in one case bilaterally.

At the highest level of expressivity, reached before selection was terminated, often more than one limb showed reductions of the preaxial long bones. The tibia now also exhibited terminal reductions and tibia hypoplasia became more frequent than radius hypo- or -aplasia. All combinations of radial and tibial reductions within a sample of 18 litters (122 animals) from this level of selection are summarized in Fig. 4: 95 individuals (78%) show reductions of the preaxial element of the zeugopod. Its realization is symmetrical in 7 cases and asymmetrical in 88 cases. 82 of these developed aplasias which were located according to the rule found in the manifestation of the trait of the py-mutant on the preceding levels of the selection. Only 6 cases were not in accordance with this rule.

Hence, side preference and crossed asymmetry were of the same kind and strictness at the end of selection as they were in the beginning.

Side preference of spontaneous preaxial polydactylism in the inbred strain C57BL/6J

The inbred strains CBA/JKch and C57BL/6JKch were investigated over a longer period of time for the occurrence of spontaneous malformations. Each animal was inspected right after birth and at weaning. A total of 3530 animals of the CBA strain and 4135 of the C57BL strain was examined. The CBA animals showed no malformations. In the C57BL strain, however, 16 animals (= 0.39%) had preaxial hyper- or polydactylism. In 15 cases the right hind limb was affected and in only 1 case the left hind limb. Thus, the side preference of spontaneous preaxial polydactylism is within the same order of magnitude as that of the py-mutant.

Apart from polydactylism, 2 of the investigated animals of the C57BL strain showed postaxial ectrodactylism of the fore limbs. Other malformations observed are not considered in this context. py-Heterozygotes, which resulted from crosses of homozygous py-males of high and maximum expressivity with CBA or C57BL females, developed a higher percentage of spontaneous polydactylism and hyperdactylism than the inbred strain C57BL. Maximum expressivity of the father and a C57BL-genome of the mother had the greatest effect (KOCHER, 1977).

In 1457 py-heterozygotes 36 cases of preaxial hyper- or polydactylism were found (inspection shortly after birth, re-inspection at weaning): in 26 cases the right hind limb was affected and in 7 cases the left hind limb, 2 animals showed a broadening of the first ray of the left fore limb, 1 animal had preaxial polydactylism of the right fore limb. Hence, 2/3 of the heterozygous hyper- or polydactyls exhibited the same type of side preference as the py-mutant.

Bilateral differences with and without side preference

The polydactylous malformation pattern of the py-mutant could be copied by treating genetically normal embryos with the alkylating substances TEM (KOCHER, 1967) and cyclophosphamide (Endoxan) (KOCHER et al., unpublished) on day 10 of gestation. In py-heterozygotes considerably lower doses of TEM or cyclophosphamide produced the polydactylous malformation pattern than was the case in homozygotes for the normal allele with comparable maternal genomes (KOCHER, 1972, 1977 and unpublished).

Irrespective of the dosage of the applied substance, the majority of the material from the TEM experiment was pooled in groups according to the genetic constitution of the parents and the distribution pattern of polydactylism (Fig. 5).

Polydactylism was only induced, if one of the parents was C57BL or py/py. In the inbred strain CBA, TEM did not produce polydactylism on day 10 of gestation, even in high doses (up to the embryonal LD 100). Figure 6 shows the proportion of cases with side preference of the py-mutant, with bilateral manifestation, and with a side preference different from that of the py-mutant.

In py-heterozygotes from CBA mothers a clear-cut side preference is recognizable. Such a side preference may be obscured in the case of the py-heterozygotes from C57BL mothers, where the percentage of polydactylism is highest and the manifestation is bilateral in the majority of the animals.

None of the three +/+ constitutions exhibit side preference.

The fetuses of the cyclophosphamide experiment were - like the fetuses of the TEM experiment - divided into groups according to the genetic constitution of the parents and examined for symmetry and asymmetry in the realization of polydactylism (Figures 7 and 8, Table 1). As in the TEM experiment, the reciprocal hybrids do not display a side preference in the realization of polydactylism ($\chi^2 = 0.11$; $p > 0.05$). However, a pronounced side preference occurred in the heterozygotes ($\chi^2 = 13.09$; $p < 0.01$), not only in CBA ($\chi^2 = 4.10$; $p < 0.05$), but also in C57BL ($\chi^2 = 9.80$; $p < 0.01$) mothers, again in accordance with the side preference of the py-mutant.

In this experiment only two of the treated animals showed bilateral manifestation of polydactylism in the fore limbs, whereas the hind limbs were normal. However, bilateral manifestation of polydactylism in the hind limbs with fore limbs being normal, was often observed. Part of these animals showed differences in expressivity of polydactylism in both hind limbs (Fig. 9). Here again, only in the py-heterozygotes a preponderance of higher expressivity was found on the right side.

DISCUSSION:

The causal background of asymmetrical realization of limb malformations has hitherto merely been subject to conjectures. Differences between embryonic systems, as between those of birds and mammals, or physiological side differences based on asymmetries in developmental anatomy, such as the asymmetry of blood circulation, may be mentioned in this connection.

Details on side preference in the realization of limb malformations in various mouse mutants are summarized in a monograph by GRÜNEBERG (1963). In connection with corresponding facts of malformations caused by teratogens (see below) and our own investigations, it seems to be possible to establish some rules for side preferences of polydactylous and hemimelic malformations:

In mutants, which, like polydactyly, produce preaxial polydactylism or hemimelia (Tail-short , luxate; Dominant hemimelia in heterozygous condition) the fore limbs are affected preferentially on the left side, the hind limbs on the right side (an exception is the peculiar behaviour of the homozygotes of Dominant hemimelia, which exhibit a side preference contralateral to that of the heterozygotes). The oppositely crossed side preference (right fore limb, left hind limb) is realized in the mutant postaxial hemimelia and a strain producing postaxial polydactylism.

A corresponding attribution of the side preference to preaxial or to postaxial hemimelia is also found in limb malformations caused by certain drugs: According to WILLERT and HENKEL (1969), in dysmelia caused by thalidomide in the human arm, with the radial fingers and the radius being affected in the first place, the more pronounced defects occurred more often on the left than on the right side. In contrast to this, rats whose mothers had received diets containing acetazolamide showed a variable deficiency of postaxial elements of the right fore limb (LAYTON and HALLESY, 1965). Similar results were obtained in the rat by WILSON et al. (1968), in the mouse by GREEN et al. (1973) and by CASTRO-CORREIA et al. (1974). The latter authors found postaxial polydactylism and postaxial ectromelia again mainly on the right side.

The strict side preference, which is observed in the crossed asymmetrical realisation of preaxial polydactylism of the py-mutant from the lowest to the highest level of expressivity, requires experimental investigations on the dependency of this type of asymmetry on more primitive conditions. Those investigations are underway.

SUMMARY:

Limb malformations of various causation were investigated with regard to the bilateral symmetry of the vertebrate body. The following patterns of distribution could be established:

1.) strict symmetry in treatment-phase-specific defects of the chick limb after treatment with triethylenemelamine (TEM) during different phases of organogenesis;

2.) strict symmetry in terminal reductions of the chick limb after treatment with the pentosanpolysulfoester SP54 during later phases of organogenesis;

3.) side preference in crossed asymmetry of the manifestation of the polydactyly (py) gene effect on various levels of selection breeding for maximum expressivity in the mouse;

4.) side preference in the occurrence of spontaneous polydactylism in a subline of the inbred strain C57BL and in py-heterozygotes of the mouse;

5.) bilateral differences without side preference in the realization of preaxial polydactylism in +/+ mouse embryos treated on day 10 with TEM or cyclophosphamide, but side preference in equally treated +/py-embryos.

Table 1:

Genotype of treated animals	Number of polydactylous animals with side preference: unlike py-mutant	like py-mutant
+/+	13	15
+/py	13	48

Side preference of polydactylism after cyclophosphamide (Endoxan) treatment on day 10 of gestation.

ACKNOWLEDGEMENTS

This work was supported by grants from the Deutsche Forschungsgemeinschaft to the Sonderforschungsbereich 29, Berlin. The experiments were performed in part with equipment lent by the Kultusministerium Baden-Württemberg.

The authors are indebted to Mrs. B. STEYN for translation of the manuscript, Mrs. J. KLEIN-FRIEDRICH for layout and typing, Dr. B. GROVER for useful criticism, Mrs. L. BECKER and Mrs. A. KLEIN-GABSKY for drawing the figures and to Mrs. I. WOLFF for photographic work.

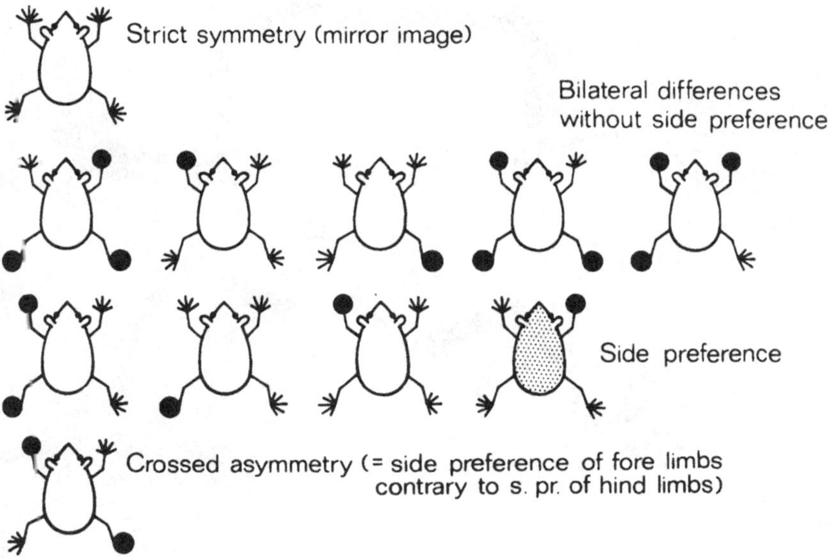

Fig. 1: Possibilities of the realization of limb malformations with regard to the sagittal plane of tetrapods. Lines 1 to 4 illustrate the distribution patterns I to IV in the text. Identical formation of preaxial polydactylism in the 4 limbs (first line) is a hypothetic case. Black circles (2nd to bottom line) indicate limbs which are malformed in a defined manner.
Dotted mouse: exception to the rule.

Fig. 2:

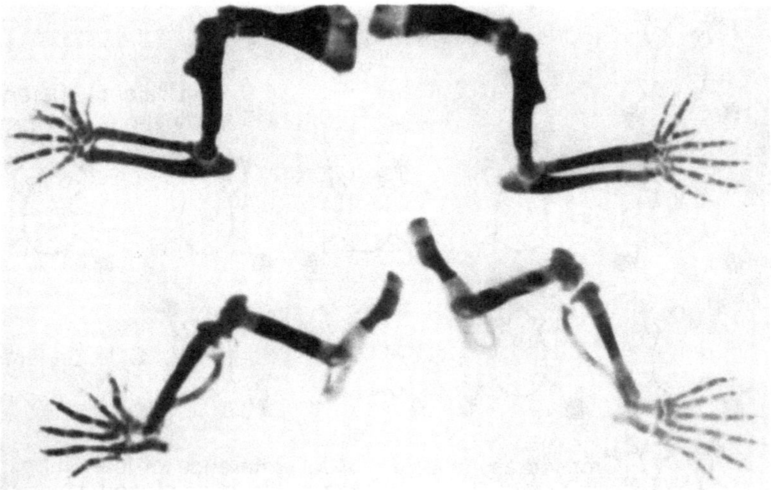

Fig. 3:

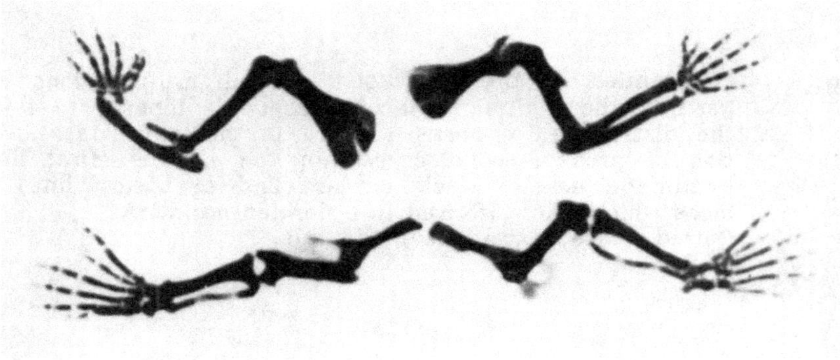

Figures 2 and 3: Limbs and girdles of polydactyly (py/py) mice (double stained whole mounts from 18 day fetuses) exhibiting polydactylism at high levels of expressivity. Note duplication of the 2nd ray in the left hand in Fig. 2 and hypoplasia of the left radius in Fig. 3.

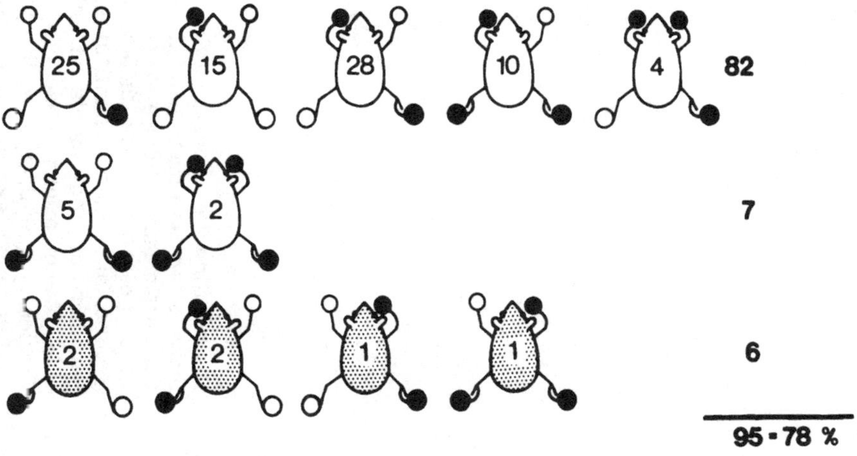

Fig. 4: Distribution of secondary preaxial reductions of the zeugopod and autopod after the highest level of expressivity in the + selection line has been reached (number of individuals of all side combinations observed). Empty circles indicate polydactylous autopods on normal zeugopods, black circles polydactylous autopods (with secondary reductions) on hemimelic zeugopods. First line: asymmetrical combinations with py side preference, second line: symmetrical combinations, third line (dotted mice): asymmetrical combinations, not in agreement with py side preference.

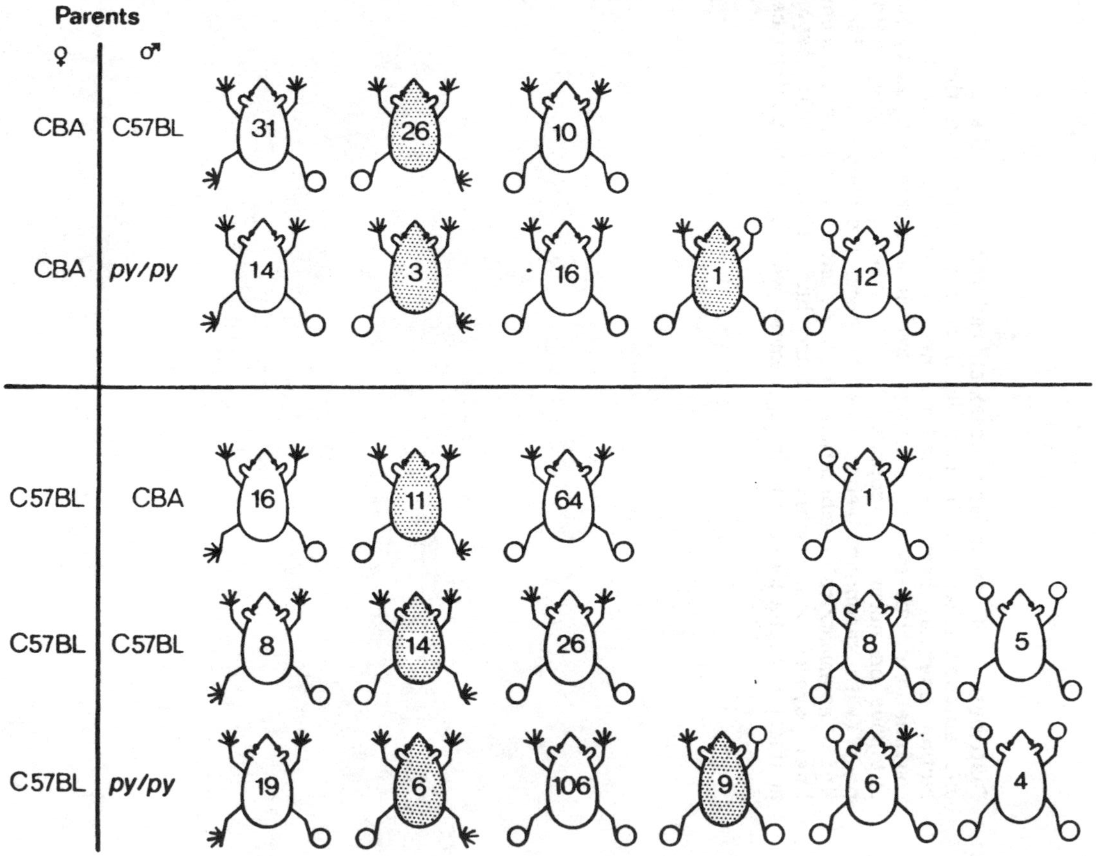

Fig. 5:

Distribution of polydactylous limbs after treatment with triethylenemelamine (TEM) on day 10 of gestation in the different groups of genetic constitution (number of individuals of all side combinations observed). Circles = polydactylous limbs. Dotted mice: exceptions to the py-rule of side preference.

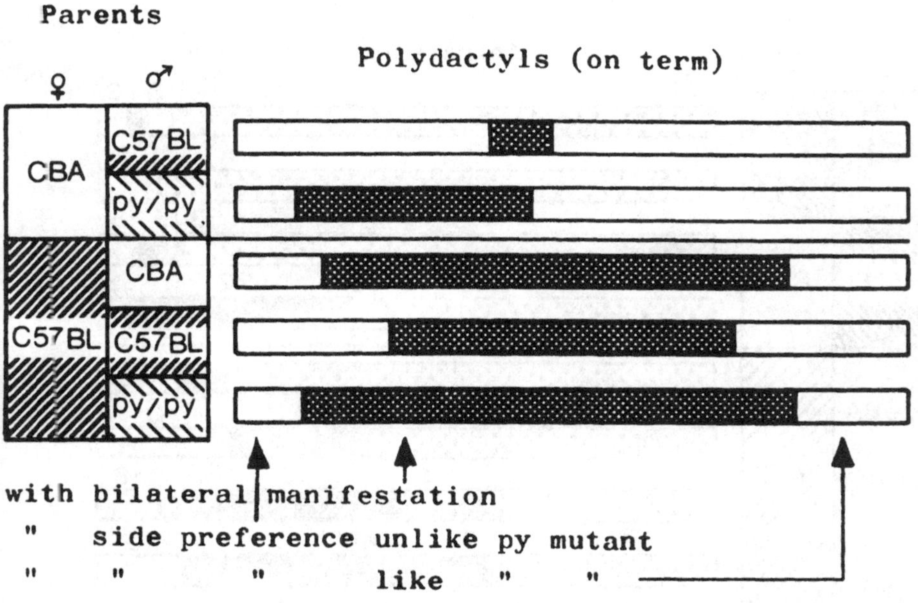

Fig. 6: Proportions of polydactyls with bilateral manifestation (cross hatching), side preference like py-mutant and side preference unlike py-mutant after TEM treatment on day 10 of gestation. The total of polydactyls of each type of cross is put equal to 100% (total length of bars).

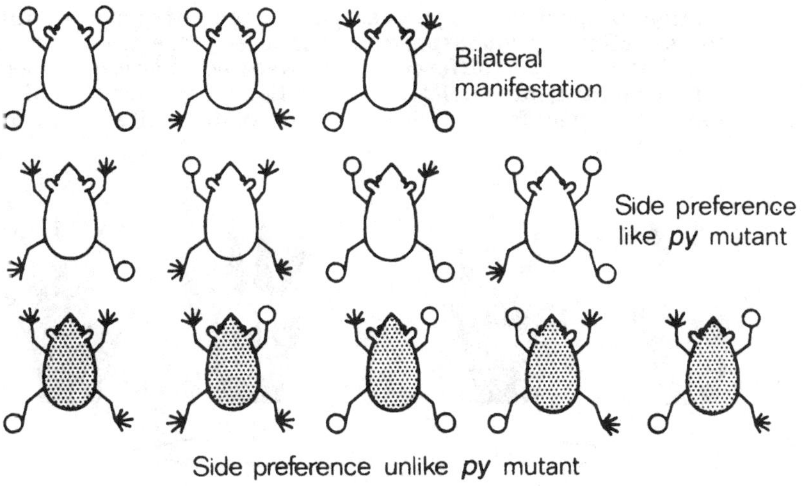

Fig. 7: Manifestation of polydactylism after treatment with cyclophosphamide (Endoxan) on day 10 of gestation. Circles = polydactylous limbs. For percentage and numbers see Fig. 8.

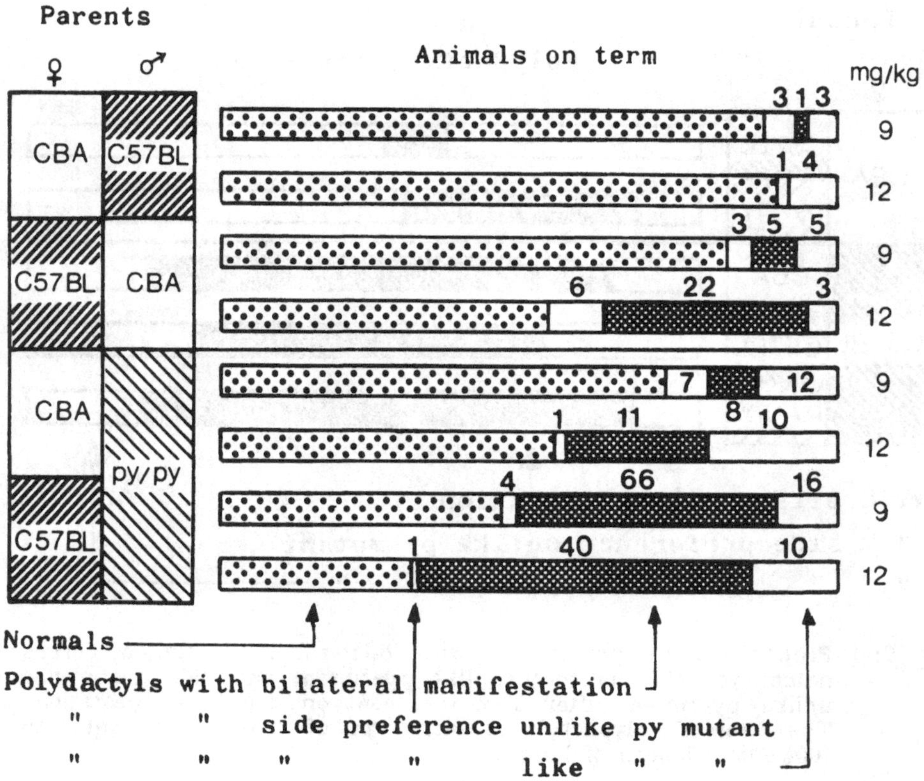

Fig. 8: Relative proportion of polydactyls in the offspring of different crosses after cyclophosphamide (Endoxan) treatment on day 10 of gestation. Two different doses were administered to each genetic constitution. Relative proportions and number of individuals are given for the different modes of manifestation of polydactylism.

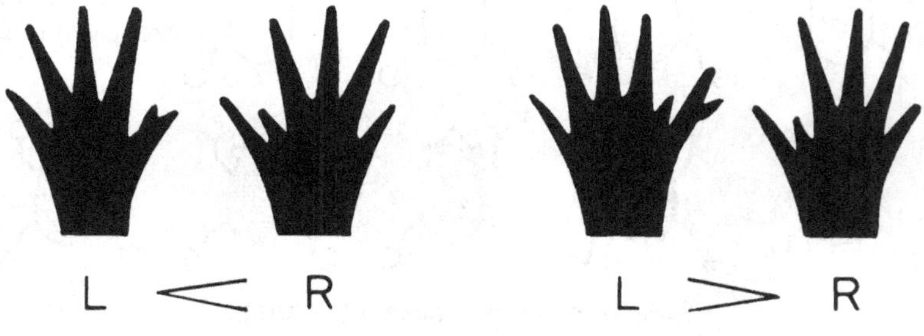

Fig. 9: Schematic representation of two pairs of hind limbs with bilateral manifestation of polydactylism showing different degrees of expressivity (right side preference, left side preference) after cyclophosphamide (Endoxan) treatment on day 10 of gestation.

REFERENCES

Castro-Correia, J., Sousa-Nunes, A., Silva-Bacelar, A., 1974, Teratogenic action of acetazolamide in mice, Teratology, 10, 221 - 226.

Green, M.C., Azar, C.A., Maren, T.H., 1973, Strain differences in susceptibility to the teratogenic effect of acetazolamide in mice. Teratology, 8, 143 - 146.

Grüneberg, H., 1963, The Pathology of Development, Blackwell Scientific Publications, Oxford.

Kocher, W., 1967, Genetisch und chemisch verursachte praeaxiale Polydactylie bei der Maus, Verh. Dtsch. Zool. Ges., Göttingen 1966, Zool. Anz., Suppl. 30, 412 - 422.

Kocher, W., 1969, Die Wirkungsmuster des Triäthylenmelamin (TEM) und ihre Behandlungsphasen-Spezifität während der Organogenese des Hühnerkeimes. I. Veränderungen der Körpermaße, der äußeren Form und der Oberflächenstrukturen, Wilh. Roux's Arch. Entwickl. Mech. Org., 162, 161 - 196.

Kocher, W., 1970, Die Wirkungsmuster des Triäthylenmelamin (TEM) und ihre Behandlungsphasen-Spezifität während der Organogenese des Hühnerkeimes. II. Veränderungen des knorpeligen Primordialskelettes der Extremitäten und des Rumpfes, Wilh. Roux's Arch. Entwickl. Mech. Org., 165, 53 - 86.

Kocher, W., 1972, Chemoteratologisch-genetische Experimente zur Gestaltungsanalyse der Wirbeltierextremität, Rev. suisse Zool., (Suppl.), 79, 153 - 164.

Kocher, W., 1977, Action and interaction of chemical and genetic factors in teratogenesis of the limb, in: "Morphogenesis and Malformation of the Limb", Birth Defects, 13, 1 - 18.

Kocher-Becker, U., Kocher, W., Merker, H.-J., 1978, Morphogenetic effects of the pentosanpolysulfoester SP54 on the chick embryo, in: "Role of Pharmacokinetics in Prenatal and Perinatal Toxicology", Third Symposium on Prenatal Development, Berlin 1978, Georg Thieme Publ., Stuttgart, pp. 595 - 610.

Layton, W.M. Jr., Hallesy, D.W., 1965, Deformity of forelimb in rats: association with high doses of acetazolamide, Science, 149, 306 - 308.

Wilson, J.G., Maren, T.H., Takano, K., Ellison, A., 1968, Teratogenic action of carbonic anhydrase inhibitors in the rat, Teratology, 1, 51 - 60.

Willert, H.-G., Henkel, H.-L., 1969, Klinik und Pathologie der Dysmelie, Springer-Verlag, Berlin, Heidelberg, New York.

Immunofluorescent Microscopic Investigations of Intercellular Substances during Limb Development

H.-J. Barrach, K. Grundmann, N. Hinz, A. Felies

Institut für Toxikologie und Embryonal-Pharmakologie, Freie Universität Berlin, Garystraße 9, D-1000 Berlin 33

INTRODUCTION:

During the development of the extremity of the mammalian embryo, mesenchymal cells differentiate into fibrocytes, chondrocytes, myocytes and bone cells. In the mouse, these events take place during the phase of organogenesis (days 11 to 14). The differentiation process manifests itself first on the cellular level. Cells of the homogeneous mesenchyme change their phenotype and start to produce the same proteins as the adult cells. This involves cell proliferation and presumptive intermediate stages of cells (HOLTZER, 1978; ABBOTT et al., 1974).

In order to discover if a cell has differentiated, one can look for a marker protein produced by the adult cell. We choose to purify those proteins and to raise antibodies against them. With this tool, it is possible to follow the differentiation process and we hope to detect the mechanism of malformation caused by specific drugs.

METHODS:

Table 1 summarizes the marker proteins used in this study and their origin. For the source of type II collagen and the chondroitin sulfate proteoglycans, we used the SWARM rat chondrosarcoma (SMITH et al., 1975). For the isolation of type II collagen, we followed the method described by SMITH (SMITH et al., 1975). Proteoglycans were isolated according to HASCALL and HEINEGARD (1975), HEINEGARD (1972), and OEGEMA et al. (1975). Antibodies against link protein were a gift from ROBIN POOL, Montreal (POOL et al., 1980).Type I collagen and procollagen type III were isolated from skin of fetal or newborn mice. Type I collagen was extracted and purified according to the method described by BORNSTEIN and PIEZ (1966), and MILLER et al. (1967). Procollagen type III was prepared as described by SMITH et al. (1977), GRUNDMANN (1979), and TIMPL et al. (1975). The source of type IV collagen was human placenta. For methods, see SAGE et al. (1979) and GLANVILLE et al. (1979). The glycoprotein laminin was extracted and purified from a transplantable ENGELBERT-HOLM-SWARM sarcoma grown intramuscularly in NMRI mice (TIMPL et al., 1979). The proteoglycan BM1 was also prepared from this tumor (HASSELL et al., 1980). All these proteins except BM1 were proven to be pure by sodium dodecyl sulfate (SDS) polyacrylamide gel electrophoresis.

The procedure, starting with the antigen and resulting in a specifically stained picture, is demonstrated in Table 2. The antigens (500 µg) were suspended in 50 µl phosphate buffered saline (PBS) and mixed with 50 µl complete FREUND'S adjuvant. These mixtures were injected directly into

Teratology of the Limbs

the surgically exposed lymph node of the hind limb of rabbits. For booster injections, the proper antigen (500 µg) was mixed with incomplete FREUND'S adjuvant. These injections were given three times - after three, six and nine weeks - into the same lymph node of the previously operated upon leg. The lymph node was easy to palpate at this stage.

After the second booster injection, the animals were bled weekly from the ear. The titer and the specificity of the antibodies in the sera were tested by ELISA assay (GOSSLAU and BARRACH, 1979). Sera with high specific titers were purified by cross immunoadsorption on antigen bound SEPHAROSE 4B columns (CUATRECASAS, 1970; v. d. MARK et al., 1976). The ELISA assays and the immunofluorescence blocking studies showed that the purified antibodies reacted only with the specific antigen and did not cross-react with other antigens.

For the staining, we used the so-called "sandwich" technique. First, frozen sections were incubated with the specific antibody. After washing off the non-reactant antibodies, in a second step, we incubated the section with anti-IgG antibodies which were labeled with fluorescein isothiocyanate (FITC). For the observation of the staining, we used a ZEISS fluorescence microscope.

RESULTS:

In a previous paper, we have reported studies on the development of the long bone with respect to cartilage and bone formation (BARRACH and ANGERMANN, 1977). We used antibodies against type I and type II collagen. In this report, we will present some data we have obtained by using antibodies against the collagen types I, II, pro III, IV, cartilage specific proteoglycans, link protein, the glycoprotein laminin, and the basement membrane proteoglycan, BM1.

We put several pictures together to show the entire front limb of the mouse. Figures 1 through 4 show serial sections cut from the front limb of a day 18 mouse. The staining with the antibodies against type I collagen, type II collagen, procollagen type III and proteoglycan allow a comparison of the protein components in different tissue structures. Type I collagen antibodies stain the bone anlagen of the humerus, ulna and radius (Fig. 1). The periost and the periostal bone sheath and the enchondral bone trabeculae show a strong fluorescence. Here, the tendons are stained with type I antibodies, but some tendons, membranes and aponeuroses also stain with other antibodies besides type I collagen. One example of those is the membrana interossea between the radius and ulna (see below, Figs. 2 and 4). The perichondrium reacts with the type I antibodies while the cartilage shows no staining.

The perichondrium and the periost contain type III collagen (Fig. 2). We also have evidence that the periostal bone sheath has some type III collagen (see also Fig. 13), and at this stage of development, day 18 of gestation, the tendon and again the membrana interossea are stained. The region of cartilage and the enchondral bone did not react with the type III antibodies. By comparing the staining in Figs. 1 and 2, more and different structures can be seen to be stained with procollagen type III antibodies. The perimysium and the fasciae of the muscles and also the corium and the subcutis of the skin are stained. This result is in agreement with biochemical data (e.g., SMITH et al., 1977) that fetal skin contains high amounts of type III collagen.

Type II collagen antibodies stained only the cartilaginous parts of the bone anlagen (Fig. 3). At day 18 of gestation, the staining is limited to the proximal and distal extremes of the long bones. The calcified cartilage in the hypertrophic zone shows good reaction with the antibodies.

The cartilage-specific proteoglycans are other specific markers for chondroblasts or chondrocytes (Fig. 4). Prior to the reaction with the antibodies, there was no pretreatment of the frozen sections with an enzyme. Mainly, the cartilaginous parts of the bone anlagen are stained. In addition, again the membrana interossea between the radius and ulna and some other tendons are stained. We know that the antibodies are directed against the core protein of large chondroitin sulfate proteoglycan monomers and here, preferentially, against the hook region which attaches this molecule to the hyaluronic acid. The reaction of these antibodies in those structures of tendons, membranes or aponeuroses needs some more investigation. These structures show no metachromatic staining which would appear when normal chondroitin sulfate proteoglycans are present.

The figures 5 through 7 show sections from skeletal muscle in higher magnification which are stained with different antibodies. Staining results show that it is possible to differentiate between structures as close as the reticulin fibers around the muscle cells and the basement membranes with a light microscope. Procollagen type III antibodies stain the collagen fibers around the cells in the sarcolemma and the fibers in the perimysium (cross section, Fig. 5 a). The myotubes inside are not stained (longitudinal section, Fig. 5 b).

Collagen type IV (Figs. 6 a and b) and also the glycoprotein laminin (Figs. 7 a and b) and the preoteoglycan BM1 (not shown) are constituents of basement membranes. The antibodies against these substances stain the sarcolemma and the basal membranes of blood vessels in these sections. In the longitudinal sections 6 b and 7 b, there is some staining inside the myotubes. The drawing of a myotube explains this finding (Fig. 8). The sarcolemma forms a tranversal tube system and sections through these structures give the impression of staining inside the myotubes.

Antibodies against the glycoprotein laminin in a cross section (Fig. 7 a) and in a longitudinal section (Fig. 7 b) show the same staining patterns as the type IV collagen staining. Comparing the procollagen type III staining (Fig. 5) with the laminin staining, one can see the distribution of the reticulin fibers - type III collagen - and the basement membrane component - laminin - in the sarcolemma.

The first section from mouse skin day 18 shows unspecific staining with antibodies against type II collagen (Fig. 9). The cornified epithelium has a high affinity to the FITC-labeled anti-rabbit antibodies. There is no other structure stained with collagen type II antibodies.

Type I collagen is found in the corium and subcutis of the skin (Fig. 10). The "holes" are cross sections of hair follicles. Procollagen type III antibodies stain the same structures of the skin (Fig. 11). Collagen type I and type III are in the same locations. This technique does not allow the quantification of the amount of collagen (in this case, type I and type III collagen). It is only possible to show the existence and the distribution of the protein in tissue sections.

The antibodies against BM1, laminin and type IV collagen visualize the structures containing basement membranes. The basement membrane under-the epithelium, under the endothelium of the blood vessels, and around muscle cells are stained. In this section which is stained with antibodies against the basement membrane proteoglycan BM1, one can see in addition the basement membrane of the hair follicle and hair papilla and sweat glands (Fig. 12).

The following pictures show some sections from the region of the enchondral ossification in the humerus of a day 18 mouse. As was also seen in the first immunofluorescent picture (Fig. 1), type I antibodies indicate the type I collagen in the periost, periostal bone, and the enchondral bone (Fig. 13). Type III staining is missing in the trabeculae of the bone, but there is staining in the periostal bone sheath, in the periost, and in the perichondrium (Fig. 14). There is a distinct difference between enchondral and periostal bone formation. The enchondral bone contains type I collagen only, whereas the periostal bone stains with antibodies against type I collagen and procollagen type III. The cartilage stains specific with type II collagen antibodies (Fig. 15). After treatment with hyaluronidase, there is no difference in the intensity of staining in the different areas of the cartilaginous bone anlage. The type II collagen is present in the hypertrophic cartilage which undergoes calcification and also in the first bone trabeculae.

The staining of the cartilage with the antibodies against chondroitinsulfate proteoglycan monomers was of interest because it was reported that in the region of hypertrophic cartilage the amount of large proteoglycan aggregates shifts to small aggregates and non-aggregating forms of small proteoglycans (KUETTNER et al., 1975). This is thought to be connected with the calcification in this hypertrophic cartilage. In vitro experiments of BLUMENTHAL et al. (1979) showed that cartilage proteoglycan A_1-fraction (aggregates) and proteoglycan D_1-fraction (monomers) were inhibiting the hydroxyapatite formation. These authors postulated that breakdown of the aggregates into subunits is not sufficient to allow the hypertrophic cartilage to calcify there has to be a decrease in the proteoglycan concentration. Proteoglycan antibodies were found to stain the region of calcified cartilage and one can find these proteoglycans along with type II collagen also in the first bone trabeculae (Fig. 16). This method shows the presence of the complete core protein of the proteoglycans. The cartilage stained uniformly through the cartilage in the proliferative area and in the calcified hypertrophic area. If there are smaller non-aggregating proteoglycans (KUETTNER et al., 1975), or a decreased concentration of cartilage specific proteoglycans in the calcified cartilage (BLUMENTHAL et al., 1979) compared to the proliferative area, one would expect a weaker staining. However, it is possible that a lower concentration of the proteoglycans in the calcified cartilage is compensated for by the fact that these proteoglycans are more reactant with the antibodies than in other parts of the cartilage.

Treating the frozen section with chondroitinase ABC removes some PG staining from the lacunae and exposes the PG in the cartilage matrix to the antibodies (Fig. 17). The distribution and the intensity of the staining throughout the cartilage look very much like the type II collagen staining (Fig. 15). Another evidence that this proteoglycan is present in the calcified cartilage is the staining result with the antibodies against link protein (Fig. 18). So far, there is no doubt that there is core protein and link protein to hook the proteoglycans to hyaluronic acid along with type II collagen in the calcified cartilage.

With the aid of these antibodies, we now have a good knowledge of the development of the skeleton of the extremities of the mouse from day 13 until after birth. We are in the process of overcoming technical problems in cutting frozen sections of the early stages days 10 to 13 of gestation. These stages are the most sensitive to many drugs inducing abnormalities of the limb. With these sections of treated and untreated limbs, it will be possible to follow the differentiation process (Table 3) from the mesenchymal cells into chondroblasts, osteoblasts, or fibroblasts by the detection of the newly-formed proteins.

Table 1: Listing of the marker proteins and their origin. These proteins were used to raise antibodies in rabbits.

TISSUE	MARKER PROTEIN	ORIGINATES FROM
CARTILAGE	TYPE II COLLAGEN	RAT CHONDROSARCOMA
	LARGE CHONDROITINSULFATE PROTEOGLYCANS	RAT CHONDROSARCOMA
	LINK	BOVINE NASAL CARTILAGE (GIFT FROM ROBIN POOL, MONTREAL)
BONE	TYPE I COLLAGEN	FETAL MOUSE SKIN
	PRO TYPE III COLLAGEN	FETAL MOUSE SKIN
MUSCLE	TYPE I COLLAGEN	FETAL MOUSE SKIN
(FASCIAE)	PRO TYPE III COLLAGEN	FETAL MOUSE SKIN
	TYPE IV COLLAGEN	HUMAN PLACENTA
	LAMININ	EH - SARCOMA (MOUSE) (ENGELBERT-HOLM-SARCOMA)
	B M I	EH - SARCOMA (MOUSE)
TENDON	TYPE I COLLAGEN	FETAL MOUSE SKIN
LIGAMENTS	PRO TYPE III COLLAGEN	FETAL MOUSE SKIN
MEMBRANES	LARGE CHONDROITINSULFATE PROTEOGLYCANS	RAT CHONDROSARCOMA
BASEMENT MEMBRANES	TYPE IV COLLAGEN	HUMAN PLACENTA
	LAMININ	EH - SARCOMA (MOUSE)
	B M I	EH - SARCOMA (MOUSE)

Table 2: Proteins were isolated from adult tissues and tested for purity. The protein preparations were then injected into rabbits after mixing with complete Freund's adjuvants. After the second booster injection, the animals were bled and the sera were tested for antibodies against the injected protein with the ELISA assay. In order to purify the antibodies, the serum was passed over a series of antigen columns to remove cross-reacting antibodies, and, in the last step, the antibodies were bound to the specific antigen. Antibody preparations with the highest specific titer were used to stain 6 - 8 μ cryostat sections.

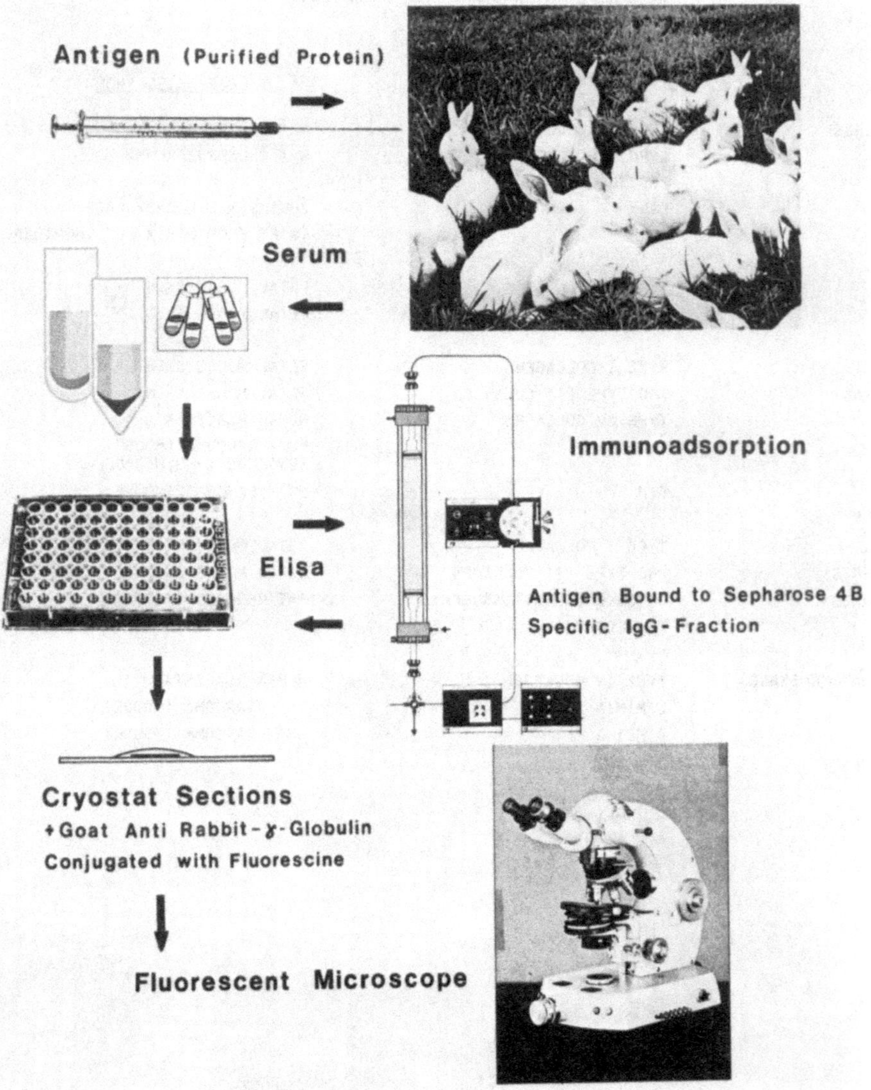

Table 3: Differentiation of mesenchymal cells into tissue specific cells of cartilage, bone, muscle and tendons. The cell specific proteins can be detected by specific antibodies in tissue sections or by ELISA assay.

CARTILAGE		
MESENCHYMAL CELLS	CHONDROBLASTS	TYPE II COLLAGEN PROTEOGLYCANS
BONE		
MESENCHYMAL CELLS	OSTEOBLASTS	TYPE I COLLAGEN (TYPE III COLLAGEN)
MUSCLE (FASCIAE)		
MESENCHYMAL CELLS	MYOBLASTS FIBROBLASTS	TYPE I COLLAGEN PRO TYPE III COLLAGEN TYPE IV COLLAGEN LAMININ B M I
TENDONS, LIGAMENTS, MEMBRANES		
MESENCHYMAL CELLS	FIBROBLASTS	TYPE I COLLAGEN PRO TYPE III COLLAGEN PROTEOGLYCANS

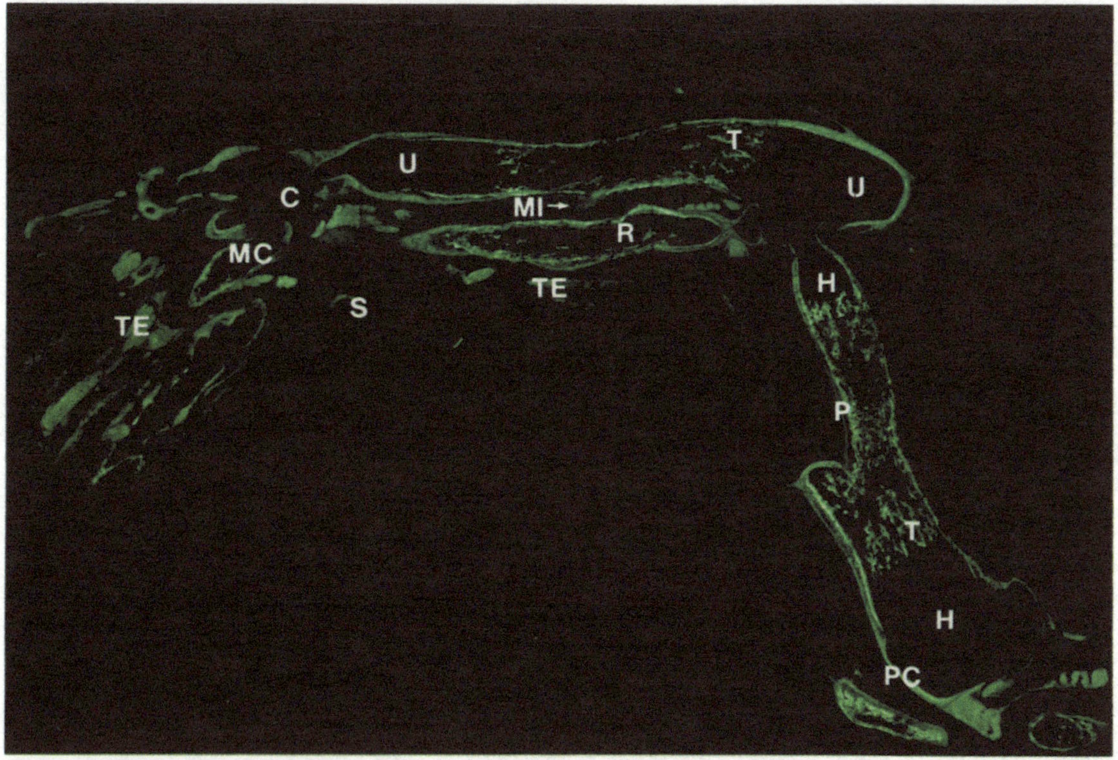

Fig. 1: The section from the front limb of a day 18 mouse. For the immunohistological staining, highly purified antibodies against type I collagen were used. Only structures containing type I collagen show strong fluorescence. The bone trabeculae (T) of the humerus (H), ulna (U), and radius (R); the periost (P) and perichondrium (PC) of these bone anlagen; the perichondrium of the carpals (C) and metacarpals (MC) of the hand; the tendons (TE); and the skin (S) are stained. The cartilaginous parts of the bone anlagen show no staining. Membrana interossea (MI). x 18.

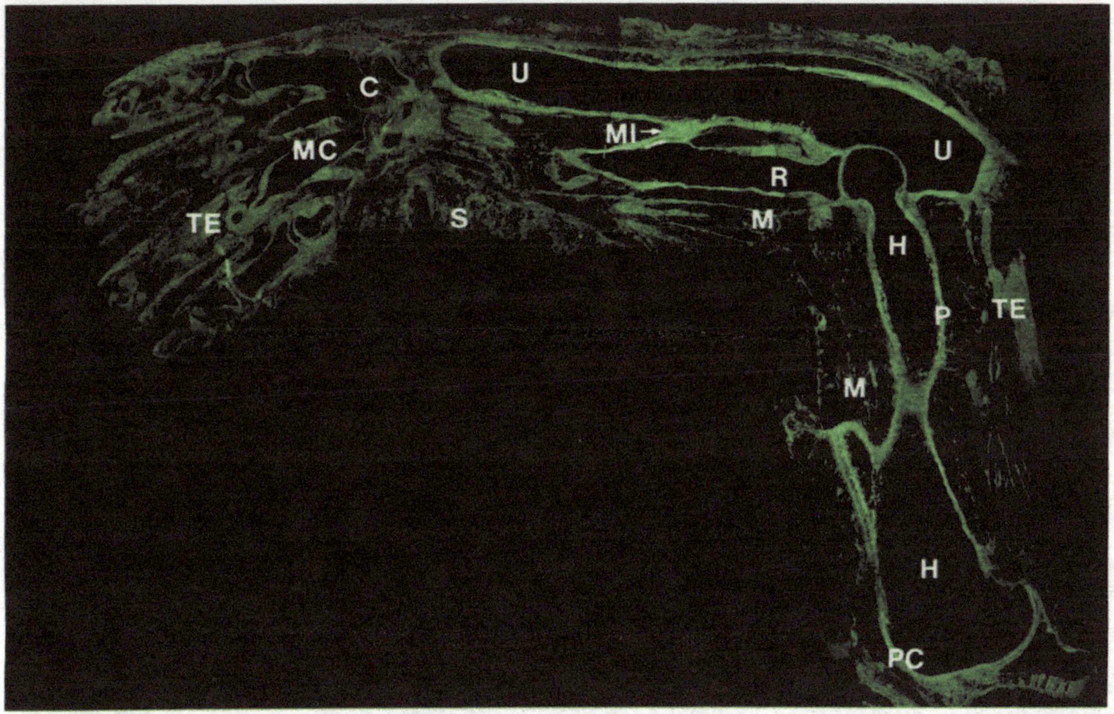

Fig. 2: An adjacent section was stained with type III procollagen antibodies. The periost (P) and the perichondrium (PC) of the long bones, the carpals (C) and the metacarpals (MC) are stained. The tendons (TE), fasciae of the muscles (M) and the corium of the skin show strong fluorescence. Membrana interossea (MI). x 18.

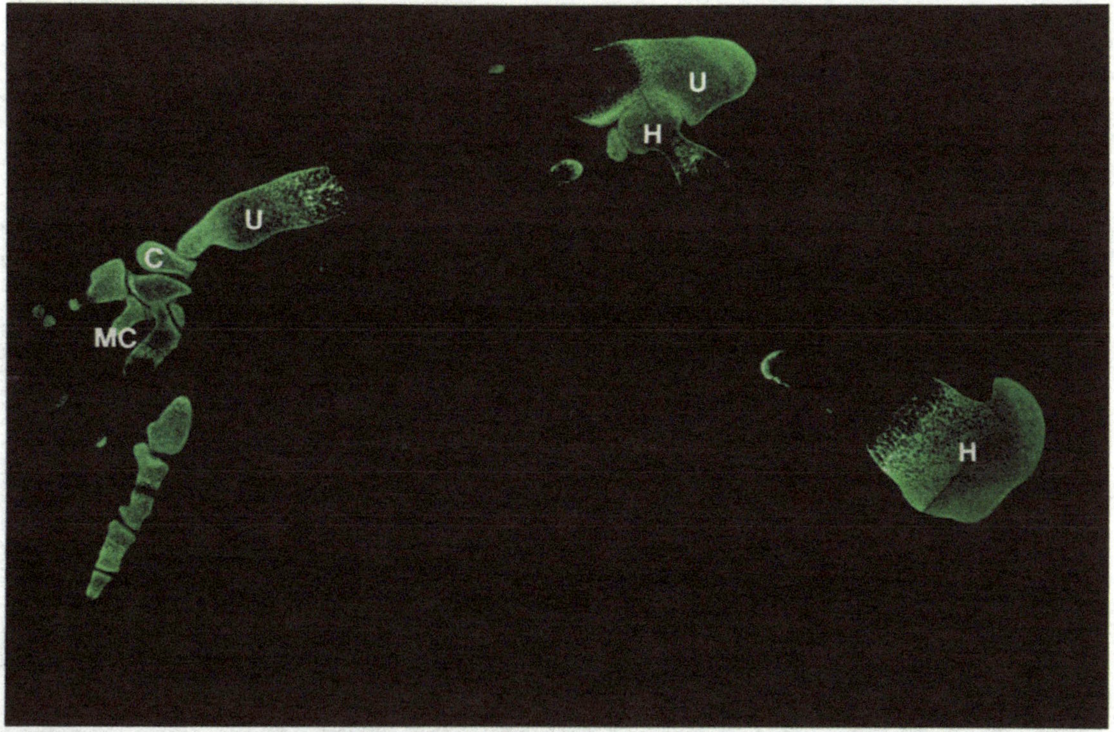

Fig. 3: Only the cartilaginous extremes of the long bone anlagen [humerus (H) and ulna (U)], the carpals (C), metacarpals (MC), and phalanges are stained with type II collagen antibodies. x 18.

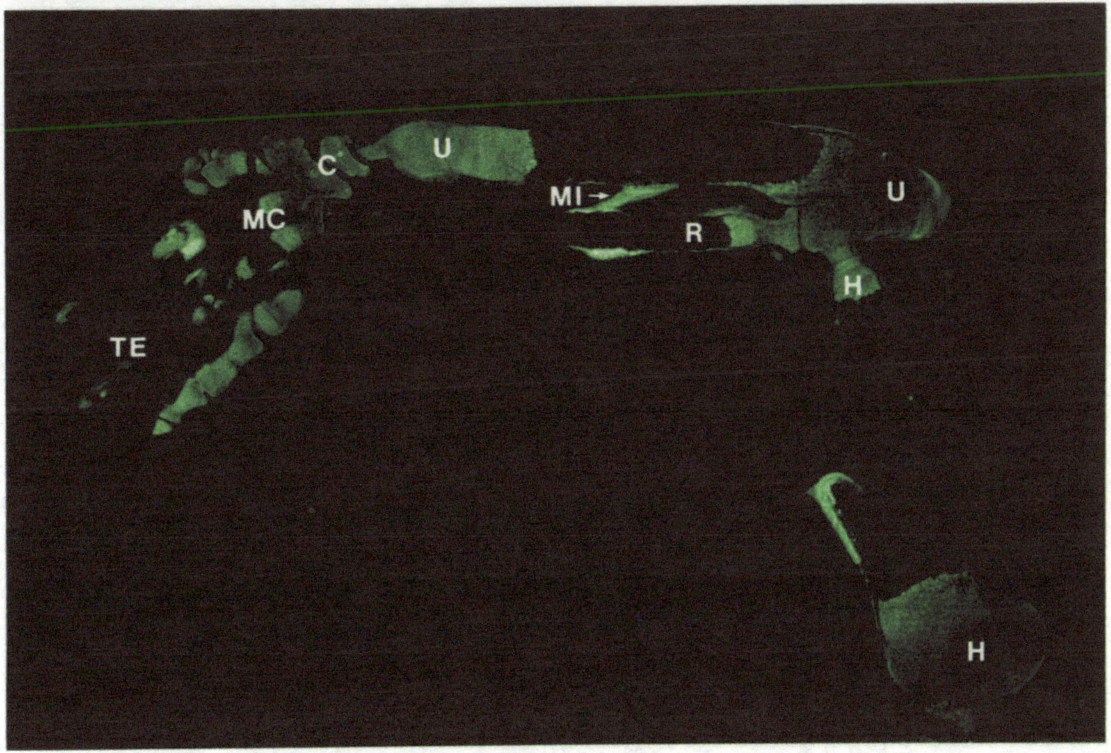

Fig. 4: A similar section from the forelimb shows the staining with antibodies against the monomer proteoglycan isolated from cartilage of the rat chondrosarcoma. The frozen section is not enzyme treated prior to the antibody reaction. The staining is in the cartilage of the bone anlagen, preferentially in the lacunae of the cartilage cells, in some tendons (TE) and in the membrana interossea (MI). x 18.

Fig. 5: Sections of skeletal muscle from a day 18 mouse stained with antibodies against procollagen type III. The staining is located around the myotubes (MY) in the reticulin fibers: endomysium (EN), in the perimysium (PE), and connective tissue septum (CO)
a. Cross section,
b. Longitudinal section.
x 200.

Fig. 6: Similar section stained with collagen type IV antibodies. The surrounding membrane - the sarcolemma (SA) of the muscle cells is stained, but not the perimysium. In addition, membranes of the blood vessels (BL) are stained.
a. Cross section,
b. Longitudinal section with staining of the transversal tube system.
x 200.

Fig. 7: Antibodies against laminin indicate the distribution of this glycoprotein in the membranes of the myotubes (MY). The staining results are comparable with those in Fig. 6 stained with collagen type IV.
a. Cross section,
b. Longitudinal section.
x 200.

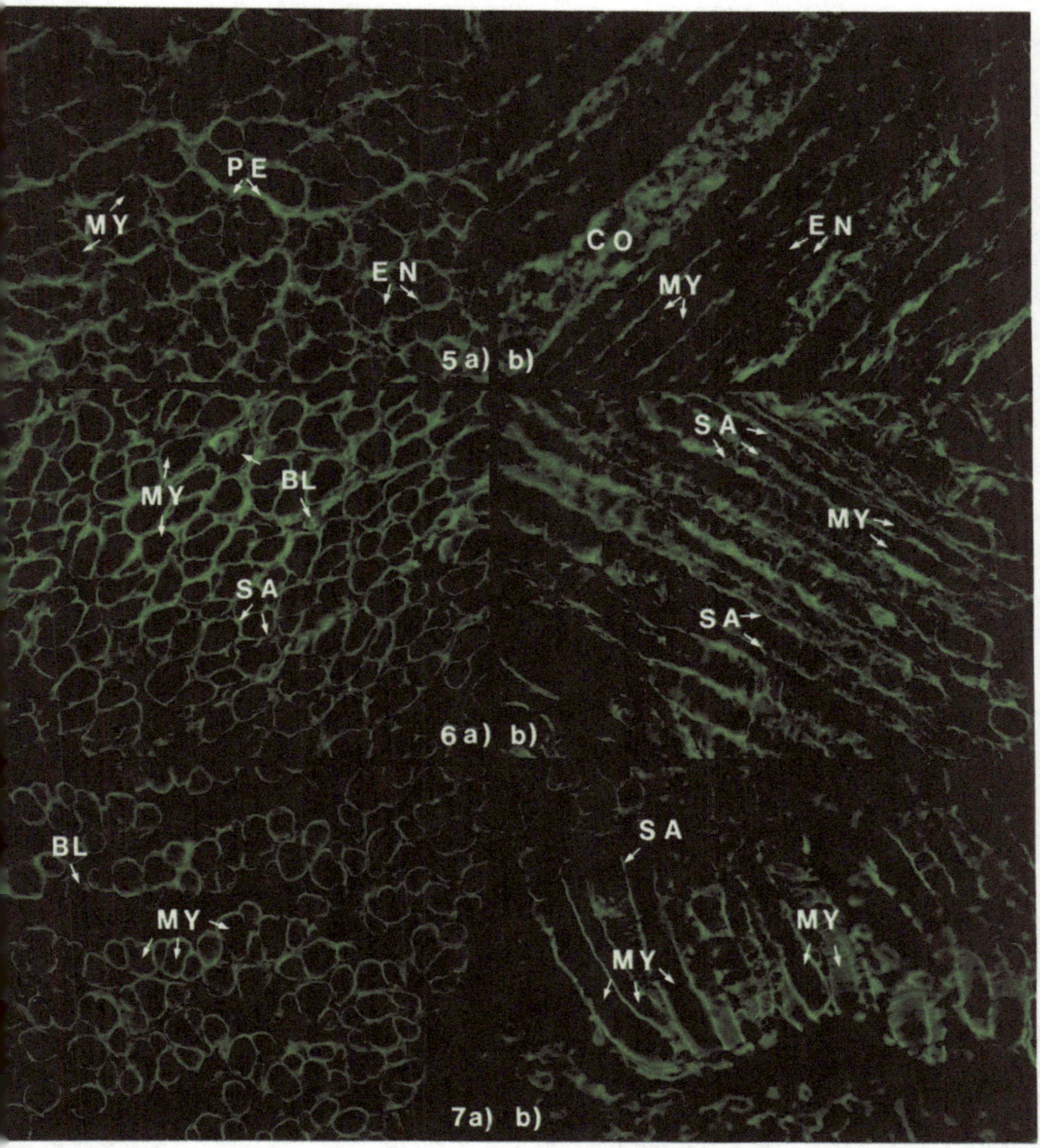
PE
MY
EN
CO
EN
MY
5 a)
b)
MY
BL
SA
SA
MY
SA
6 a)
b)
BL
MY
SA
MY
MY
7a)
b)

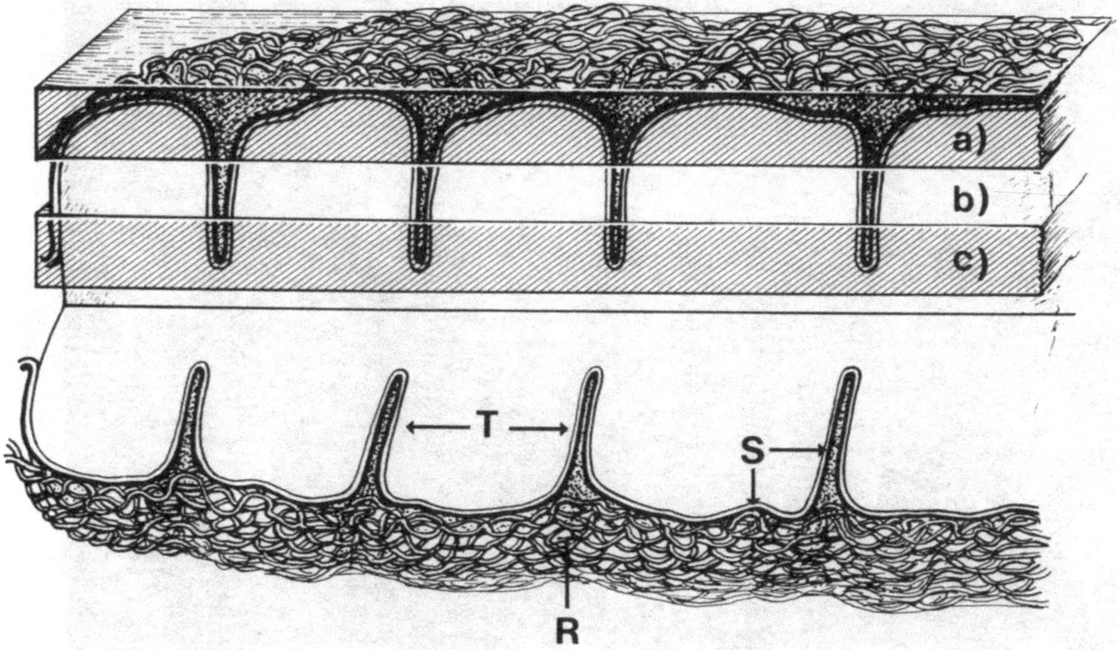

Fig. 8: This drawing shows the possible longitudinal section through the myotubes. After staining with different antibodies the sections show:

a. riticulin fibers (R) and sarcolemma (S),
b. sarcolemma of the transversal tube system (T),
c. the same structures as (b) or no structures inside the myotube.

Fig 9: Section from the skin of a day 18 mouse, stained with type II collagen antibodies. Only the cornified upper layer of the epithelium (E) picked up some unspecific staining. x 110.

Fig. 9 Fig. 10

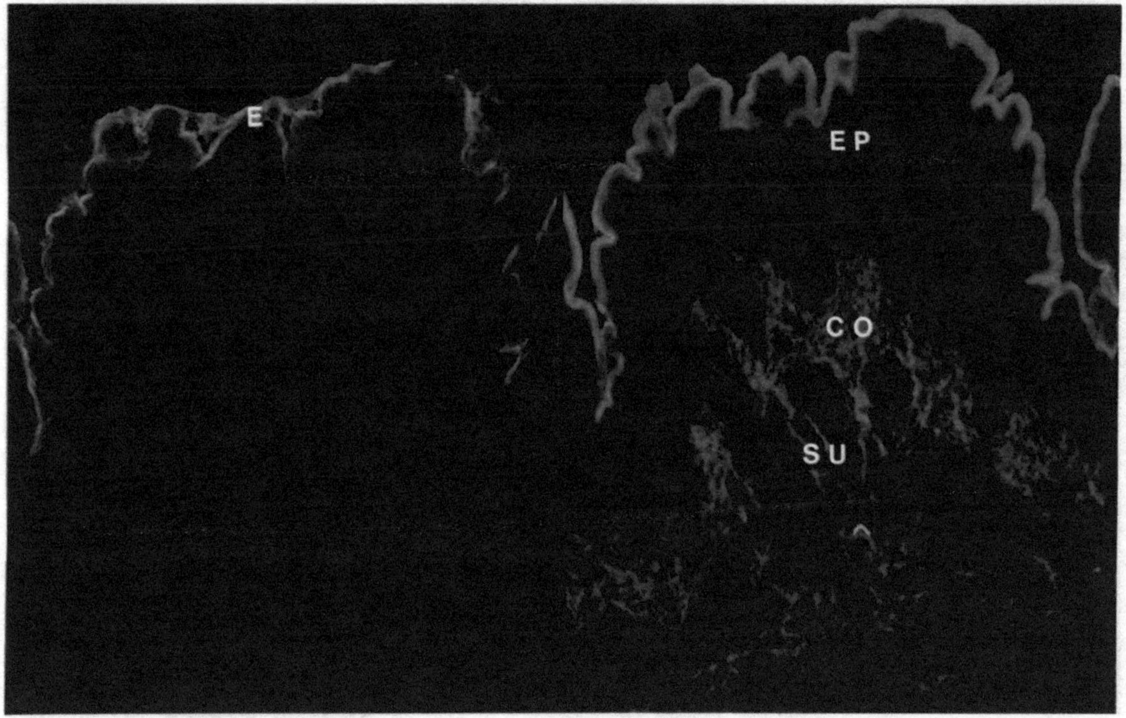

Fig. 10: In the very next section from the same area of skin, type I collagen antibodies were used for staining. There is fluorescence in the skin starting under the epidermis (EP) in the chorium (CO), and subcutaneous (SU) tissue.
x 110.

Fig. 11: This section of mouse skin was incubated with antibodies against type III procollagen. The same structures as in Fig. 10 show specific staining: epidermis (EP); corium (CO); subcutis (SU); hair follicle (HF), cross section.
x 110.

Fig. 11

Fig. 12

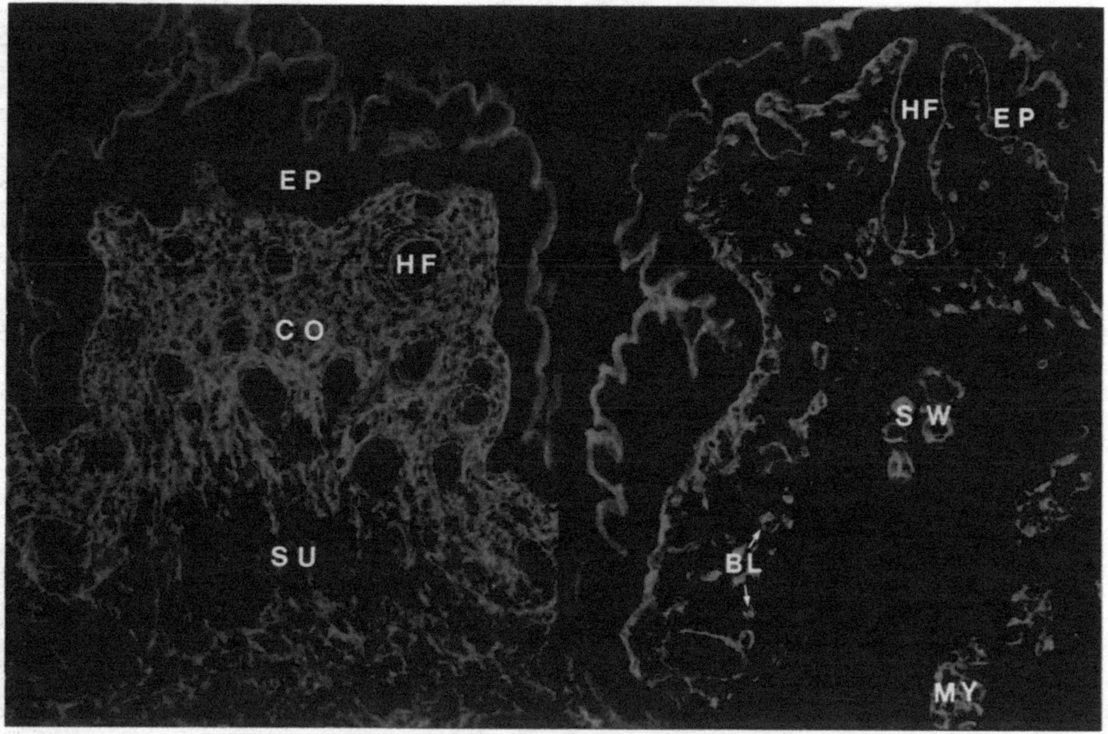

Fig. 12: For the staining with antibodies against basement membrane constituents, this picture shows the staining result when the proteoglycan (BM1) antibodies were used. The membrane under the epidermis (EP), under the endothelia of the blood vessels (BL) and the sweat glands (SW) are strongly stained. The same fluorescence shows around the hair follicles (HF) and myotubes (MY).
x 110.

Figures 13 and 14: Enlargements of the transition zone from cartilage to bone in the humerus of a day 18 mouse.

Fig. 13. Fig. 14.

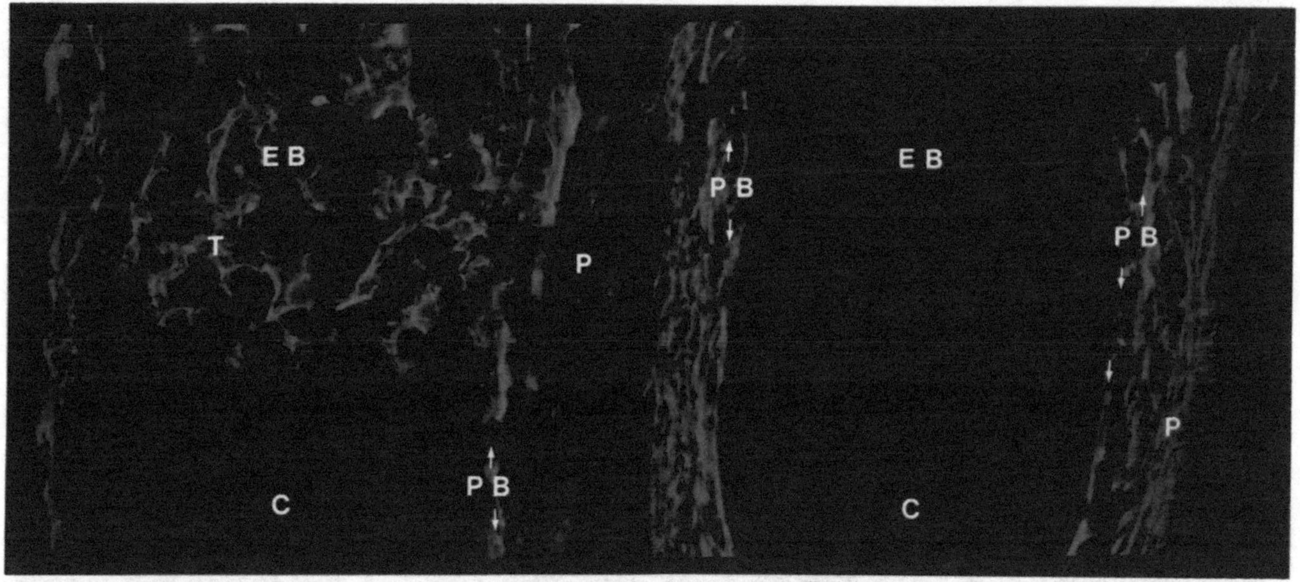

Fig. 13: Antibodies against type I collagen were used to stain this section. The enchondral bone (EB), perichondral bone (PB), and the periost (P) are visible. Bone trabecula (T), cartilage (C). x 110.

Fig. 14: This section shows the staining with antibodies against type III procollagen. There is staining in the periostal bone (PB) and in the periost (P), enchondral bone (EB), cartilage (C). x 110.

Figures 15 and 16 These pictures show sections from the humerus of a day 18 mouse taken from the same region as in Figs. 13 and 14.

Fig. 15. Fig. 16.

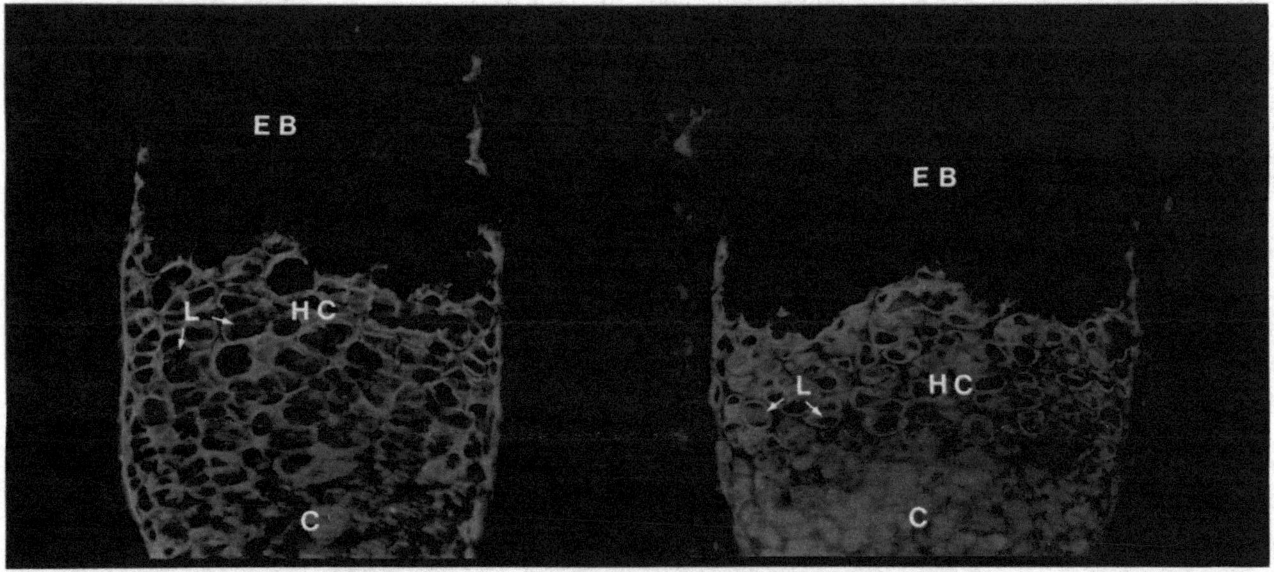

Fig. 15: The frozen section was pretreated with hyaluronidase and then incubated with antibodies against type II collagen. The antibodies stain the cartilaginous part of the transition zone. Cartilage (C), calcified hypertrophic cartilage (HC), lacuna of the hypertrophic cartilage (L), enchondral bone (EB). x 110.

Fig. 16: When stained with antibodies against cartilage specific proteoglycans, the cartilage in the proliferative area and the calcified hypertrophic area (HC) is visible. Most of the staining is in the lacunae (L). This section was not pretreated with an enzyme. x 110.

Figures 17 and 18: Similar sections taken from the humerus in the same region as that shown in the last four figures.

Fig. 17. Fig. 18.

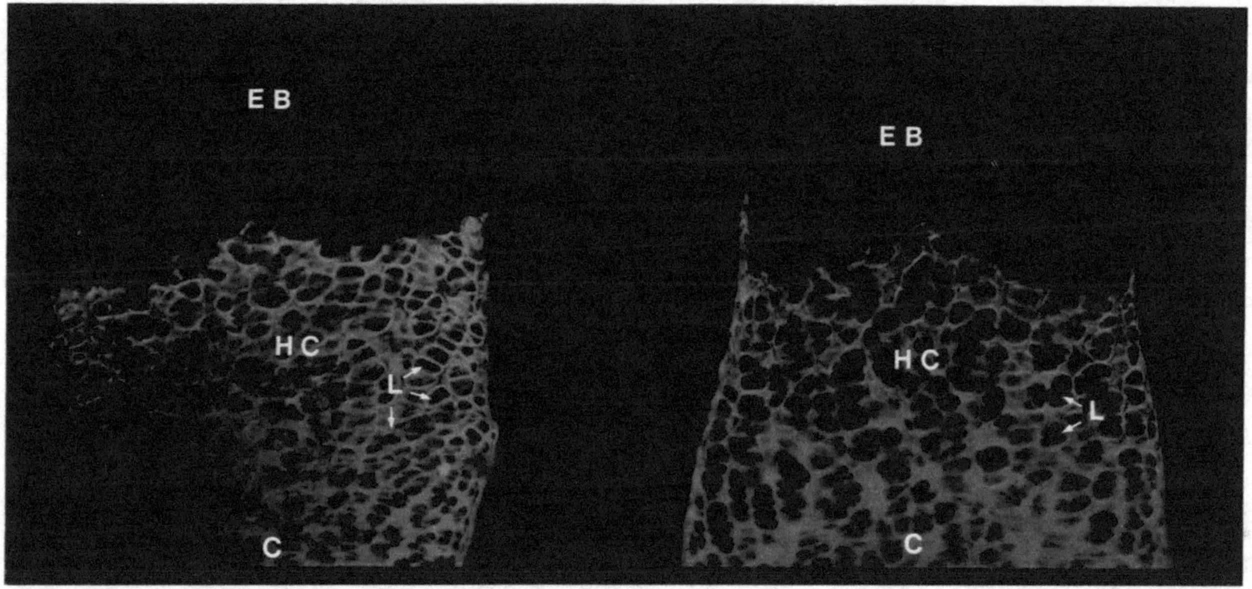

Fig. 17: This section was pretreated with chondroitinase ABC and then incubated with cartilage specific proteoglycan antibodies. Comparing this staining result with the staining in Fig. 16, the matrix preferentially reacted with the antibodies and the lacunae (L) have no staining inside. Cartilage (C), calcified hypertrophic cartilage (HC), enchondral bone (EB). x 110.

Fig.18: The cartilaginous part of this section was stained with antibodies against link protein. After treatment with chondroitinase ABC, the antibodies reacted with the link protein in the matrix of the calcified hypertrophic cartilage (HC) and the proliferative area of the cartilage (C). Enchondral bone (EB). x 110.

REFERENCES

Abbott, J., Schiltz, J., Dienstmann, S., Holtzer, H., 1974, The phenotypic complexity of myogenic clones, Proc. Nat. Acad. Sci., USA, 71, 1506 - 1510.

Barrach, H.-J., Angermann, K., 1977, Immunofluorescence as a tool in teratological research (Localization of collagen types in fetal tissues by immunofluorescence), in: "Methods in Prenatal Toxicology", (D. Neubert, H.-J. Merker, T.E. Kwasigroch, eds.), pp. 332 - 347.

Blumenthal, N.C., Posner, A.S., Silverman, L.D., Rosenberg, L.C., 1979, Effect of proteoglycans on in vitro hydroxyapatite formation, Calcif. Tiss. Internat., 27, 75 - 82.

Bornstein, P., Piez, K.A., 1966, The nature of the intramolecular cross-links in collagen. The separation and characterization of peptides from the cross-link region of rat skin collagen, Biochemistry, 11, 3460 - 3473.

Cuatrecasas, P., 1970, Protein purification by affinity chromatography, J. Biol. Chem., 245, 3059 - 3065.

Glanville, R.W., Rauter, A., Fietzek, P.P., 1979, Isolation and characterization of a native placental basement membrane collagen and its component α-chains, Eur. J. Biochem., 95, 383 - 389.

Goßlau, B., Barrach, H.-J., 1979, Enzyme-linked immunosorbent microassay for quantification of specific antibodies to collagen type I, II, III, J. Immunol. Meth., 29, 71 - 77.

Grundmann, K., 1979, Präparation und Anwendung von spezifischen Collagen-und Procollagen- Antikörpern zur Immunfluoreszenz-Färbung von embryonalen Mäuseextremitäten und Zellkulturen, Thesis, Freie Universität, Berlin.

Hascall, V.C., Heinegård, D., 1975, The structure of cartilage proteoglycans, in: Extracellular Matrix Influences on Gene Expression, (H.C. Slavkin, R.C. Greulich, eds.), pp. 423 - 433, Academic Press, New York.

Hassell, J.R., Gehron Robey, P., Barrach, H.-J., Wilczek, J., Rennard, S., J., Martin, G.R., 1980, Isolation of a heparansulfate containing proteoglycan from basement membrane, Proc. Nat. Acad. Sci., USA, 77, 4494 - 4498.

Heinegård, D., 1972, Extraction, fractionation and characterization of proteoglycans from bovine tracheal cartilage, Biochem. Biophys. Acta, 285, 181 - 192.

Holtzer, H., Okayama, M., Biehl, J., Holtzer, S., 1978, Chondrogenesis in chick limb buds and somites, Experientia, 34, 281 - 284.

Kuettner, K.E., Pita, J.C., Howell, D.S., Sorgenta, N., Einstein, R., 1975, Regulation of epiphyseal cartilage maturation, in: Extracellular Matrix Infuences on Gene Expression, (H.C. Slavkin, R.C. Greulich, eds.), pp. 435 - 440, Academic Press, New York.

von der Mark, K., von der Mark, H., Gay, S., 1976, Study of differential collagen synthesis during development of the chick embryo by immunofluorescence. I. Preparation of collagen type I and type II specific antibodies and their application to early stages of the chick embryo, Develop. Biol., 48, 237 - 249.

Miller, E.J., Martin, G.R., Piez, K.A., Powers, M.J., 1967, Characterization of chick bone collagen and compositional changes associated with maturation, J. Biol. Chem., 242, 5481 - 5489.

Oegema, T.R., Jr., Hascall, V.C., Dziewiatkowsky, D.D., 1975, Isolation and characterization of proteoglycans from the Swarm rat chondrosarcoma, J. Biol. Chem., 250, 6151 - 6159.

Pool, A.R., Pidoux, J., Reiner, A., Tamg, L.-H., Choi, H., Rosenberg, L., 1980, Localization of proteoglycan monomer and link protein in the matrix of bovine articular cartilage: an immunohistochemical study, J. Histochem. Cytochem., 28, 621 - 635.

Sage, H., Woodbury, R.G., Bornstein, P., 1979, Structural studies on human type IV collagen, J. Biol. Chem., 254, 9893 - 9900.

Smith, B.D., Martin, G.R., Miller, E.J., Dorfman, A., Swarm, R., 1975, Nature of collagen synthesized by a transplanted chondrosarcoma, Arch. Biochem. Biophys., 166, 181 - 186.

Smith, B.D., McKenney, K.H., Lustberg, T.J., 1977, Characterization of collagen precursors found in rat skin and rat bone, Biochemistry, 16, 2980 - 2985.

Timpl, R., Glanville, R.W., Nowack, H., Wiedemann, H., Fietzek, P.P., Kühn, K., 1975, Isolation, chemical and electronmicroscopical characterization of neural-salt-soluble type III collagen and procollagen from fetal bovine skin, Hoppe-Seyler's Z. Physiol. Chem., 365, 1783 - 1792.

Timpl, R., Rohde, H., Gehron Robey, P., Rennard, S.J., Foidart, J.-M., Martin, G.R., 1979, Laminin - a glycoprotein from basement membranes, J. Biol. Chem., 254, 9933 - 9937.

An Analysis of the Asymmetric Response of the Developing Limb to Embryotoxic Agents

Richard G. Skalko, Thomas E. Kwasigroch

East Tennessee State University, College of Medicine, Department of Anatomy, P.O. Box 19960A, Johnson City, Tennessee 37601, U.S.A.

In 1965, Layton and Hallesy showed that the carbonic anhydrase inhibitor, acetazolamide, had a unique embryotoxic effect when administered to pregnant rats throughout gestation. The response produced was a high percentage of postaxial defects in the right forelimbs and this observation presented a completely different perspective to our attempts to analyze chemically-induced malformations of the limbs. Since the appendages are bilaterally symmetrical, it is a reasonable assumption that any toxic response will reflect this fact and, indeed, the collective experience of many laboratories tends to support this assumption. Thus, for most agents that have been studied in the past several years, defects of the limbs tend to occur bilaterally or, if unilateral, are randomly distributed between right and left sides.

The asymmetric response of the developing limbs to teratogens is not an isolated effect of acetazolamide but has also been shown to occur in response to theophylline (FUJII and NISHIMURA, 1969; TUCCI and SKALKO, 1978) and the heavy metal, cadmium (BARR, 1973; LAYTON and LAYTON, 1979). The phenomenon of asymmetric development, while rare, also occurs as a natural process (e.g., in the ovaries of birds) and as a specific disease state in humans referred to as congenital asymmetry (PARKER and SKALKO, 1969).

The effects of acetazolamide have been most extensively studied and have been shown to produce defects in other systems in addition to those of the forelimbs (WILSON et al., 1968). This review, however, will be restricted to an analysis of defects of the forelimb. In both rats (LAYTON and HALLESY, 1965; WILSON et al., 1968) and mice (GREEN et al., 1973; BIDDLE, 1975), the principle response of the forelimb is a postaxial reduction deformity on the right side (Table 1). This response is unique in its constancy and, on first examination, appears to be independent of both strain and species. However, upon careful analysis there is a strain-dependent and a stage-dependent sensitivity, particular in mice.

GREEN et al. (1973) showed that if various inbred strains were treated with 750 mg/kg acetazolamide twice a day on either days 9 or 10, the CBA/J strain was the most sensitive with the peak response occurring after treatment on day 10. The C57BL/6J strain, while slightly less sensitive, demonstrated maximal effect after a similar treatment on day 9. The response of the A/J strain, however, was less than that of the other two and was independent of the day of treatment. The apparent influence of the genetic makeup of exposed fetuses on the embryotoxic response was further documented by the observation of SCOTT et al. (1972) that, in rats, the effect was more prevalent in female than in male embryos.

With respect to the production of forelimb defects, the embryotoxic response to treatment with cadmium is similar to that seen after exposure to

Teratology of the Limbs

acetazolamide (Table 2). In a study of two stocks of Wistar rats, BARR (1973) demonstrated that the developing limbs of the C stock were totally resistant (although other malformations were produced) while with the S stock, the limbs were sensitive to cadmium with the predominant effect occurring on the left side. In mice, LAYTON and LAYTON (1979) have documented a distinct strain-specificity of response to treatment on day 9 with some strains showing no specific side preference (A/J) while others (e.g., DBA) were effected on the right side primarily (Table 2).

Attempts to explain this response in mechanistic terms have, so far, been unsuccessful. WILSON et al. (1968) have discounted the role of carbonic anhydrase as the principal site of the embryotoxic action of acetazolamide since the sensitive period in rats (days 10, 11 ; Table 1) precedes the appearance of measurable quantities of the enzyme by two days. LAYTON and LAYTON (1979) suggest that both cadmium and acetazolamide produce their effect by "inhibiting enzymes involved in morphogenesis" but, as has been shown (NEUBERT et al., 1970), the biochemical complexity of the developing mammalian embryo is such that the definition of "critical" pathways involved in normal and abnormal development is a formidable task. Thus, we are faced with yet another developmental enigma. How can the highly specific response of the forelimb to both acetazolamide and cadmium be explained satisfactorily? More importantly, what insight can be provided to aid in the design of meaningful experiments to resolve this problem? In the same way that we are beginning to appreciate that neuronal elements may have a critical role to play in normal limb morphogenesis (McBRIDE, 1979), it is equally reasonable to expect that the development of the vasculature may be critical to our understanding of how limb asymmetries arise. This view is particularly relevant since the main arterial supply to the forelimbs develops asymmetrically due to developmental changes in the aortic arch system with the left subclavian artery originating from the arch of the aorta and the right artery being a branch of the innominate. The role of differential vascularization in limb development has been discussed before (CAPLAN and KOUTROUPAS, 1973) and these observations may be of some relevance in any systematic attempt to explain the differential response documented above.

In the chick wing bud at stage 20 many small lateral offshoots of the aorta (the primary subclavian capillary plexus) supply circulation to the wing. By stage 21, a recognizable central artery, the primary subclavian artery, is seen. At stage 22, marginal collecting vessels form and the presumptive cartilage-forming areas become less vascularized than the prospective muscle-forming areas. By stage 24, the basic pattern of limb circulation is established with a central brachial artery and a peripheral marginal vein. Coincident with this, the mesodermal core is essentially avascular while the peripheral muscle-forming areas are highly vascularized. These morphological stages are equivalent to the period of mouse development when the embryo progresses from 30 - 48 somites (KOCHHAR, 1977) and the definitive aortic arches form (THIELER, 1972). This anatomical relationship is shown in Table 3.

Since both acetazolamide (Table 1) and cadmium (Table 2) are maximally effective in mice between those periods of development encompassing 13 - 34 somites, it is possible that the primary lesion is produced in the developing vasculature and, through a series of intermediate steps, leads to the postaxial defects which have been reported. While we recognize and accept the speculative nature of this interpretation, it is amenable to experimental analysis and it is supported by a recent study (HOOTNICK et al., 1980) which showed that skeletal dysplasias of the lower limb (shortening or absence of the fibula) are associated with the persistence of an embryonic vascular pattern. While it is not possible to develop a causal relationship on the basis of present evidence, it is apparent that abnormal limb development is associated with abnormal vasculature. Well-designed and critical experiments should be capable of resolving this apparent and intriguing relationship and should aid in our understanding of the asymmetric response of the developing limb to specific teratogens.

Table 1:

Asymmetric response of the forelimb to acetazolamide.

SPECIES	STRAIN/ STOCK	DAY(S) OF TREATMENT	SOMITE NUMBER	PRINCIPAL EFFECT	PREDOMINANT SIDE
RAT[1]	SHERMAN	ALL	-	POSTAXIAL	RIGHT
RAT[2]	WISTAR	10; 11	5 - 25	POSTAXIAL	RIGHT
MOUSE[3]	CBA/J	10	30 - 34	POSTAXIAL	RIGHT
	C57BL/6J	9	13 - 20	POSTAXIAL	RIGHT
	A/J	9; 10	13 - 34	POSTAXIAL	RIGHT
MOUSE[4]	CBA/J	10	30 - 34	POSTAXIAL	RIGHT

[1]Layton and Hallesy, 1965
[2]Wilson et al., 1968
[3]Green et al., 1973
[4]Biddle, 1975

Table 2:

Asymmetric response of the forelimb to cadmium.

SPECIES	STRAIN/ STOCK	DAY(S) OF TREATMENT	SOMITE NUMBER	PRINCIPAL EFFECT	PREDOMINANT SIDE
RAT[1]	C (WISTAR)	10	5 - 12	-	-
	S (WISTAR)	10	5 - 12	POSTAXIAL	LEFT
MOUSE[2]	A/J	9	13 - 20	POSTAXIAL	-
	DBA	9	13 - 20	POSTAXIAL	RIGHT

[1]Barr, 1973
[2]Layton and Layton, 1979

Table 3:

Relationship between aortic arch development in the mouse with limb development in the chick and the mouse.

STAGE OF CHICK DEVELOPMENT[1]	SOMITE NUMBER[1] (MOUSE)	AORTIC ARCH FORMATION[2] (MOUSE)
19	30	II and III
22	36	IV
23	42	VI
24	48	

[1]Kochhar, 1977
[2]Thieler, 1972

REFERENCES

Barr, M., Jr., 1973, The teratogenicity of cadmium chloride in two stocks of Wistar rats, Teratology, 7, 237 - 242

Biddle, F.G., 1975, Teratogenesis of acetazolamide in the CBA/J and SWV strains of mice, 1. Teratology, Teratology, 11, 31 - 36.

Caplan, A.I., Koutroupas, S., 1973, The control of muscle and cartilage development in the chick limb; the role of differential vascularization, J. Embryol. exp. Morph. 29, 571 - 583.

Fujii, T., Nashimura, H., 1969, Teratogenic action of some methylated xanthines in mice, Okajimas Fol. Anat. Jap., 46, 167 - 175.

Green, M.C., Azar, C.A., Maren, T.H., 1973, Strain differences in susceptibility to the teratogenic effect of acetazolamide in mice, Teratology, 8, 143 - 146.

Hootnick, D.R., Levinsohn, E.M., Randall, P.A., Packard, D.S., Jr., 1980, Vascular dysgenesis associated with skelatal dysplasia of lower limb, J. Bone Joint Surgery, (in press).

Kochhar, D.M., 1977, Abnormal organogenesis in the limbs, in: "Handbook of Teratology", vol. 2, (J.G. Wilson, F.C. Fraser, eds.), pp. 453 - 479, Plenum Press, New York.

Layton, W.M., Jr., Hallesy, D.W., 1965, Deformity of forelimb in rat: association with high doses of acetazolamide, Science, 149, 306-308.

Layton, W.M., Jr., Layton, M.W., 1979, Cadmium induced limb defects in mice: strain associated differences in sensitivity, Teratology, 19, 229 - 236.

McBride, W.G., 1979, The inductive influence of neurons in limb development, in: "Advances in the Study of Birth Defects", vol. 1, (T.V.N. Persaud, ed.), pp. 129 - 139, Univ. Park Press, Baltimore.

Neubert, D., Merker, H.-J., Köhler, E., Krowke, E., Barrach, H.J., 1970, Biochemical aspects of teratology, in: "Advances in the Biosciences", vol. 6, (G. Raspé, ed.), pp. 575, - 621, Pergamon Press, Oxford.

Parker, D.A., Skalko, R.G., 1969, Congenital asymmetry: report of 10 cases with associated developmental abnormalities, Pediatrics, 44, 584 - 589.

Scott, W.J., Butcher, R.E., Kindt, C.W., Wilson, J.G., 1972, Greater sensitivity of female than male rat embryos to acetazolamide teratogeneticity, Teratology, 6, 239 - 240.

Thieler, K., 1972, "The House Mouse. Development and Normal Stages from Fertilization to 4 Weeks of Age", Springer-Verlag, Berlin.

Tucci, S.M., Skalko, R.G., 1978, The teratogenic effects of the theophylline in mice, Toxicology Letters, 1, 337 - 341.

Wilson, J.G., Maren, T.H., Takano, K., Ellison, A., 1968, Teratogenic action of carbonic anhydrase inhibitors in the rat, Teratology, 1, 51 - 60.

Resistance of the Rat to Certain Specific Limb Teratogens

H. Tuchmann-Duplessis

Laboratoire d'Embryologie, Faculté de Médecine,
45, rue des Sts. Pères, F-75270 Paris Cédex 06, France

Limb malformations are of special interest not only in human pathology but also for the analysis of embryonic mechanisms. According to SAXÉN et al., 1974, talipes and malformations of the musculo-skeletal system in humans are approximately three times more frequent than those of the central nervous system and of the digestive tract.

Some limb malformations are of genetic origin, others can be experimentally produced in a large variety of species ranging from the chick to the primate embryo. The general pattern of limb organogenesis is quite similar in all vertebrates. The differences are of chronological nature according to the specific timing of the general development.

In this presentation, the main events of normal limb development will be discussed. Then we will consider the impairments leading to malformations and describe the unexpected reactions we have observed in Wistar rats treated with thalidomide or azathioprine.

The normal development:

The first indication of limbs is characterized by a mesodermal thickening covered by the ectoderm in the region of the embryonic flanc. The primitive thickening increases rapidly through active cellular multiplication and undergoes an elongation in the proximo-distal direction. When the bud has achieved a certain length the mesodermal cells begin to differentiate into cartilage, muscles and bones.

In humans, the development of the limbs is quite similar. From the lateral mesoderm of the somatopleure a longitudinal thickening originates which is covered by the surface ectoderm. This is the Wolffian crest. The middle portion disappears rapidly leaving only two nods in the region of the future upper and lower limb bud. The upper limb bud appears opposite somites 8 - 12 about the 26th day when the crown rump length of the embryo is about 4 - 5 mm. The lower limb buds appear two days later opposite somites 24 - 29.

The essential basic constituents can already be distinguished at 34 days. The limb aquires its distal segment in the 7th week. A groove divides the proximal segment leading to the formation of the three definitive segments. During the 8th week, the limbs undergo changes in orientation. The middle segment buds at an angle of 90° to the proximal segment, thus forming the elbow of the upper limb and the knee of the lower limb. A final torsion causes the elbow to point dorsally and the knee ventrally.

During the initial morphogenesis of limbs there is no special zone of the bud which could be considered as a growth centre. The rate at which the bud lengthens is quite similar to the rate of cell division. In the chick the proximal limb bud regions grow with a doubling time of approximately 10 hours and the length of the cell cycle is also 10 hours.

Teratology of the Limbs

However, despite these morphological similarities, important differences in the susceptibility to specific teratogens can be observed between two animal species, the rat and the rabbit.

The influence of the two antimetabolites, 6-mercaptopurine and azathioprine.

The well known anti-tumor drug, 6-mercaptopurine, is embryotoxic and teratogenic in the rat. Very early treatments are mainly embryotoxic. During days 6 - 12 of pregnancy daily doses ranging from 0.50 to 0.75 mg/kg result in a large number of resorptions (20 to 80%), and (10 to 15%) congenital malformations. Higher doses induce complete resorptions.

In the mouse, doses of 0.50 to 1 mg/kg given after implantation result in limb, central nervous system, and eye malformations.

The rabbit is much more susceptible to 6-mercaptopurine. Doses of 1 mg/kg given between day 6 and 12 induce 40 - 50% resorptions and 10 - 15% malformations. With administration of this drug between day 10 - 14 of pregnancy, a high proportion (20 to 70%) of limb deformities is observed: syndactylia, ectromelia, phocomelia and amelia. A related compound, azathioprine 6-[(1-methyl-4-nitroimidazol-5-yl)thio]purine which also has anti-tumor and immunosupressive properties is not teratogenic in the rat or mouse (TUCHMANN-DUPLESSIS and MERCIER-PARAT, 1964). However, an important teratogenic effect could be observed in the rabbit. Doses of 5 to 15 mg/kg produce 40 - 50% obvious limb and musculo-skeletal malformations. Eye and central nervous system malformations are less frequent.

We investigated the reasons for these unexpected reactions.

In a first series of experiments a large range of doses of azathioprine was administered to the rat with the hope to find a teratogenic dose. In fact, with increasing doses ranging from 1 to 10 mg/kg per day the abortion rate increased to 100% in some groups, but no malformations were observed.

Since 6-mercaptopurine and azathioprine are both antitumor drugs, we investigated to ascertain whether the teratogenic action observed in the rabbit was directly related to antitumor activity. It has been shown that the antitumor activity of azathioprine can be abolished by a previous administration of glutathion or cysteine. Therefore, experiments were repeated in the rabbit by a combined treatment (TUCHMANN-DUPLESSIS and MERCIER-PARAT, 1966).

As shown in Table 1, which summarizes the main results, the pretreatment by either of these two compounds did modify the teratogenic potential of azathioprine in the rabbit.

Although this experimental approach does not explain why azathioprine is devoid of a teratogenic action in the rat, it indicates that there is not a direct relationship between the antitumor and the teratogenic activity of this antimetabolite.

We will discuss later the hypothesis which could be put forward to explain the lack of susceptibility of the rat to azathioprine. But at this point, the two series of experiments performed by the groups NEUBERT and MERKER; LESSMÖLLMANN et al., 1975, should be evaluated. They developed an organ culture system of mammalian limb buds.

In one experiment, 6-mercaptopurine or azathioprine was added to normal limb buds differentiating in organ culture. In the other experiment mice were treated on day 10 of gestation with 6-mercaptopurine or azathioprine. The limb buds were then removed and cultured according to the routine technique. The authors observed the following clear-cut results:

Abnormalities were observed when either of these antimetabolites, 6-mercaptopurine or azathioprine were added to limb buds differentiating in culture.

These in vitro experiments indicate that the mouse embryo is susceptible to the teratogenic action of azathioprine.

However, when azathioprine was injected subcutaneously on the 10th day of pregnancy, no malformations were observed when limb buds of these azathioprine-treated mice were cultured in vitro, beginning 24 hours after the injection. In the same experimental conditions, limb buds from 6-mercaptopurine-treated animals showed malformations.

From these experiments the authors concluded that in pregnant mice azathioprine did not reach the developing embryo in a concentration sufficient to trigger the teratogenic effects. This explanation does not seem entirely satisfactory since when we used a very large dose range of azathioprine, we could not produce malformations in the rat.

We experienced a similar situation with thalidomide. The rat is not susceptibile to this agent either (GIROUD et al., 1962). While in the rat doses ranging from 50 to 500 mg/kg given before or after implantation produced a high resorption rate but no malformation, similar treatments determined 25 to 40% obvious anomalies in the rabbit.

It should be mentioned also that in certain strains of mice, particularly in the A/Jax strain, eye and facial malformations can be observed. From our experience we conclude that the rat is resistant to the dysmorphogenic action of thalidomide as compared to many other animal species like cats, dogs, pigs and monkeys, which are highly susceptible to this drug.

DISCUSSION:

Three problems deserve consideration:

a) The mechanism of action of agents which produce limb defects;
b) the reason for the lack of susceptibility of the rat to potent teratogens;
c) the significance of negative results in one or several animal species.

The precise mechanism of control of the growth and differentiation of the limbs is still a matter of discussion. There is little doubt that the apical ectodermal ridge (AER), which covers the extremity of the mesenchyme, plays a major role in the limb bud morphogenesis.

However, it is not clear if the AER is an inductor stimulating the mesenchymal outgrowth or if it acts as a protector of mesenchymal proliferations, since it has been shown that the mesoderm underlying the AER has properties different from those of the proximal mesenchyme.

At the beginning, the proliferation index in all parts of the mesenchyme is virtually 100%. Afterwards, the mitotic index decreases drastically in the regions of prospective cartilage and subsequently in the region of future muscle, but remains constant in the distal part of mesenchyme.

It has been suggested by STARK and SEARLS (1974) that when the cell proliferation begins to fall in central proximal regions preceding the formation of the humeral cartilage, a "progress zone" with high cell proliferation is maintained in a narrow band of mesenchyme directly under the AER.

Therefore, impairment of limb growth and differentiation can result from various mechanisms: lack of cellular interaction between the mesenchyme and the AER, increased or premature cell destruction and modifications of the reaction of limb mesenchyme with subsequent impairment of chondrogenesis.

Since it has been shown that X-rays, which cause important cell death, determine a large variety of limb defects, it seems likely that cytotoxic drugs like 6-mercaptopurine which produce a wide-spread cell death in the entire embryo, as evidenced by the general growth retardation of the foetus, might induce limb malformations through cell destruction.

The mechanism of action of teratogens which have only a low cytotoxicity like thalidomide, is probably more complex. The drug may interfere with the normal interrelationships between the mesenchyme and AER. The compound might also act specifically on cells undergoing chondrogenic differentiation through a biochemical modification of macromolecules during differentiation of the cartilage.

Other hypothesis have been proposed involving an injury of the epithelial lining of the axial artery of the limb bud (JURAND, 1966) or a lesion of the sensory peripheral nerves (McCREDIE, 1973). It has also been suggested that the nerves act on the vascular system, their lesions or denervation would prevent vascularization of the blastema (SMITH and WOLPERT, 1975). However, as far as thalidomide is concerned, any of these hypotheses must be verified by morphological or biochemical investigations.

The second question was raised by experiments performed with azathioprine and thalidomide. The lack of susceptibility of the rat to potent limb teratogens is quite unexpected. Since the general pattern of limb morphogenesis is quite similar in most vertebrates, the basic reactions to specific exogenous agents should also be similar.

The explanation proposed by the NEUBERT, MERKER groups, suggesting an insufficient concentration of the teratogen in the embryo, does not seem entirely satisfactory since with both azathioprine and thalidomide a very large range of doses were used, without obtaining positive results.

The existence of a particular detoxification mechanism seems more likely and should be investigated.

Finally, there is also a practical problem when one deals with chemicals which could be used as therapeutic agents.

Should one consider a compound as safe for humans if it does not induce malformations in the rat and in the mouse? Do the positive results in the rabbit constitute proof of a potential teratogenicity for the human embryo?

The two examples chosen in this presentation, azathioprine and thalidomide lead to contradictory interpretations. While the teratogenic potential of thalidomide is well established there is no proof from clinical data that azathioprine is a teratogen for humans.

One wonders therefore which morphological or biochemical criteria should be used to reach a valid prospective conclusion.

Table 1: Influence of glutathion and cysteine on the teratogenic potential of azathioprine.

	Day of Treat.	Resorp. %	Malform. %
Azathioprine 10 mg/kg	6 - 14	30	23
+ Glutathion 30 mg/kg	8 - 14	0	21
Azathioprine 10 mg/kg	6 - 14	25	20
+ Cysteine 50 mg/kg	8 - 14	0	15
Azathioprine 10 mg/kg	6 - 14	12	35
+ Cysteine 100 mg/kg	6 - 14	37	10

REFERENCES

Cairins, J.M., 1975, The functions of the apical ectodermal ridge and distinctive characteristics of the adjacent mesoderm in the avian wing bud, J. Embryol. exp. Morph., 341 - 354.

Giroud, A., Tuchmann-Duplessis, H., et Mercier-Parat, L., 1962, Observations sur les répercussions teratogènes de la thalidomide chez la souris et le lapin, C.R. Soc. Biol., 156, 765 - 768.

Jurand, A., 1966, J. Embryol. exp. Morph., 16, 289 - 300.

Kochhar, D.M., 1977, Abnormal organogenesis in the limbs, in: Handbook of Teratology, pp. 453 - 479, Plenum Press.

Lessmöllmann, U., Neubert, D., Merker, H.-J., 1975, Mammalian limb buds differentiating in vitro as a test system for the evaluation of embryotoxic effects. 2nd Symposium on Prenatal Development. G. Thieme Publ., pp. 99 - 113.

McCredie, J., 1973, Lancet, 2, 1058 - 1061.

Saxén, L., Klemetti, A., Haro, A.S., 1974, A matched-pair register for studies of selected congenital defects, Am. J. Epidem., 3, Vol. 100, 297 - 306.

Smith, A.R., Wolpert, L., 1975, Nature, 257, 224 - 225.

Stark, R.J., Searls, R., 1974, The establishment of the cartilage pattern in the embryonic chick wing and evidence for a role of the dorsal and ventral ectoderm in normal wing development, Develop. Biol., 38 - 51.

Tuchmann-Duplessis, H., Mercier-Parat, L., 1964, Production de malformations des membres chez le lapin par administration d'un anti metabolite l'Azathioprine, C.R. Acad. Sci., Paris, 259, 3648.

Tuchmann-Duplessis, H., Mercier-Parat, L., 1966, Réactions provoquées chez l'embryon par deux antimetabolites chimiquement voisins, Bull. Acad. Suisse, Sci. Méd., 22, 153 - 165.

Observations on Human Digits 'In Vitro' and its Possible Role in Evaluating Teratogens

K. T. Rajan, H.-J. Merker, M. Wilkins
East Glamorgan General Hospital, Church Village,
Nr. Pontypridd, Mid. Glam., U.K.

Abstract:

The growth and differentiation of human digits was investigated 'in vitro'. Human foetal fingers were maintained in culture for periods of 12 days. The digits grew rapidly in culture and after 6 days had elongated by 60%. The amount of intercellular matrix increased, joint formation was noted and articular cartilage matured together with the formation of joint capsule. In explants maintained in vitamin A, growth was arrested, the digits were shorter and thinner and histological sections demonstrated a reduction in metachromasia and compression of the growth area. Electron microscopical inspection of cartilaginous tissue revealed a decrease in collagen fibrils and proteoglycan granules, an alteration in their thickness and diameter, lesion of cell organelles and deformation of chondrocytes. Mineralisation in collagen-free areas and phagocytosis of apatite crystals were observed in the perichondral bone sheath. The results indicate that human digits are extremely vulnerable to hypervitaminosis A. It might therefore, be advantageous to use human material in the "in vitro" testing of teratogenic drugs.

INTRODUCTION:

In the last decade there has been increasing awareness of teratogenic effects of drugs and as a consequence numerous experimental models have been used to produce congenital anomalies (WADDINGTON and CARTER, 1952; DURAISWAMI, 1955; TUCHMANN-DUPLESSIS and MERCIER-PAROT, 1959; BECK et al., 1960; RAJAN, 1974). Apart from one model (RAJAN, 1974; REYNOLDS, 1972) the work was accomplished in animals and it is therefore not surprising that even among the optimists some scepticism regarding the applicability of these studies to human subjects still remains. TUCHMANN-DUPLESSIS clearly demonstrated (1971) that there were variations in the response to drugs between the same species. Primates have been used (WILSON et al., 1968) and it is of interest that spontaneous malformations are less frequent than in humans. Therefore some doubts still remain regarding the predictability of the results and their applicability to the human species.

In this contribution, an alternative method, using organ culture of human skeletal tissue is discussed and the use of a known teratogen - Vitamin A - has been explored.

MATERIAL and METHODS:

Human foetal fingers of week 11 to 16 of gestation were used, obtained either at hysterotomy for the termination of pregnancy, or spontaneous abortions, the latter within 30 minutes of the event. The digits were washed in chemically defined medium BGJ (BIGGERS, GWATKIN and HEYNER, 1961) supplemented with 15% foetal calf serum (Flow Labs) and 100 µg of

Teratology of the Limbs

Vitamin C per ml. The vitamin was added fresh since it is very unstable. Following TROWELL'S procedure (1954), the explants were placed on a metal grid and the tissue culture medium was injected beneath the grid to moisten the tissue but not to immerse the digits. The explants were maintained in an atmosphere of 5% carbon dioxide, 20% oxygen and 70% nitrogen. The medium was changed at 2 day intervals and used medium was sucked off with a syringe for future biochemical analysis.

Fixation: The digits were fixed in ZENKER'S fluid and 5 µ sections were stained with toluidine blue and Azan aniline blue. For electron microscopy the tissues were fixed immediately after removal in 3% glutaraldehyde in cacodylate buffer and post-fixed in 1% osmium tetroxide containing 1.5% ruthenium red (LUFT, 1971).

Vitamin A: An ethanolic solution of Retinol (Koch-Light Laboratories, Colnbrook, Bucks) was utilised in a final concentration of 3 and 6 IU/ml. An equal amount of ethanol was added to the control cultures. The digits and the medium were collected in acetone for biochemical analysis, the results of which have been published elsewhere (SCHIMMELPFENNIG et al., 1974).

RESULTS:

In all, 120 human digits were cultured with and without Vitamin A (60 controls and 30 each in 3 and 6 IU/ml of Retinol). All the digits maintained in Vitamin A were shorter and thinner than controls. This effect was evident even in as small a dose as 3 IU/ml (compared with post-foetal mice where a dose 3 times as high was essential to produce a similar effect (RAJAN, 1969). At 6 IU/ml there was marked tissue necrosis and the chondrocytes were fragmented. There was well marked loss of metachromasia and compression of the growth zone in all the digits treated with Vitamin A (Figs. 1 - 6). As electron microscopical studies have shown, the cartilage matrix consists of collagen structures and proteoglycan granules. The collagen fibrils are 100 - 200 Å thick and run singly and irregularly. Slight cross-striation is seen only rarely and at high magnification. The proteoglycan granules are 300 - 600 Å in diameter. They are located freely in the interfibrillar spaces or are resting directly on the collagen fibrils.

After vitamin A treatment the number of matrix structures, especially that of proteoglycans, decreases at varying degrees. In certain areas only few collagen fibrils are still present and PG granules are absent altogether. In some areas, however, the matrix seems to be unchanged. Preferential localization of these alterations in certain cartilaginous areas is not demonstrable. Moreover, after vitamin A treatment the morphology of collagen and PG also changes. In areas with only few PG granules fibrils are observed which exhibit a thickness of up to 500 Å and distinct cross-striation. Thin filaments of approximately 100 Å in diameter form bundles. The PG granules also show variations in size or merge to form larger units. In the compressed layer, which corresponds to the growth zone or the columnar cartilage, the intercellular spaces are very small. Many thick collagen fibrils arranged in a parallel fashion and only few PG granules occur.

The cells of phalangeal cartilage are also influenced by vitamin A treatment. A great number of the chondrocytes in the epiphyseal region, which exhibit a round or polygonal shape in controls, are stretched and deformed by invaginations. They often resemble fibroblast-like cells. These changes are especially pronounced in the compressed growth zone.

In the cytoplasm of cartilaginous cells vacuoles of varying size are observed. It cannot be stated with certainty whether these originate from lysosomes, mitochondria or other membrane-bordered organelles. Number and length of the cavities of the rough endoplasmic reticulum as well as the number of free ribosomes are decreased.

Other alterations induced by vitamin A treatment occur in the region of the perichondral bone sheath. Despite technical difficulties two findings were observed in a large number of preparations:

1. a change in the mineralized matrix (osteoid) and
2. a change in the cell - matrix relationship.

In the control digits the first apatite crystals are deposited in a matrix, which consists of 200 - 300 Å thick collagen fibrils. In the vitamin A treated bone anlagen, however, large areas fail to show collagen fibrils and the apatite crystals are located in a collagen-free matrix. The morphology of the crystals and their aggregates is normal. Therefore, a close spatial relationship could not be detected between collagen fibrils and apatite crystals, as has been observed in control preparations.

Collagen fibrils do not occur between fully mineralized sections and adjacent cells. Often small, densely mineralized trabeculae project into these cells, are surrounded by processes or are recognizable in membrane-bordered inclusions of the cytoplasm. An increase in the phagocytosis of apatite aggregates can therefore be assumed.

DISCUSSION:

Vitamin A is a known teratogen, especially in excess. COHLAN (1953) reported its marked teratogenic effect in pregnant rats. When this vitamin is given throughout pregnancy, numerous skeletal malformations including cleft palate are common (COHLAN, and STONE, 1961, GEELEN, 1979). Other investigators (GIROUD, and MARTINET, 1959; KOCHHAR, 1968, 1976) have stressed the importance of the critical period for producing deformities even when exposing the embryo to the teratogen for a very short period when the development of the skeletal tissue is affected. Vitamin A is obviously able to disturb skelettogenesis in several critical phases. A number of findings suggest an influence on cell migration during the development of the mesoderm (MORRIS, 1975) or for a cytotoxic reaction in the somites. Other findings indicate a change in the mesenchyme or an influence on blastema formation (GEELEN, 1979; KOCHHAR, 1968, 1976; KWASIGROCH and KOCHHAR, 1975; NAKAMURA et al., 1973). These effects can be attributed to a change in the cell membrane under the influence of vitamin A (LEWIS et al., 1978). On the other hand, vitamin A is able to trigger teratogenic effects very late during development, i.e. after the onset of chondrogenesis. In this case the cartilage matrix is changed in such a way that it cannot pass on the stored information on size and shape of the bone anlagen. Subsequent chondral osteogenesis is disturbed (MERKER, 1977).

It has been suggested that in these late developmental phases Vitamin A acts as a teratogen by virtue of its specific action on the lysosomes (ROELS, 1970; LLOYD and BECK, 1970). The released enzymes are supposed to damage the cells and disintegrate the matrix. There are, in addition, the potentiating effects of agents such as cortisone and methylthiouracil (WOOLLAM and MILLAN, 1960); thyroxin and insulin, on the other hand, antagonise the action of hypervitaminosis A. However, many other workers have been unable to demonstrate this effect in their experimental models (COHLAN and STONE, 1961). This may be due to the fact that there are species differences, in addition to the route of administration, which may influence the outcome of the experiment. The decreased number of matrix structures and the changes in the cytoplasm observed in our experiments after vitamin A treatment may be interpreted as an effect on an activation and release of lysosomal enzymes. The influence of the morphology of collagen fibrils and PG granules is the result of this disintegration. The PGs regulate the aggregation of collagen (MERKER et al., 1978 a, b; LILJA and BARRACH, 1980). A change results in different fibril thickness. The variation in the size of PG granules and their merging are due to the breakdown of the three-dimensional network and its subsequent aggregation. The changes in the cell shape and cell density may also be attributed to a lesion of the matrix. Since vitamin A also influences the direction of cell differentiation, the occurrence of an other, fibroblast-like cell type has to be taken into account (HASSEL et al., 1979; LEWIS et al., 1978). A decrease in PG synthesis (PENNYPACKER et al., 1978; NAKAMURA, 1975) and a synthesis of other collagen types would be expected. These ideas also help explain changes in the matrix during mineralization. The onset of mineralization in the desmal bone is obviously independent of collagen (see also MERKER et al., 1975). The mechanism of a putative stimulation of apatite phagocytosis has not as yet been elucidated.

The use of the "in vitro" technique to test the effect of teratogenic drugs as an alternative method would obviously reduce the number of animal experiments and to this effect alternative methods have been investigated and have proved useful (BARRACH and NEUBERT, 1980). The effect of vitamin A on growth and the possible induction of malformation has been well documented (HASSEL et al., 1978, 1979; KOCHHAR and AYDELOTTE, 1974; LEWIS et al., 1978; NAKAMURA, 1977; PENNYPACKER et al., 1978). It has been possible to demonstrate this effect on growth in human skeletal tissue in culture with specific reference to vitamin A. Species specificity of teratogenic drugs and extra-polation from animal experiments to human tissue poses an important problem in experimental teratology. The use of human materials for the "in vitro" screening of various drugs with specific reference to the teratogenic action under controlled conditions might be rewarding.

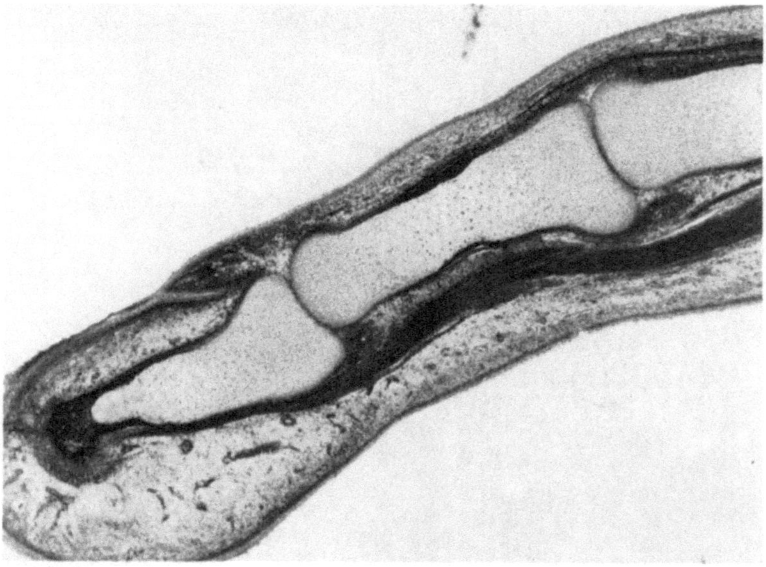

Fig. 1: Foetal digit before culture. Azan aniline blue. Mag. x 41.

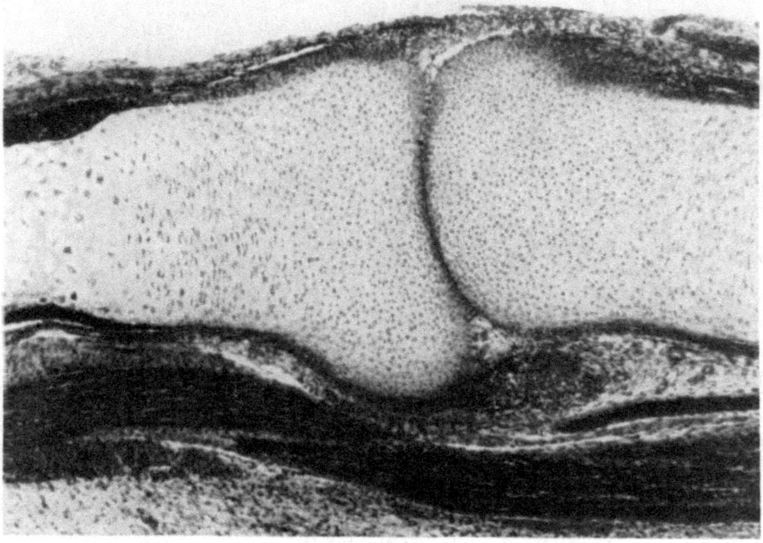

Fig. 2: As Fig. 1. Mag. x 100.

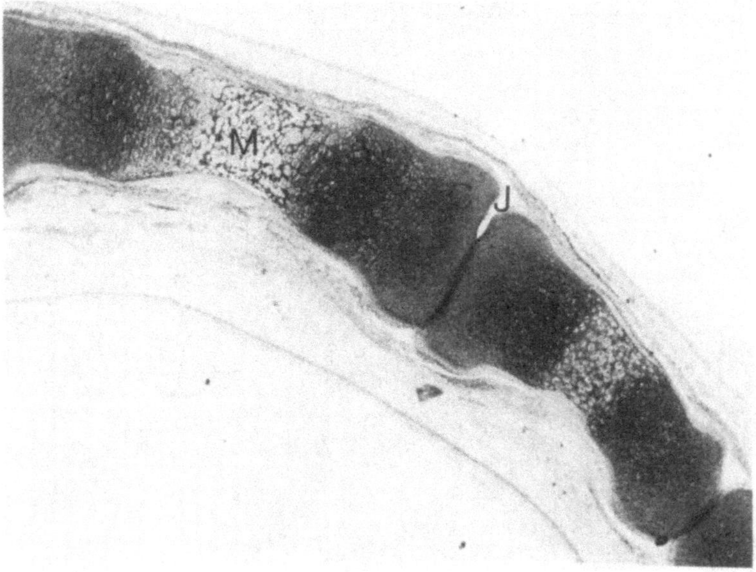

Fig. 3: Foetal digit after 6 days in culture. Toluidine blue. Mag. x 41.

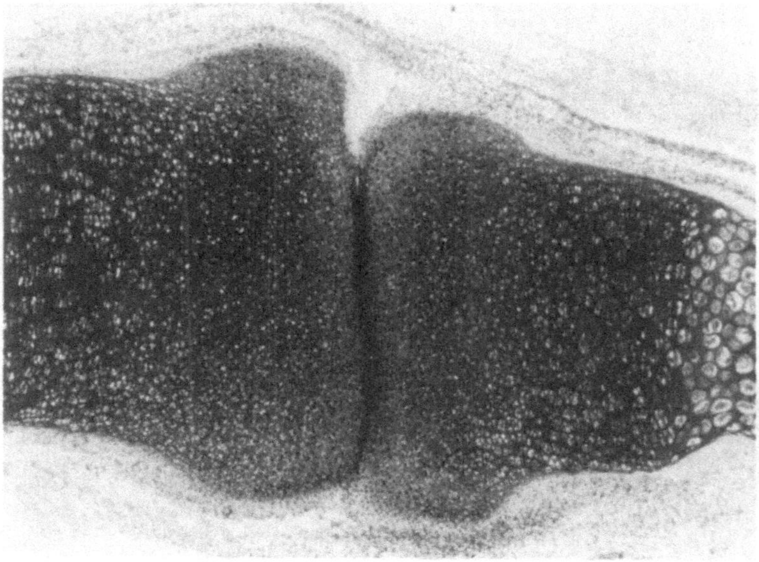

Fig. 4: As Fig. 3. showing normal cartilage and joint formation. Mag. x 10

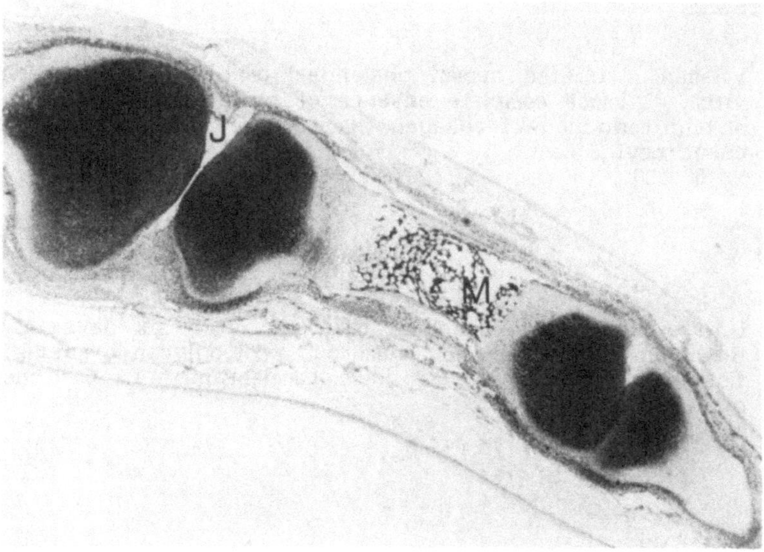

Fig. 5: Foetal digit after culture with Vitamin A (3.5 IU/ml). Toluidine blue. Mag. x 41.

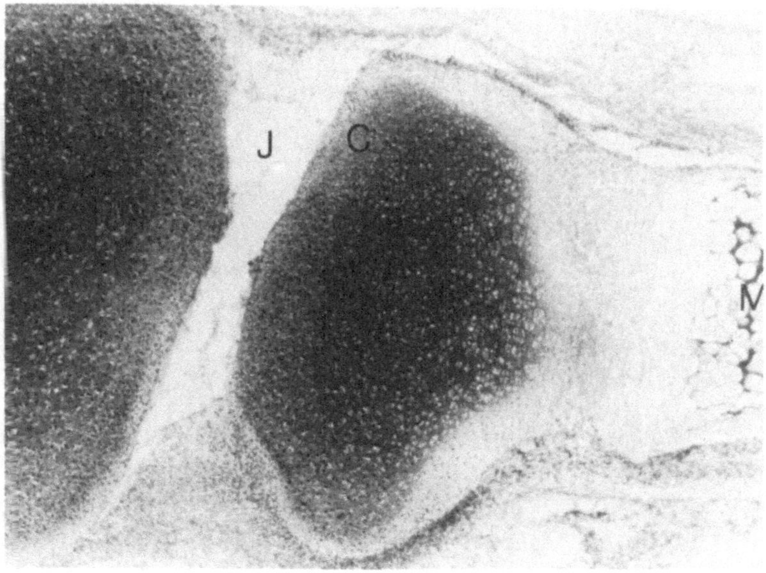

Fig. 6: As Fig. 5, showing loss of metachromasia and compression of the growth zone. Mag. x 100.

Fig. 7 A, B, C:

Fig. A: Vitamin A treated human phalangeal cartilage after six days in vitro. Almost complete absence of proteoglycan granules (O), strong reduction of collagen filaments (↓). C = periphery of a chondrocyte.
x 60 000.

Fig. B: Untreated human phalangeal cartilage after six days in vitro. Ruthenium red staining. Numerous proteoglycan granules, particularly in the vicinity of the cell membrane (↓). C = chondrocyte.
x 25 000.

Fig. C: Vitamin A treated human phalangeal cartilage after six days in vitro. Ruthenium red staining. Clearly decreased number of proteoglycan granules (O), unchanged number and structure of collagen filaments (↓).
x 60 000.

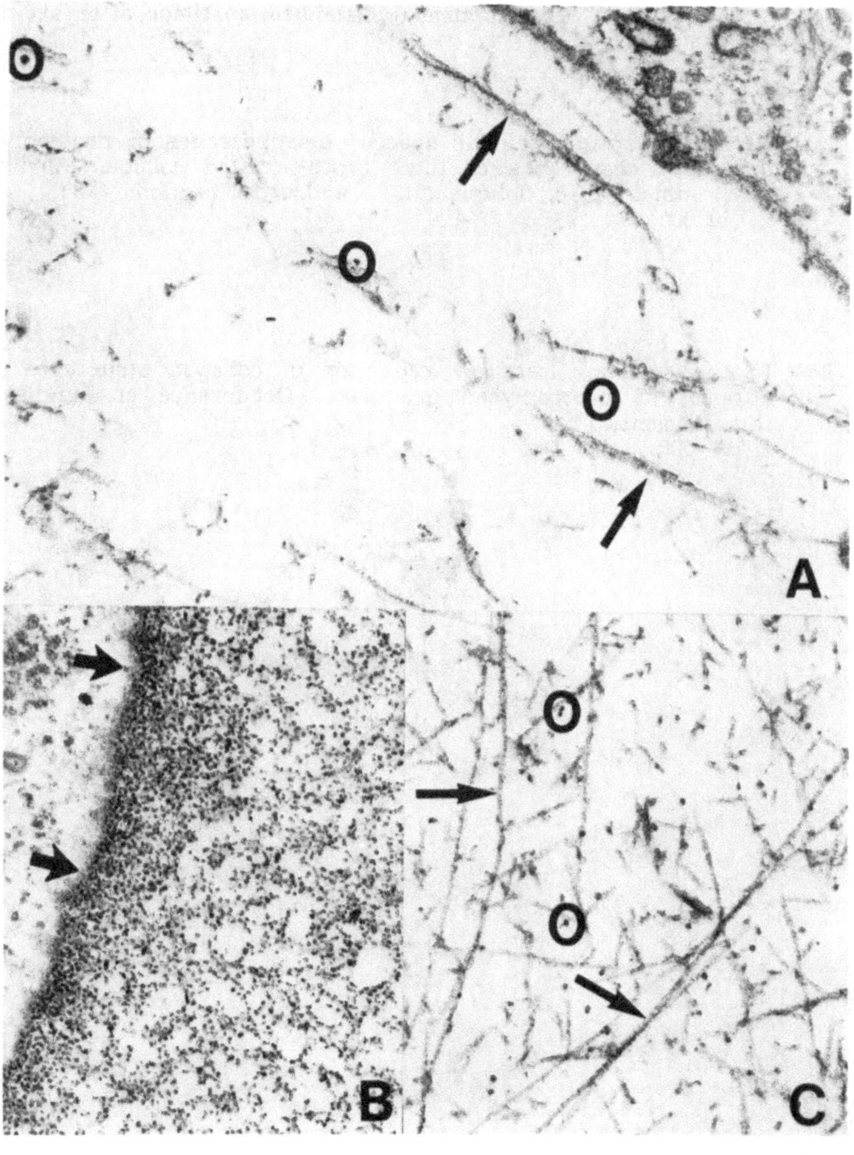
A
B
C

Fig. 8 A, B: Vitamin A treated human phalangeal cartilage after six days in vitro.

Fig. A: Narrowing of intercellular spaces, disappearance of proteoglycan granules, occurrence of thick cross-striated collagen fibrils in longitudinal (↓1)-, oblique (↓2)-, and cross sections (↓3).
x 20 000.

Fig. B: In the cartilage matrix - reduction of collagen structures (↓), absence of proteoglycan granules. Occurrence of bundles of thin filaments (*).
x 60 000.

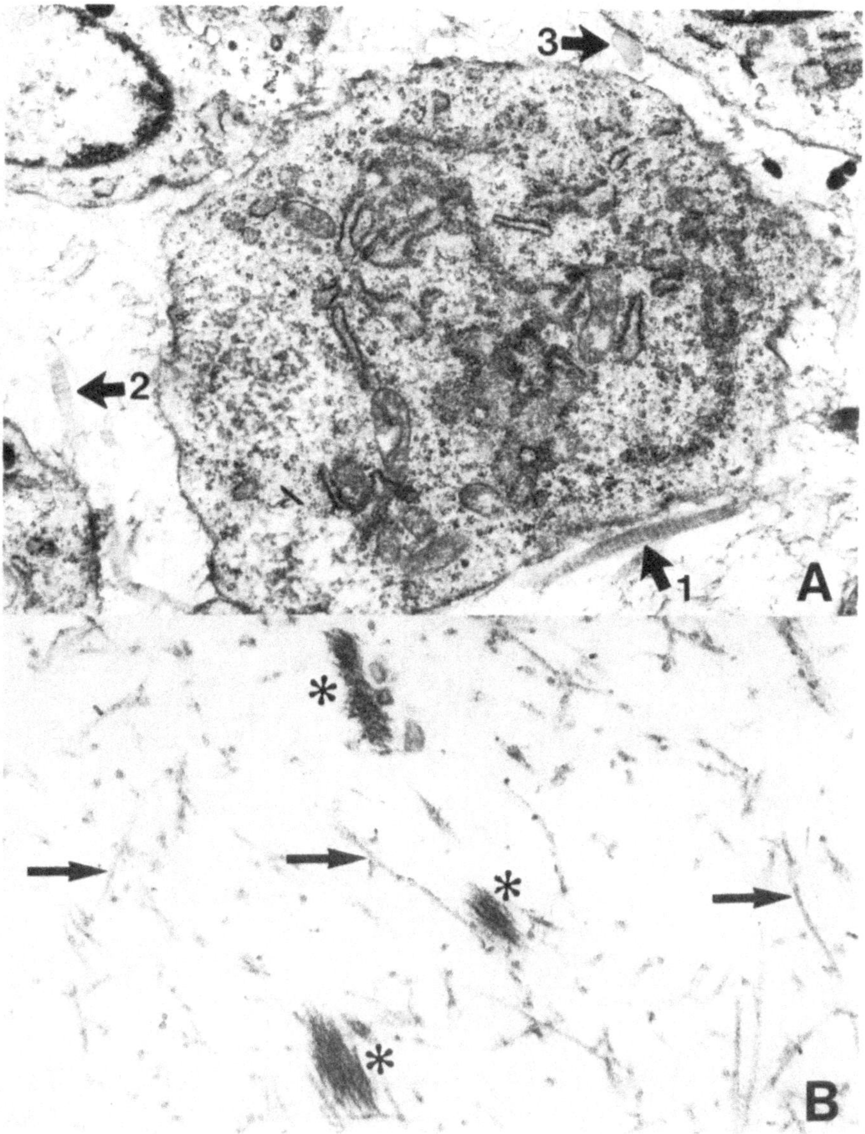
3
2
1
A
*
*
*
B

Fig. 9 A, B: Vitamin A treated human phalangeal cartilage after six days in vitro.

Fig. A: Strong deformation of chondrocytes by deep invaginations (*). Occurrence of vacuoles (↓). Decrease in number and size of the cavities of the rough endoplasmic reticulum.
x 12 000.

Fig. B: Cells from the beginning of the growth zone with fat (↓) inclusions and vacuoles of differing size (*). Reduced number of cell organelles.
x 9 000.

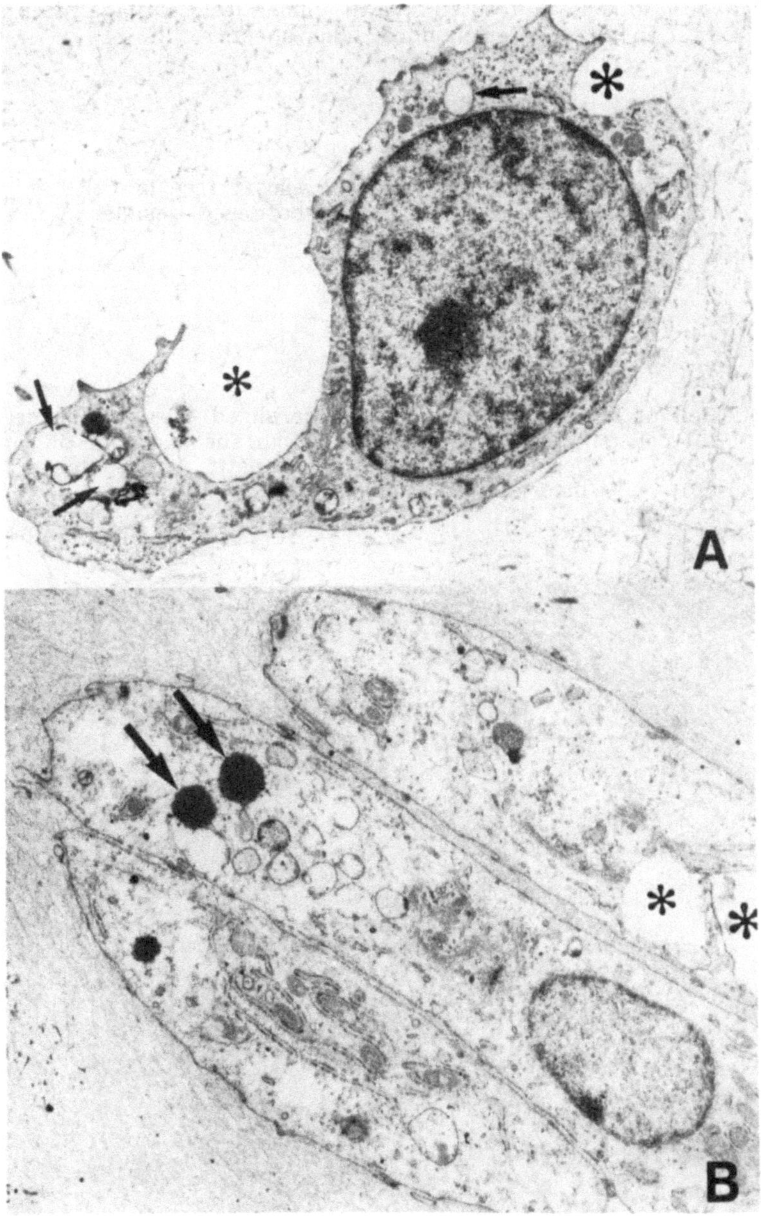
A
B

Fig. 10 A, B: Vitamin A treated human phalangeal cartilage after six days in vitro. Perichondral bone sheath.

Fig. A: Apatite aggregates in a matrix almost free of collagen (*). In the vicinity numerous membrane-bordered vesicles (↓). P = cell processes. M = cartilage matrix.
x 60 000.

Fig. B: Cell at the margin of a fully mineralized area. Absence of typical collagen fibrils between cell membrane and zone of mineralization (*). Deep invaginations of an apatite aggregate into the cell (1), fully incorporated aggregate (2).
x 60 000.

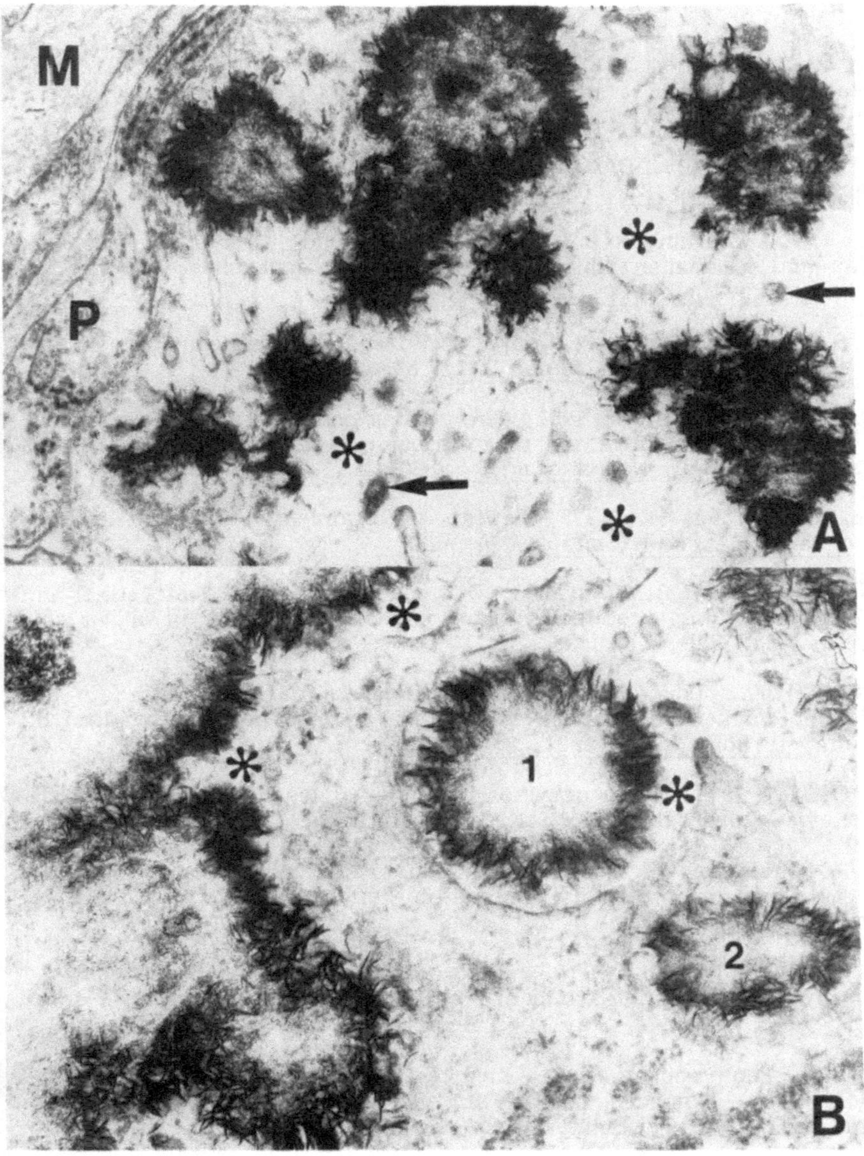
M
P
A
B
1
2

REFERENCES

Barrach, H.-J., Neubert, D., 1980, Significance of organ culture techniques for evaluation of prenatal toxicity, Arch. Toxicol., 45, 161 - 187.

Beck, F., Spencer, B., Baxter, J.S., 1960, Effect of trypan blue on rat embryos, Nature, 187, 605.

Biggers, J.D., Gwatkin, R.B.L., Heyner, S., 1961, Growth of embryonic avian and mammalian tibiae on a relatively simple chemically defined medium, Exp. Cell Res., 25, 41.

Cohlan, S.Q., 1953, Excessive intake of Vitamin A as a cause of congenital anomalies in the rat, Signs, 117, 535.

Cohlan, S.Q., Stone, S.M., 1961, Obervations on the effect of experimental endocrine procedures on the teratogenic action of hypervitaminosis A in the rat, Biol. Neonatorum, 3, 330.

De Luca, H.F., Zile, M., 1975, Aspects of teratology of Vitamin A acid, Acta Derm. Venoreal., suppl., 74, 13.

Dingle, J.T., Fell, H.B., Goodman, D.S., 1972, The effect of retinol and of retinol-binding protein on embryonic skeletal tissue in organ culture, J. Cell Sci., 11, 393.

Duraiswami, P.K., 1955, Comparison of congenital defects induced in developing chickens by certain teratogenic agents with those caused by insulin, J. Bone Joint Surg., 37 a, 277.

Geelen, J.A.G., 1979, Hypervitaminosis A induced teratogenesis, in: Critical Reviews in Toxicology, C.R.C. Press, pp. 351 - 375.

Giroud, A., Martinet, M., 1959, Extension to several species of mammals of embryonal malformations due to hypervitaminosis A, Compt. Rend. Soc. Biol., 153, 201.

Hassel, J.R., Pennypacker, J.P., Lewis, C.A., 1978, Chondrogenesis and cell proliferation in limb bud cell cultures treated with cytosin-arabinoside and vitamin A, Exp. Cell Res., 112, 409.

Hassel, J.R., Pennypacker, J.P., Kleinman, H.K., Pratt, R.M., Yamada, K.M., 1979, Enhanced cellular fibronectin accumulation in chondrocytes treated with vitamin A, Cell, 17, 821.

Kochhar, D.M., 1968, Studies on the vitamin A-induced teratogenesis: Effects on embryonic mesenchyme and epithelium, and incorporation of H^3-thymidine, Teratology, 1, 299.

Kochhar, D.M., 1976, Transplacental passage of label after administration of H^3-retinoic acid to pregnant mice, Teratology, 14, 53.

Kochhar, D.M., Aydelotte, M.B., 1974, Susceptible stages and abnormal morphogenesis in developing mouse limb, analysed in organ culture after transplacental exposure to vitamin A (retinoic acid), J. Embryol. exp. Morph., 31, 721.

Kwasigroch, T.E., Kochhar, D.M., 1975, Locomotory behavior of limb bud cells. Effects of excess vitamin A in vivo and in vitro, Exp. Cell Res., 95, 269.

Lewis, C.A., Pratt, R.M., Pennypacker, J.P., Hassel, J.R., 1978, Inhibition of limb chondrogenesis in vitro by vitamin A: alterations in cell surface characteristics, Develop. Biol., 64, 31.

Lilja, S., Barrach, H.-J., 1980, An electron microscopical study of the influence of different glycosaminoglycans on the fibrillogenesis of collagen Type I and II in vitro, Virch. Arch., (A), (in press).

Lloyd, J.B., Beck, F., 1970, Teratogenesis, in: "Lysosomes in Biology and Pathology", (J.T. Dingle and H.B. Fell, eds.), pp. 433, North Holland, Amsterdam, London.

Luft, J.H., 1971, Ruthenium red and violet, II. Fine structural localisation in animal tissues, Anat. Rec., 171, 369.

Merker, H.-J., 1977, Considerations on the problem of critical period during the development of limb skeleton, in: Morphogenesis and malformation of the limb. Birth Defects: original article series, Vol. XIII, No. 1, pp. 179 - 202, A.R. Liss, Inc., New York.

Merker, H.-J., Franke, L., Günther, Th., 1975, The effect of D-penicillamine on the skeletal development of rat foetuses, Naunyn-Schmied. Arch. Pharmacol., 287, 359 - 376.

Merker, H.-J., Lilja, S., Barrach, H.-J., Günther, Th., 1978 a, Formation of an atypical collagen and cartilge pattern in limb bud cultures by highly sulfated GAG, Virch. Arch., (A), 380, 11 - 30.

Merker, H.-J., Günther, Th, Krüger, V., 1978 b, Effects of 4-methylium-belliferyl-ß-D-xylopyranosid on morphology of embryonic cartilage in limb bud cultures, Teratology, 18, 291 - 310.

Morris, G.M., 1975, Abnormal cell migration as a possible factor in the genesis of vitamin-A-induced craniofacial anomalies, in: New approaches to the evaluation of abnormal embryonic development, (D. Neubert, H.-J. Merker, eds.) pp. 678 - 687, G. Thieme-Verlag, Stuttgart.

Nakamura, H., 1975, Analysis of limb anomalies induced in vitro by vitamin A in mice, Teratology, 12, 61.

Nakamura, M., 1977, Digital anomalies in the embryonic mouse limb cultured in the presence of excess vitamin A, Teratology, 16, 195.

Nakamura, H., Yamawaki, H., Fujisawa, H., Yasuda, M., 1973, Effects of hypervitaminosis A on developing mouse limb buds: Ultrastructural observations, Teratology, 8, 100.

Pennypacker, J.P., Lewis, C.A., Hassel, J.R., 1978, Altered proteoglycan metabolism in mouse limb mesenchyme cell cultures treated with vitamin A, Arch. Biochem. Biophys., 186, 351.

Rajan,K.T., 1969, The cultivation of post foetal mammalian cartilage and its response to hypervitaminosis A, Exp. Cell Res., 55, 419.

Rajan, K.T., 1974, "Experimental embryology and teratology" Vol. 1, (Woollam and Morriss, eds.) pp. 65 - 89.

Rajan, K.T., Hopkin, A.M., 1970, Human digits in organ culture, Nature, 227, 621.

Reynolds, J.J., 1972, in: "The Biochemistry and Physiology of Bone" Vol. 1, pp. 69 - 126, Academic Press, New York.

Roels, O.A., 1970, The influence of vitamin A and E on lysosomes, in: "Lysosomes in Biology and Pathology" (J.T. Dingle, B. Fell, eds.), pp. 254, North Holland, Amsterdam, London.

Schimmelpfennig, K., Rajan, K.T., Evans, P., Kaufmann, C.H., 1974, A study of glycosaminoglycans from organ culture of human embryonic digits. Effect of Vitamin A, in: "Proceedings of the Symposium of Tissue Culture in Medical Research", pp. 24 - 31, Heinemann, London.

Trowell, O.A., 1954, A modified technique for organ culture in vitro, Exp. Cell Res., 6, 246.

Tuchmann-Duplessis, H., 1971, Teratogenic drug screening, present procedures and requirements, Teratology, 4, 480.

Tuchmann-Duplessis, H., Mercier-Parot, L., 1959, A propos. D. Malformations Produites par les Bleu-Trypan, J. Biol. Med., 48, 238.

Waddington, C.H., Carter, T.C., 1952, Malformations in mouse embryos induced by trypan blue, Nature, London, 169, 27.

Wilson, J.G., Fradkin, R., Hardmann, A.A., 1968, Progress report on teratogenic testing in rhesus monkeys, Teratol. Soc. 8th Ann. Meet.

Woollam, D.H.M., Millan, J.W., 1960, The modification of the cativity of certain agents exerting a deleterious effect on the development of the mammalian embryos, in: CIBA Found. Symp. Congenital Malformation, pp. 158.

The Effects of Sodium Salicylate, Cytosine Arabinoside, and Eserine Sulphate on Rat Limb Buds in Culture

Dr. O. P. Flint

8F27, Pathology Safety of Medicines, ICI Pharmaceuticals Division,
Mereside Alderley Park, Macclesfield, Cheshire SK10 4TG, U.K.

Mesodermal cells from the developing chick limb bud can be easily isolated and cultured. When chick limb mesoderm which has not yet undergone chondrogenesis is cultured at just post-confluent densities for at least three days, small discrete foci of chondromucopolysaccharide secreting cells are formed (UMANSKY, 1966; CAPLAN, 1970; see Fig. 2 a). AHRENS et al. (1977, 1979) describe a simple micro-mass culture technique which produces a large number of post-confluent cultures from a relatively small number of limb buds, permitting a more quantitative study of differentiation in vitro and of the effects of teratogens on differentiation. Whole limb buds cultured as organ cultures have also been used to examine the effects of teratogens (KOCHHAR, 1977; MERKER et al., 1978).

I have brought these ideas together, first to make a comparison between limbs cultured as dissociated cells or as organ cultures, secondly to extend the use of post-confluent cultures (micro-mass) to mammalian cells, in this case the rat, and thirdly to make a comparison between micro-mass cultures where the drug is administered directly into the culture or indirectly before the culture by an in vivo route. Two of the three drugs whose effects are described, cytosine arabinoside (CA) and sodium salicylate (SAL), are well known teratogens in the rat (CHAUBE and MURPHY, 1965, 1968; GOLDMAN and YAKOVAC, 1963). The third, eserine sulphate or physostigmine (ES) is only known as a teratogen in the chick (BUEKER and PLATNER, 1956) at concentrations of 1.0 - 15.0 mg per egg. The lethal dose of ES in the rat is so low (about 1 - 2 mg/kg i.p.) that its possible teratogenic effect on mammalian embryos is more easily studied in vitro. All three teratogens affect skeletal development.

Preparative Methods:

13.5 day embryos were removed from pregnant Alderley Park outbred rats. Limb buds were either explanted whole onto millipore filter rafts or dissociated to form micro-mass cultures largely according to the technique described by AHRENS et al. (1977). The medium in both cases was Ham's F12 supplemented with 10% fetal calf serum, L-glutamine and antibiotics. Micro-mass cultures were dispensed at 4 x 10^5 cells per 20 µl drop, left for two hours to allow cells to adhere to the culture dish as a 10 - 12 mm spot then topped up with excess medium, and drugs in the case of treated cultures. In a separate experimental series drugs were administered i.p. to the pregnant mother 12 hours before removal of the embryos and no drugs later added to the cultures.

Culture Assay:

Organ cultures were measured with a micrometer measuring eyepiece in a dissecting microscope. Micro-mass cultures were assayed for changes of cell number, protein mass (LOWRY et al., 1951), ^{35}S- sulphate incorporation, ^{3}H-thymidine incorporation and, after staining for sulphated chondromucopolysaccharides with Alcian Blue at pH 1.0 (LEV and SPICER, 1964) the number and total area of foci per spot on day five of culture were measured with an ARTEK 980 colony counter adapted to a dissecting microscope.

Reference to significance in this paper implies statistical significance with probability $p < 0.05$.

Organ Cultured Limb Buds:
Though cultured on Ham's F12, development of control limb buds (Fig. 1 a) was at least as good as that obtained by AYDELOTTE and KOCHHAR (1972) with Biggars BGJ medium. Differences in the growth of treated and control limbs were assessed by measurement, prior to culture and just before fixation on day five of culture (Tables 1, 2) of both limb length from tip to flank and limb breadth at the flank-limb junction. Above a certain concentration all three compounds reduced growth of the explant. ES reduced length and breadth from 1 μg/ml, CA reduced length from 100 ng/ml and breadth from 1 μg/ml, and salicylate reduced length from 100 μg/ml and breadth from 1 mg/ml. Except in the case of CA limb growth was inhibited at lower concentrations than cartilage formation when examined in cartilage clearances or sectioned material (SAL > 500 μg/ml, Fig. 1 d; CA > 100 ng/ml, Fig. 1 c; ES - no inhibition up to 100 μg/ml, Fig. 1 b). More cell death was found in sections of treated limbs than in controls in all three cases, probably accounting for reduced growth.

Micro-mass Cultures: Drug by in vitro route:

1. Fixed and Stained Preparations (Fifth day of culture):
   ES does not inhibit cartilage formation in the concentration range up to 100 μg/ml but from 50 μg/ml appears to either increase the size of the foci or cause fusions between adjacent foci or both (Fig. 2 b). SAL reduces cartilage formation from about 500 μg/ml (Fig. 2 c, d) and CA from about 50 ng/ml (Fig. 2 e, f).

2. Quantitative Measurements:
   a.) Development of controls (Fig. 3):
   A steady increase in the size of the pool of dividing cells from day 1 to day 5 is only accompanied to day 3 by an increase in cell number, which then falls suggesting that from day 3 replacement by division is being overtaken by cell loss of some kind. Other aspects of growth in the culture do not suggest cell death as a result of poor culture health. There is another source of cell loss intimately connected with the formation of chondrogenic foci. By day 3 these are secreting quantities of intercellular matrix material that can be easily recognized after staining with Alcian Blue at low pH (see also AHRENS et al., 1977). A typical focus forms by a centripetal aggregation of cells (Ede et al., 1977) followed by differentiation of (at first) the central cells into chondrocytes which actively manufacture extracellular materials. These pass both into the medium and beneath the cell sheet, lifting the cell sheet from the substrate in the region of the focus. Cells are then lost from both the upper and lower surface of this differentiated area (see for example, Fig. 5 in EGUCHI and OKADA, 1971). Those cells lost from the upper surface of the many foci may account for reduction in cell number after day three. There is no significant change in the quantity of protein per spot between day one and five. Cell growth in just subconfluent cultures and cultures plated out at postconfluent densities is inversely proportional to cell number. Incorporation of ^{35}S-sulphate does not rise above background level (about 10 CPM/μg protein, in Fig. 3) until day two when, in close agreement with the observed pattern of Alcian Blue staining, there is a steady rise until day five.

b.) Comparison of treated with control cultures (see Fig. 4, 5): Between day one and day five treated cultures become divided into two groups. These are the ES cultures which develop chondrogenic foci and the SAL and CA cultures which do not. Protein (Fig. 4) is strongly reduced in SAL and CA treated cultures on day five but there is no difference from controls in ES treated cultures. In their development up to day five SAL treated cultures show an immediate and significant reduction on day one in protein mass, but CA treated cultures are not significantly different from controls and do not reduce to SAL treated culture level until day three. Response to CA is therefore delayed, but to SAL immediate. Protein in ES treated cultures appears to rise slightly above controls on days three, four and five.

^{35}S-sulphate incorporation in CA treated cultures does not rise significantly above background levels on any day of culture (Fig. 4), and in fact no foci are seen to develop in cultures treated with 100 ng/ml of this drug (Fig. 2 b, Table 3). Nor do foci develop in cultures treated with SAL at 750 µg/ml even though incorporation on day one is strongly above control levels and does not fall below control to background level until day five. This suggests that CA and SAL act in two different ways. It is most likely that CA inhibits cell division and possibly movement but is not immediately cell lethal (see also HASSELL et al., 1978). SAL produces much more debris and dead cells from day one accounting for the reduced protein assay. Dying cells have leaky membranes and adsorb the isotope explaining the high levels of ^{35}S-sulphate incorporation in cultures which have otherwise low protein and no chondrogenic expression (Fig. 2 d, Table 3). As cells break down after death and isotope is returned to the medium, counts return to a background level. ^{35}S-sulphate incorporation in eserine treated cultures rises above controls on days three, four and five, particularly (significantly) on day four. Increased isotope incorporation and protein mass on these days seem to account for the observed increase in chondrogenic focus size (Fig. 2 b), which can also be sensitively measured and demonstrated by colony counting techniques (Table 3).

Micro-mass Cultures: Drug by in vivo route:

ES was excluded from this group, first because comparison of effective doses by in vivo and in vitro routes in SAL and CA treatments suggested that the effective in vivo ES dose would be at least one hundred times the lethal dose, and secondly because sublethal ES doses had no effect on subsequent cultures. Dose ranges used for CA and SAL were known to correspond to ranges within which a teratogenic effect could be produced, at the highest dose by a single injection and at the lowest dose by injections over several days. The CA dose range was 20 - 400 mg/kg (CHAUBE and MURPHY, 1968) and the SAL dose range was 10 - 600 mg/kg (GOLDMAN and YAKOVAC, 1963; LARSSON and ERIKSSON, 1966). A single injection was given 12 hours before embryo removal.

Protein was reduced on day one in SAL at 600 mg/kg and subsequently by half the control value on day five with no effect at lower doses (Table 4). CA protein remained at control values on day one up to 400 mg/kg, but at this dose and only this dose, was reduced to half the control value on day five. ^{35}S-sulphate incorporation was significantly reduced from control values by day five in both SAL and CA treated cultures at the lower doses of 100 mg/kg (Table 5). Isotope incorporation in all CA treated cultures and the lower doses of SAL treated cultures did not differ on day one from control values. But at the highest SAL dose incorporation was higher on day one than in controls. Both CA and SAL treated cultures respond to the highest in vivo dose by patterns of protein and ^{35}S-sulphate incorporation which are similar to those observed in in vitro dosed cultures. What is not similar is that SAL cultures produced some recognizable chondrogenic foci after treatment in vivo at 600 mg/kg, whereas CA cultures did not after doses of 400 mg/kg. This may reflect too low a dosing regime in in vivo SAL treatment. These results are confirmed by colony counting techniques (Table 6).

DISCUSSION:

All three drugs reduce limb growth in organ culture, most severely in the case of CA and SAL. Cell death is a partial explanation but the precise mechanism is not clear from these experiments. Micro-mass cultures are more informative than organ cultures. First, comparisons of the effective dose levels in vivo and in vitro tell us something about the in vivo metabolism of the drugs. Effective in vivo dose ranges, 100 - 600 mg/kg, were similar for both CA and SAL. But when the drugs were directly applied, cultures were much more sensitive to CA (> 10^3x) than to SAL. Metabolism to non-teratogenic by-products and elimination must have a stronger effect on CA than on SAL in vivo.

Secondly, development of cultures as described by increase in protein and incorporation of ^{35}S-sulphate reveal differences of action between CA and SAL, but these differences are maintained whether administration is by an in vivo or an in vitro route. The mechanism by which these drugs act on the embryo in vivo must be similar to that in vitro and the differences of behaviour of CA and SAL treated cultures suggest what those mechanisms may be. CA has a delayed, inhibitory effect acting most probably through inhibition of cell division (HASSELL et al., 1978). SAL has a direct and rapid cell lethal effect.

ES does not inhibit chondrogenesis in organ culture though the limbs are smaller than the controls as a result of cell death. In micro-mass cultures ES potentiates differentiation producing more and larger chondrogenic foci and greater secretion of sulphated chondromucopolysaccharides. These paradoxical effects of reduction in organ culture and increase in micromass culture are both reproduced in vivo. LANDAUER (1954) observed (in chick embryos) both micromelia, corresponding to the reduction in limb size in organ culture, and syndactilism, corresponding to increased chondrogenesis and fusion between adjacent foci in micro-mass cultures.

SUMMARY:

In vitro techniques using both organ and cell culture combine to elucidate the action of three teratogens on the differentiating rat limb skeleton. Sodium salicylate has a direct cell lethal effect on the embryo, whereas cytosine arabinoside has a delayed effect probably interfering with the cell cycle. Eserine sulphate has a dual effect reducing the mass of mesoderm by causing cell death and increasing the mass of cartilage by increased chondrogenesis.

Table 1:

Limb length in mm from flank to ridge*

Treatment	Mean length	S	p	Signific.
Before culture	0.72	0.06	-	-
Day 5 control	1.76	0.24	<0.001	S
1 µg Eserine/ml	1.44	0.18	0.025<p<0.01	S
10 µg Eserine/ml	1.11	0.18	<0.001	S
100 µg Eserine/ml	1.11	0.25	<0.001	S
100 ng Cytosine arab./ml	1.23	0.09	0.01>p>0.005	S
1 µg Cytosine arab./ml	0.80	0.17	<0.001	S
10 µg Cytosine arab./ml	0.66	0.22	<0.001	S
10 µg Salicylate/ml	1.57	0.12	0.50>p>0.10	NS
100 µg Salicylate/ml	1.25	0.09	0.01>p>0.005	S
1 mg Salicylate/ml	0.85	0.09	<0.001	S

* 60 limbs cultured.

Table 2:

Limb breadth in mm at junction with flank*

Treatment	Mean breadth	S	p	Signific.
Before culture	0.80	0.06	-	-
Day 5 control	0.90	0.08	0.50>p>0.25	NS
1 µg Eserine/ml	0.78	0.17	0.05>p>0.025	S
10 µg Eserine/ml	0.70	0.06	0.005>p>0.001	S
100 µg Eserine/ml	0.73	0.10	0.01>p>0.005	S
100 ng Cytosine arab./ml	0.80	0.12	0.50>p>0.25	NS
1 µg Cytosine arab./ml	0.42	0.04	p<0.001	S
10 µg Cytosine arab./ml	0.56	0.07	p<0.001	S
10 µg Salicylate/ml	0.83	0.05	0.50>p>0.25	NS
100 µg Salicylate/ml	0.77	0.05	0.10>p>0.05	NS
1 mg Salicylate/ml	0.67	0.12	0.025>p>0.01	S

* 60 limbs cultured.

Table 3:

Counts and area of chondrogenic foci in micro-mass cultures on day 5*.

Culture	$\bar{x}$	S	p (control/treatment)
Control Number	267.20*	49.49	
Area	167.60	43.21	
Cytosine Arab. 10 µg/ml	-		
Salicylate 500 µg/ml	-		
Eserine Number	344.17	21.58	0.01>p>0.005
100 µg/ml Area	327.17	38.12	p<0.001

* Arbitrary counts. 32 'spots' assayed. Drug by in vitro route. No detectable foci developed in Ca or SAL cultures.

Table 4:

Protein assay from cultured embryonic rat limb cells after in vivo treatment*

Culture		$\bar{x}$	S	p (day 1 /day 5)	p (day 1 control/ day 5 treated
Control	Day 1	27.50	4.02	0.10>p>0.05	
	Day 5	30.42	5.44		
Cytosine Arab. 20 mg/kg	Day 1	28.50	1.47	0.50>p>0.25	0.50>p>0.25
	Day 5	22.66	5.78		
Cytosine Arab. 100 mg/kg	Day 1	28.00	2.82	0.50>p>0.25	p>0.75
	Day 5	22.66	5.78		
Cytosine Arab. 400 mg/kg	Day 1	29.10	2.78	p<0.001	0.10>p>0.05
	Day 5	15.60	2.34		
Salicylate 10 mg/kg	Day 1	31.80	5.18	0.50>p>0.25	0.25>p>0.50
	Day 5	28.80	6.72		
Salicylate 100 mg/kg	Day 1	26.40	2.60	0.50>p>0.25	0.75>p>0.50
	Day 5	29.20	6.42		
Salicylate 600 mg/kg	Day 1	17.20	2.28	0.50>p>0.28	p<0.001
	Day 5	14.80	7.16		

* 85 'spots' assayed. $\bar{x}$ is mean protein per spot in µg.
S is standard deviation.

Table 5:

CPM/μg protein $^{35}SO_4$ incorporation into rat limb bud cells after in vivo treatment*.

Culture	Day	$\bar{x}$	S	p (day 1 /day 5)	p (day 1 control/ day 1 treated)	p (day 5 control/ day 5 control)
Control	1	10.01	3.08	p<0.001		
	5	26.25	7.33			
Cyt. Arab. 20 mg/kg	1	10.05	0.35		p>0.75	
	5	26.30	5.07			p>0.75
Cyt. Arab. 100 mg/kg	1	8.15	0.95		0.75>p>0.50	
	5	6.58	1.60			p<0.001
Cyt. Arab. 400 mg/kg	1	7.84	1.42		0.50>p>0.25	
	5	8.02	2.20			p<0.001
Salicylate 10 mg/kg	1	10.06	2.67		p>0.75	
	5	26.86	2.93			p>0.75
Salicylate 100 mg/kg	1	10.43	1.55		p>0.75	
	5	22.12	3.22			0.10>p>0.05
Salicylate 600 mg/kg	1	14.02	1.08		0.10>p>0.05	
	5	11.91	4.51			p<0.001

* 85 'spots' assayed. $\bar{x}$ is mean CPM/μg protein $^{35}SO_4$ per spot. S is standard deviation.

Table 6:

Counts and area of chondrogenic foci in micro-mass cultures on day 5*.

Number:	Culture	$\bar{x}$	S	p (control/treatment)
	Control	245*	18.45	
Cyt. Arab.	20 mg/kg	245	53.47	
	100 mg/kg	-		
	400 mg/kg	-		
Salicylate	10 mg/kg	245	51.27	
	100 mg/kg	240	51.34	
	600 mg/kg	157	10.86	$p<0.001$

Area:	Culture	$\bar{x}$	S	p (control/treatment)
	Control	299*	41.71	
Cyt. Arab.	20 mg/kg	299	86.20	
	100 mg/kg	-		
	400 mg/kg	-		
Salicylate	10 mg/kg	299	98.47	
	100 mg/kg	298	45.06	
	600 mg/kg	158	71.08	$p<0.001$

* Arbitrary units. Figures adjusted against control value to account for variations in staining on different culture days. Drug by in vivo route. No detectable foci in CA 100, 400 mg/kg.

REFERENCES

Ahrens, P.B., Solursh, M., Reiter, R.S., 1977, Stage-related capacity for limb chondrogenesis in cell culture, Develop. Biol., 60, 69 - 82.

Ahrens, P.B., Solursh, M., Reiter, R.S., Singley, C.T., 1979, Position related capacity for differentiation of limb mesenchyme in cell culture, Develop. Biol., 69, 436 - 450.

Aydelotte, M.B., Kochhar, D.M., 1972, Development of mouse limb buds in organ culture: chondrogenesis in the presence of a proline analog, L-azetidine-2-carboxylic acid. Develop. Biol., 28, 191 - 201.

Bueker, E.D., Platner, W.S., 1956, Effect of cholinergic drugs on development of the chick embryo, Proc. Soc. exp. Biol. Med., 91, 539 - 543.

Caplan, A.I., 1970, Effects of the nicotinamide-sensitive teratogen 3-acetylpyridine on chick limb cells in culture, Exp. Cell Res., 62, 341 - 355.

Chaube, S., Murphy, M.L., 1965, Teratogenic effects of cytosine arabinoside (CA) in the rat fetus (Abstract), Proc. Amer. Ass. Cancer Res., 6, 11.

Chaube, S., Murphy, M.L., 1968, The teratogenic effects of the recent drugs active in cancer chemotherapy, in: Advances in Teratology, Vol. 3, (D.H.M. Woolam, ed.), pp. 204 - 205, Academic Press Publ., New York.

Ede, D.A., Flint, O.P., Wilby, O.K., Colquhoun, P., 1977, The development of pre-cartilage condensations in limb bud mesenchyme in vivo and in vitro, in: 3rd Symposium of the B.S.D.B. on Vertebrate Limb and Somite Morphogenesis, (D.A. Ede, J.R. Hinchcliffe, M. Balls, eds.), pp. 161 - 179, C.U.P. Publ.

Eguchi, G., Okada, T.S., 1971, Ultrastructure of the differentiated cell colony derived from a singly isolated chondrocyte in in vitro culture, Develop. Growth Differ., 12, 297 - 312.

Goldman, A.S., Yakovac, W.C., 1963, The enhancement of salicylate teratogenicity by maternal immobilisation in the rat, J. Pharmacol. Exp. Ther., 142, 351 - 357.

Hassell, J.R., Pennypacker, J.P., Lewis, C.A., 1978, Chondrogenesis and cell proliferation in limb bud cell cultures treated with cytosine arabinoside and vitamin A, Exp. Cell Res., 112, 409 - 417.

Kochhar, D.M., 1977, Cellular basis of congenital limb deformity induced in mice by vitamin A, Birth Defects: Original Article Series, Vol. XII, No. 1, pp. 111 - 154.

Merker, H.J., Günther, Th., Krüger, U., 1978, Effect of 4-methylumbelliferyl-ß-D-xylopyranoside on the morphology of embryonic cartilage in limb bud cultures, Teratology, 18, 291 - 310.

Landauer, W., 1954, On the chemical production of developmental abnormalities and of phenocopies in chicken embryos, Cell Comp. Physiol., 43, 261 - 305.

Larsson, K.S., Eriksson, M., 1966, Salicylate-induced fetal death and malformations in two mouse strains, Acta Paediatr., 55, 569 - 576.

Lev, R., Spicer, S.S., 1964, Specific staining of sulphate groups with Alcian Blue at low pH, J. Histochem. Cytochem., 12, 309.

Lowry, O.H., Rosenbrough, N.F., Farn, A.L., Randell, R.J., 1951, Protein measurement with folin phenol reagent, J. Biol. Chem., 193, 265 - 275.

Umansky, R., 1966, The effect of cell population density on the developmental fate of reaggregating mouse limb bud mesenchyme, Develop. Biol., 13, 31 - 56.

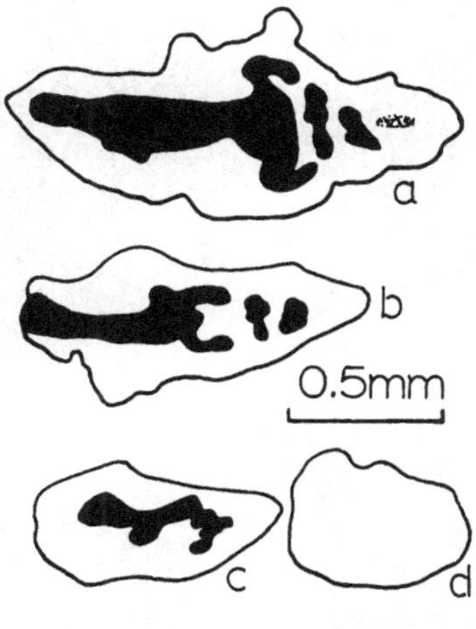

Fig. 1: Camera lucida drawings of Alcian Blue stained limbs after five days in organ culture: a) Control; b) ES 10 µg/ml; c) CA 100 ng/ml; d) SAL 1 mg/ml.

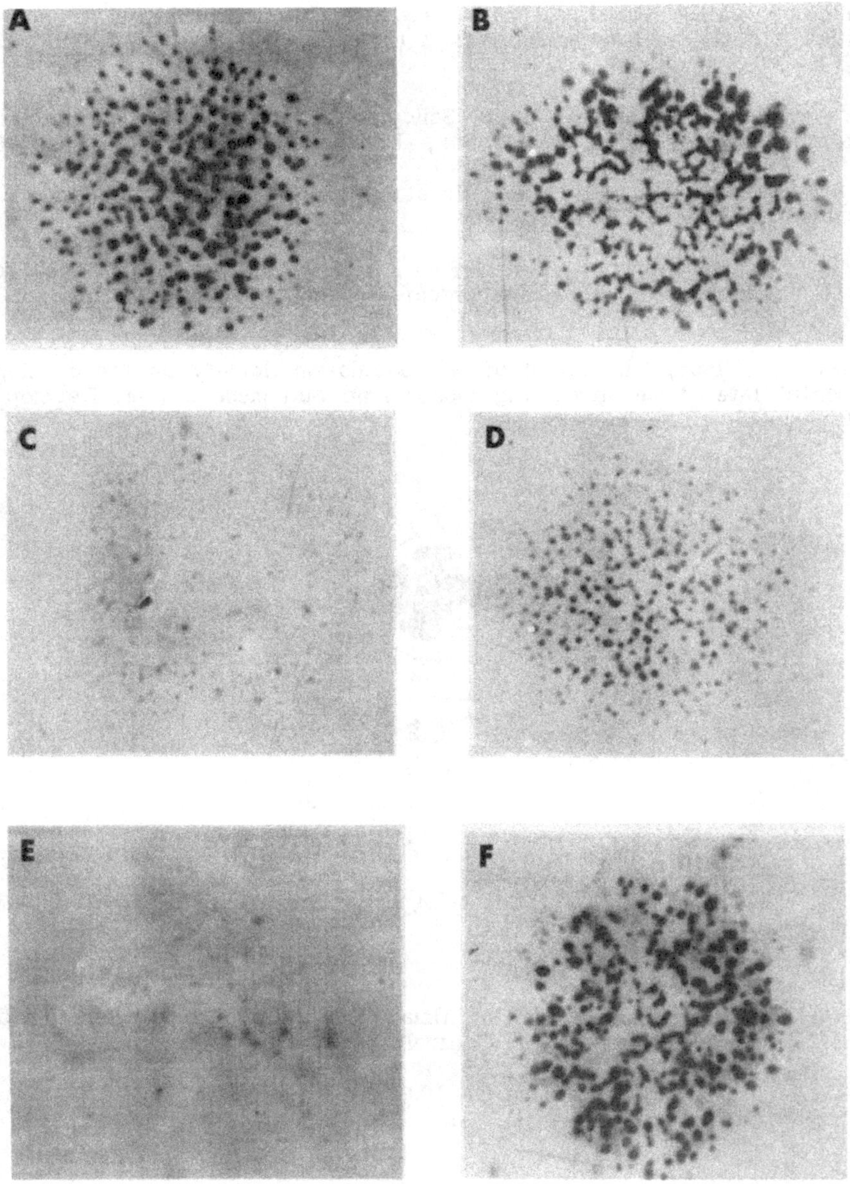

Fig. 2: Micro-mass cultures of limb mesenchyme fixed and stained with Alcian Blue at low pH on day five of culture:

a) Control;
b) ES 50 µg/ml;
c) SAL 1 000 µg/ml;
d) SAL 100 µg/ml;
e) CA 100 ng/ml;
f) CA 10 ng/ml.

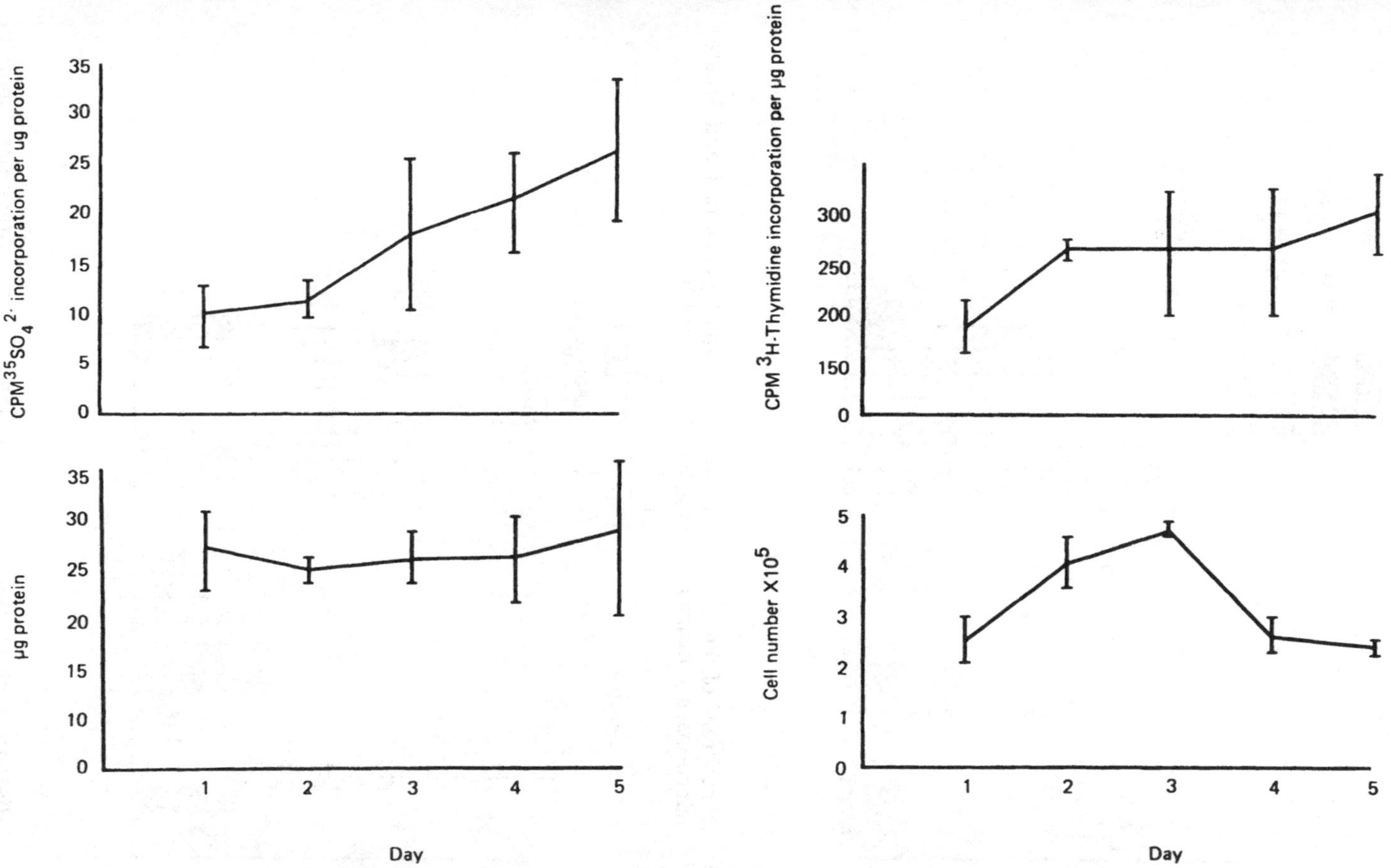

Fig. 3: Micro-mass control cultures. Change of cell number, ^{3}H-thymidine incorporation, protein assay, and ^{35}S-sulphate incorporation. All measurements per single spot plated out at 4 x 10^5 cells on day 0.

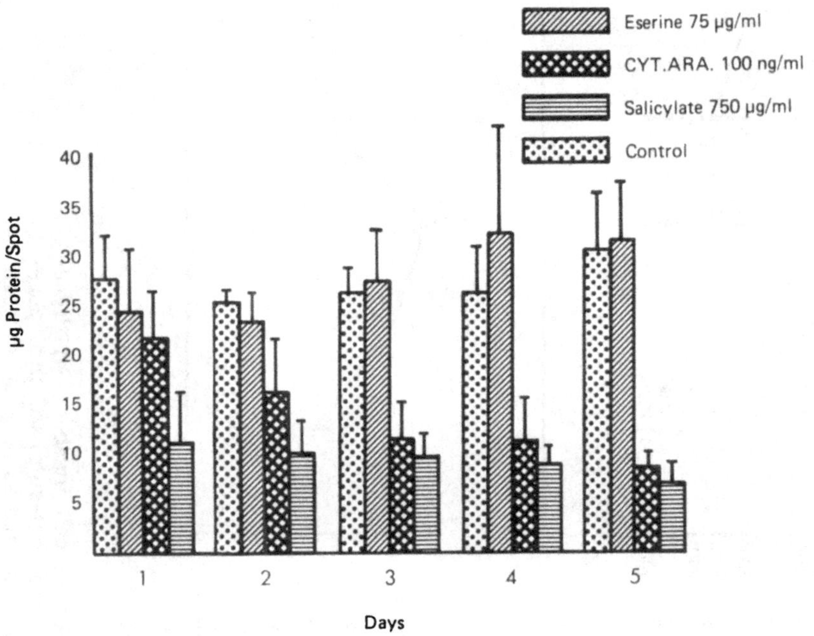

Fig. 4: Histogram of changes in protein per 'spot' in control and treated micro-mass cultures. Drug by in vitro route.

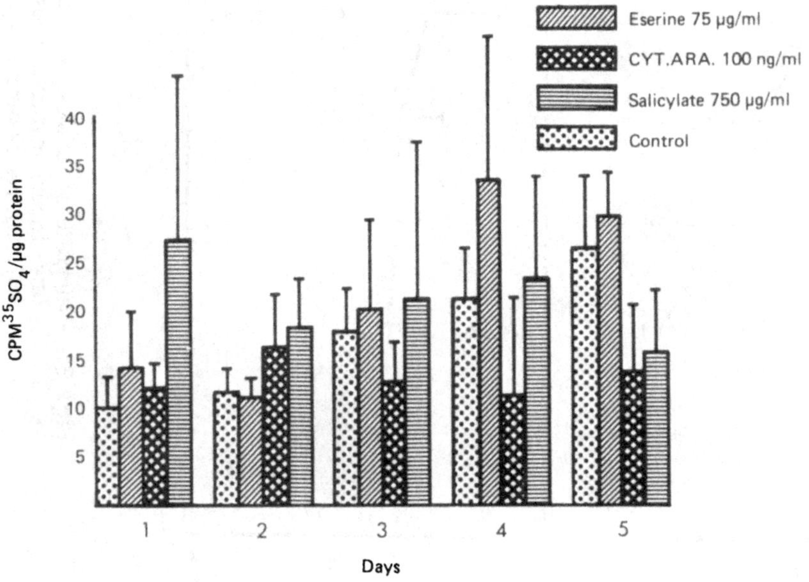

Fig. 5: Histogram of changes in ^{35}S-sulphate incorporation per 'spot' in control and treated micro-mass cultures. Drug by in vitro route.

C. Effects of Teratogenic Agents

The Transplacental Effects of Vitamin D Metabolites and Corticosteroids on the Long Bones of Rat and Mice Fetuses

A. Ornoy, B. E. Hirsch, I. Zusman, I. Atkin

Department of Anatomy and Embryology, The Hebrew University, Hadassah Medical School, P.O. Box 1172, Jerusalem, Israel

The process of bone formation involves two basic events; (a) ossification, i.e. production of bone and cartilage matrix and (b) calcification, i.e. precipitation of minerals within that matrix.

Membrane-bound matrix vesicles have been identified by electron microscopy in cartilage and bone. They are believed to serve as loci of initial calcification of epiphyseal cartilage and of bone (BONUCCI, 1971). Scanning and transmission electron microscopic studies supported by biochemical investigations have shown that these matrix vesicles originate by budding from chondrocytes and osteoblasts (ORNOY et al., 1979; ORNOY et al., 1980). Abnormalities of the developing skeleton usually involve the process of matrix formation or resorption. However, consideration must also be given to the possibility that derangement of bone calcification (as occurring in vitamin D deficient rickets) may be an important factor in pathological processes affecting bone and possibly in congenital skeletal defects.

The etiology of most congenital skeletal anomalies is obscure and theories as to the pathogenesis of these defects are based on various genetic causes (GRÜNEBERG, 1963). Skeletal defects have been produced in pregnant rats by different experimental procedures such as riboflavin deficiency, pteroylglutamic acid deficiency, zinc deficiency, manganese deficiency, or dietary imbalances (NELSON et al., 1952; HURLEY, 1977). However, the malformations of the skeleton observed in these experiments were probably caused by effects on other fetal systems, because under the experimental conditions described above multiple malformations usually occurred.

Several studies have been published in which an attempt was made to interfere with fetal skeletal development by derangements of maternal calcium and phosphorus metabolism. Usually breeding difficulties did not allow well-controlled studies. If the imbalance was not severe enough, normal offspring resulted. SONTAG et al. (1936) were able to breed rats fed a low calcium and phosphorus diet, and showed that the offspring had a lower mineral content than controls. When rats were fed a rachitogenic diet (vitamin D deficient, high calcium, low phosphorus) for two weeks, then mated and kept on the same diet throughout pregnancy, the offspring exhibited general skeletal abnormalities. Microscopic examination of the long bones showed a wide zone of hypertrophic cartilage cells in the epiphyses with persistence of hypertrophic chondrocytes in the diaphyses. These skeletal changes could be interpreted as fetal rickets (SONTAG et al., 1936; WARKANY, 1943). In our experiments two hormones, vitamin D and its metabolites and cortisone acetate known to affect bone metabolism, were administered to pregnant rats and mice, in order to assess their transplacental effects on ossification and calcification of bone in the offspring.

Teratology of the Limbs

Effects of vitamin D on fetal bone

It is well known that vitamin D (cholecalciferol) is in fact a prohormone, which gives rise to 1,25 dihydroxycholecalciferol (1,25 $(OH)_2D_3$) and to 24,25 dihydroxycholecalciferol (24,25 $(OH)_2D_3$). The 1,25 $(OH)_2D_3$ is believed to carry out many of the known biological functions of the vitamin. High doses of 1,25$(OH)_2D_3$ would cause hypercalcemia and probably bone resorption (ORNOY et al., 1979). It seems that this hormone alone is, however, unable to cure vitamin D deficient rickets (NOFF et al., 1978; Dekel et al., 1979). The other metabolite, 24,25 $(OH)_2D_3$ was shown specifically to cure rickets (ORNOY et al., 1978) and therefore, was recently used for therapeutic purposes. Because vitamin D has a direct effect on bone, and it seems to pass the rat placenta particularly when administered at high doses, it was decided to study the transplacental effects of high doses of vitamin D and its active metabolites on the fetal skeleton.

In the first experiment pregnant rats of the Hebrew University Sabra strain were treated daily from day 10 of gestation to day 21 by an oral dose of 20 000 I.U. or 40 000 I.U. of vitamin D_2. At the beginning of days 18, 20 and 22 of gestation fetuses were removed, weighed and examined for external malformations. Long bones were removed for light microscopic studies. The ash content, calcium phosphorus and magnesium content of the fetal long bones were also determined.

Hypervitaminosis D_2 reduced significantly fetal weight, net weight and ash content of fetal bones. The calcium and phosphate contents were reduced, and magnesium content was elevated (ORNOY et al., 1968). The total length of fetal tibiae and femora were reduced, mainly because of a severe reduction in the length of the diaphyses, while the length of the epiphyses was similar to that of controls (Tab. 1).

Microscopal examination of paraffin-embedded 7 µ thick longitudinal sections of long bones of the extremities showed a marked retardation in the ossification of the diaphysis. The metaphyseal line was curved. The arrangement of the cartilage columns in the epiphyses was disturbed, with many degenerating resting chondrocytes. Occasionally there was a complete disorganization of the chondrocytes, with fibrous degeneration of the intercellular matrix. The zones of hypertrophic and calcifying cartilage were narrow. The diaphysis was smaller with fewer trabeculae. On day 22, the same pathological changes persisted, with a short diaphysis and apparently fewer osteoclasts than in controls. On days 20 and 22, the zone of provisional calcification was thin when compared to controls, and the secretion of alkaline phosphatase as revealed by histochemical staining was markedly reduced (ORNOY et al., 1969).

Only 40% of the offspring of rats treated with high doses of vitamin D_2 could be raised to the age of one month. The offspring were weighed periodically, and every 3 - 5 days long bones were removed for microscopical studies. The weight of the experimental animals was reduced, and the weight decrease seemed to increase with age. By the 5th day of life the bones of experimental animals were short and distorted. The periosteal bone of the diaphysis was thin. The bone trabeculae were composed, to a large extent, of calcified cartilage that persisted in the diaphyses, surrounded by a thin layer of bone. Several fractures were found especially in the submetaphyseal area. When followed, these fractures tended to heal, forming large masses of mesenchyme and cartilage but healing was not completed and pseudoarthrosis was occasionally found. New fractures formed throughout life, and the animals also developed severe kyphoscoliosis. It seems therefore, that large doses of vitamin D_2 administered to pregnant rats caused severe, persisting skeletal defects in the offspring which resembled osteogenesis imperfecta (ORNOY et al., 1972).

We next investigated which of the metabolites of vitamin D could have been responsible for these changes, i.e. $1,25(OH)_2D_3$ or $24,25(OH)_2D_3$. Pregnant rats were treated daily during days 16 - 21 of gestation by subcutaneous injections of 0.5µg $1,25(OH)_2D_3$ (toxic doses). On day 22 of pregnancy the animals were sacrificed, fetuses were removed, weighed, femora and tibiae dissected for light microscopic studies. The long bones were measured, and the number of osteoclasts/square millimeter counted by methods described elsewhere (ORNOY, 1971). Seven thick longitudinal sections were studied by light microscopy. It was found that fetal weight was reduced to only 70% of the control weight (Tab. 1). Both fetuses and mothers exhibited hypercalcemia, and microscopical examination of fetal long bones showed marked changes when compared to controls. In the epiphyses the zone of hypertrophic cartilage was thin, and the cells disorganized (Figs. 1, 2).

VON KOSSA staining of non-decalcified sections showed calcification of both longitudinal and transverse intercartilaginous septa, throughout the zone of hypertrophic cartilage while in the controls only the longitudinal septa at the lower hypertrophic zone near the metaphysis was calcified. The metaphyseal line was curved in fetuses from experimental animals and the diaphyses were short and distorted (Fig. 1, 2). Often calcified cartilage islets surrounded by bone projected from the epiphyses deep into the diaphyses. The metaphyseal trabeculae were disorganized and sometimes appeared thick and short. The number of osteoclasts in the metaphyses and in the diaphyses was similar to that found in controls (Tab. 1).

A group of pregnant rats were similarly treated subcutaneously with 0.5 µg of $24,25(OH)_2D_3$ during days 16 - 21 of pregnancy and the fetuses removed on the 22nd day. Fetal weight on day 22 was similar to the weight of control fetuses. Although the length of tibial epiphyses and diapyses was reduced when compared to controls, this reduction was not statistically significant (Tab. 1). The maternal and fetal serum calcium concentrations were comparable to control values. Microscopic examination of fetal long bones showed that the epiphyses had a normal arrangement and structure. The diaphyses, however, had many persisting enchondral bone trabeculae. These trabeculae had a central core of calcified intercartilaginous matrix surrounded by osteoid. Control fetuses had a well developed medullary cavity in the diaphysis, with only few persisting trabeculae (Fig. 1, 4). The number of osteoclasts in the metaphyses and diaphyses was increased (Tab. 1). It can therefore be concluded that high doses of $1,25(OH)_2D_3$ cause severe abnormalities of the fetal skeleton of rats which resemble the defects found after administration of high doses of vitamin D_2. These skeletal defects seem to result from a direct toxic effect of the excess vitamin D. High doses of $1,25(OH)_2D_3$ in organ culture have been shown to cause demineralization of fetal bone (RAISZ et al., 1972). On the other hand, $24,25(OH)_2D_3$ seems to enhance bone formation by direct effects on bone forming and/or bone resorbing elements. These findings seem to support other studies which showed a direct role of this hormone in the metabolism of cartilage and bone (ORNOY et al., 1978; NOFF and EDELSTEIN, 1978).

Effects of cortisone acetate on fetal bone

High doses of corticosteroids are known to induce various bone changes. The most prominent effects include increased bone resorption and demineralization as well as slowing of bone growth (STOREY, 1963). However, in developing rats corticosteroids would induce dense bone in the metaphysis consisting of unresorbed calcified cartilage surrounded by bone (SIMMONS and KUNIN, 1967).

We therefore decided to treat pregnant rats and mice with high doses of cortisone acetate during the second half of pregnancy in order to study the transplacental effects of corticosteroids on fetal bone. Pregnant rats were treated daily by intramuscular injections of 10 mg cortisone acetate on days 10 - 21 of gestation. The fetuses were obtained on the 22nd day for morphological studies of their long bones. Other rats, similarly treated, were allowed to deliver, and the offspring examined periodically up to one month of age. The rat fetuses (22nd day) were smaller (4.92 ± 0.14 gr) when compared to controls (5.84 ± 0.12 gr). The tibial length was reduced because of a reduction in the length of the diaphyses by 30% and of the epiphyses by 15%. The ash calcium and phosphorus contents were similar to control values in spite of the smaller bones, implying that there was a higher mineral content/mg of wet bone (ORNOY and HOROWITZ, 1972).

Microscopical examinations of longitudinal sections of long bones revealed alterations in the ground substance of cartilage and bone. In the epiphyses, the zone of hypertrophic cartilage was thinner when compared to controls, being responsible for the shorter epiphyses. In the short diaphyses islets of persisting calcified cartilage were found which were surrounded by bone (Fig. 4). The trabeculae were randomly oriented, in contrast to the longitudinal orientation of bone trabeculae in control animals. The number of osteoclasts in metaphyses and diaphyses of long bones from cortisone-treated rats was three fold higher than in the controls (Fig. 4).

Cortisone-treated rats were allowed to deliver, and the long bones of the offspring studied up to one month of age. The excessive bone trabeculae gradually disappeared during the first two weeks of life. The ash calcium and phosphorus content were gradually reduced to control values, and the weight of the offspring reached the weight of control offspring by 3 weeks of age (ORNOY and HOROWITZ, 1972). It can therefore be concluded, that cortisone acetate affects transplacentally fetal bones in rats, causing short and dense bones which resemble osteopetrosis. However, this is not a true congential defect since the skeletal changes gradually disappeared after birth.

Because mice are known to react to high doses of cortisone by a reduction in bone mass, we decided to treat pregnant mice with 0.75 mg cortisone acetate by daily intramuscular injections during days 11 - 19 of gestation. The offspring were studied on days 1, 3, 5, 10, 15, 20, and 30 after birth. In these experiments we were interested to study both ossification and calcification of fetal long bones. Therefore, bones were studied by light microscopy, scanning and transmission electron microscopy.

The offspring of treated mice were smaller when compared to controls. This weight difference persisted throughout the first two weeks, and then gradually disappeared (Tab. 2). The tibiae and femora of young treated animals were shorter mainly due to shortening of the diaphyses and epiphyses, especially in the zone of hypertrophic chondrocytes. The metaphyseal and diaphyseal bone trabeculae were thinner. These changes gradually disappeared after two weeks of age, although X-rays of long bones from one month old offspring of treated mothers still showed thinner diaphyses when compared to controls. By day 10, secondary ossification centers appeared in the epiphyses of control animals, but in experimental animals these ossification centers appeared later, and ossification of the epiphyses was retarded. By day 30, microscopical examination of long bones did not reveal any significant difference between control and treated animals.

Examination of non-decalcified metacrylate embedded 2 - 3 µ thick longitudinal section of bones, stained by VON KOSSA'S stain for calcium salts revealed in treated animals calcification of longitudinal and transverse intercartilaginous septa at the zones of proliferating and hypertrophic cartilage. This was prominent during days 1 - 5 of age, and gradually disappeared thereafter. In control offspring, calcification was observed in the longitudinal septa of the zone of provisional calcification only (Fig. 5). TEM studies of the epiphyses revealed intracellular calcification in addition to calcification of the longitudinal and transverse intercartilaginous septa. This intracellular calcification was mainly confined to the mitochondria of proliferating and hypertrophic chondrocytes.

Membrane-bound matrix vesicles were observed by TEM in the interterritorial matrix of proliferating and hypertrophic cartilage in both control and experimental animals. Their shape, number and distribution was similar in controls and experimental mice. In controls hydroxyl-apatite crystals could be observed in association with matrix vesicles, mainly in the longitudinal septa of the hypertrophic zone. In experimental animals, however, mineral crystals were observed in the proliferating zone as well as in the hypertrophic zone, not necessarily associated with matrix vesicles (Fig. 6). Often crystals were observed outside matrix vesicles, or at significant distances from matrix vesicles.

SEM studies further confirmed the TEM findings. Matrix vesicles, identified as globular structures (0.1 µ in diameter) were observed in both control and experimental animals. Hydroxylapatite crystals were observed, which tended to form larger aggregates - calcospherites. The calcospherites, however, were small and non-homogeneous in treated mice, while in controls they were homogeneous, of about 1 µ in diameter (Fig. 7).

Cortisone acetate, after passing through the mouse placenta, directly affects fetal bone causing abnormal calcification of the epiphyses, thinner bone trabeculae, and small bones. These skeletal lesions do not seem to be true congenital defects, as they slowly disappear during the first two weeks of postnatal life. In this respect, they differ from the lasting skeletal defects produced by hypervitaminosis D in rats.

The experimental models for skeletal malformations described here were induced by high doses of hormones, which under certain specific conditions may be teratogenic. The skeletal defects described can be regarded as phenocopies of human genetically determined skeletal dysplasias. However, further biochemical and ultrastructural studies are needed for the proper use of these models to understand the pathogenesis of similar defects in man.

Table 1:

The transplacental effects of high doses of 1,25$(OH)_2D_3$ and 24,25$(OH)_2D_3$, on weight, tibial length and number of osteoclasts in 22 day old fetuses.

		Tibial length, mm			No. of osteoclast/mm^2	
Daily treatm.	Fetal wt. (gr.)	prox. epiph.	diaphy.	dist. epiphy.	metaphy.	diaphys.
Control.	5.47 ± 0.40	1.80 ± 0.20	2.80 ± 0.20	1.49 ± 0.18	2.7 ± 0.40	4.2 ± 0.5
0.5 µg 1,25 $(OH)_2D_3$.	3.95 ± 0.30	1.42 ± 0.10	2.27 ± 0.25	1.17 ± 0.10	2.1 ± 0.25	4.4 ± 0.26
0.5 µg 24,25 $(OH)_2D_3$.	5.07 ± 0.20	1.58 ± 0.20	2.57 ± 0.30	1.27 ± 0.20	4.0 ± 0.30	6.5 ± 0.2
40 000 I.U. Vitamin D_2.	3.07 ± 0.18	1.80 ± 0.18	2.20 ± 0.30	1.54 ± 0.20	not counted	

Table 2:

The transplacental effects of cortisone acetate on weight and tibial length in offspring of mice.

Age at sacrifice (days)	Weight of offspring (gr)		Tibial length, mm					
			Prox. epiph.		Diaphysis		Distal epiph.	
	cort.	contr.	cort.	contr.	cort.	contr.	cort.	contr.
1	1.19	1.62	1.00 ± 0.15	1.11 ± 0.16	1.85 ± 0.13	3.42 ± 0.13	0.98 ± 0.12	1.05 ± 0.13
3	----	----	1.10 ± 0.27	1.19 ± 0.29	3.16 ± 0.22	3.96 ± 0.22	1.05 ± 0.23	1.08 ± 0.24
5	2.20	3.77	1.19 ± 0.31	1.50 ± 0.41	3.81 ± 0.27	5.50 ± 0.27	1.14 ± 0.25	1.38 ± 0.31
10	4.59	6.42	1.49 ± 0.37	1.59 ± 0.45	-----	-----	1.47 ± 0.39	1.53 ± 0.42

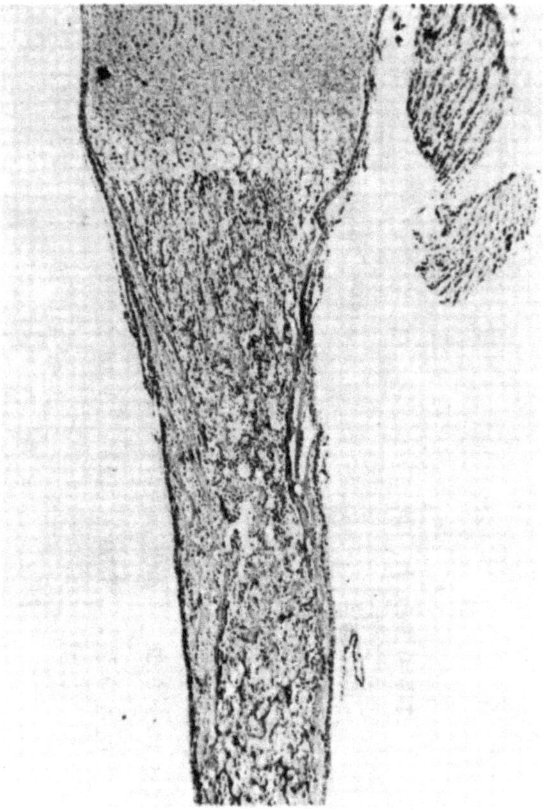

Fig. 1: Microphotograph of a longitudinal section of a tibia from a 22 day old control rat fetus. Hematoxylin and Eosine staining. x 30.

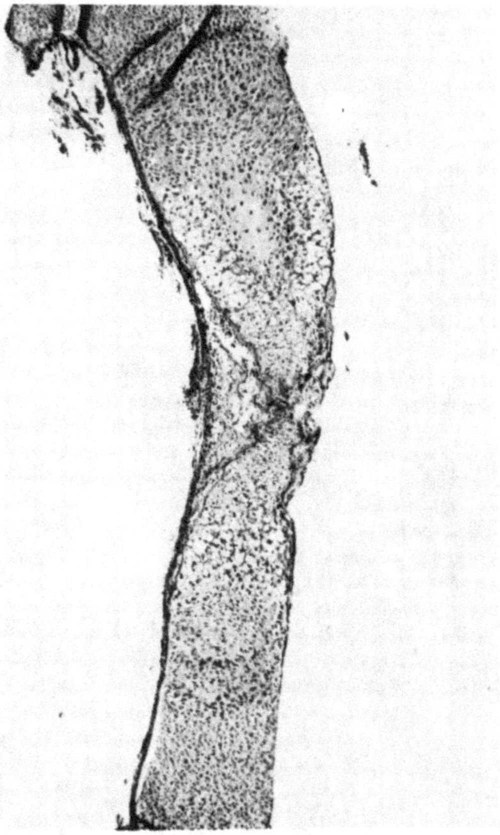

Fig. 2: Longitudinal section of a tibia from a 22 day old experimental rat fetus whose mother was treated daily with 0.5µg 1,25(OH) $_2D_3$ during days 16 - 21 of gestation. Note disorganized epiphyses, curved metaphyseal line and short distorted diaphysis. Hematoxylin and Eosine staining. x 30.

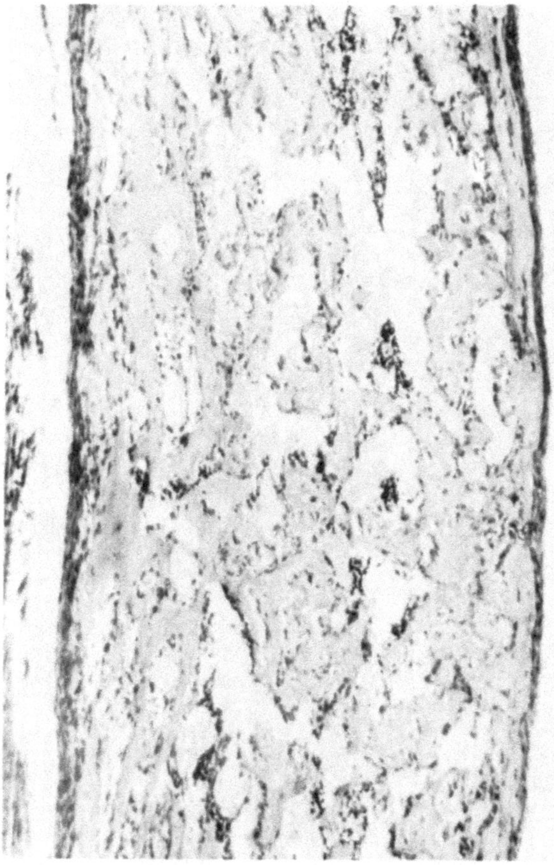

Fig. 3: Tibial diaphysis from a 22 day old experimental rat fetus whose mother was treated daily with 0.5µg of 24,25$(OH)_2D_3$ during days 16 - 21 of gestation. Note persisting bone trabeculae inside medullary cavity of the diaphysis. Hematoxylin and Eosine staining. x 90.

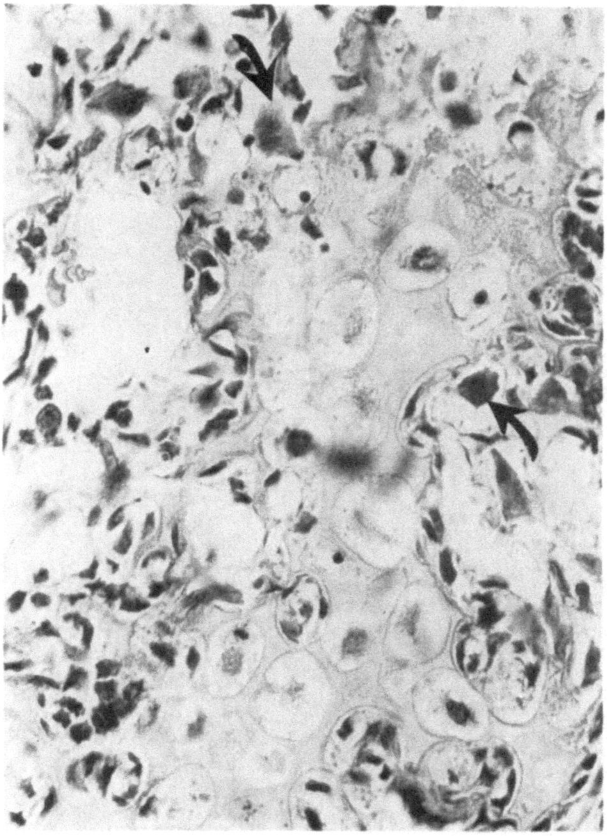

Fig. 4: Tibial diaphysis from a 22 day old experimental rat fetus whose mother was treated daily with 10 mg cortisone acetate during days 10 - 21 of gestation. Note persisting calcified cartilage surrounded by a thin layer of bone and numerous osteoclasts. Hematoxylin and Eosine staining. x 400.

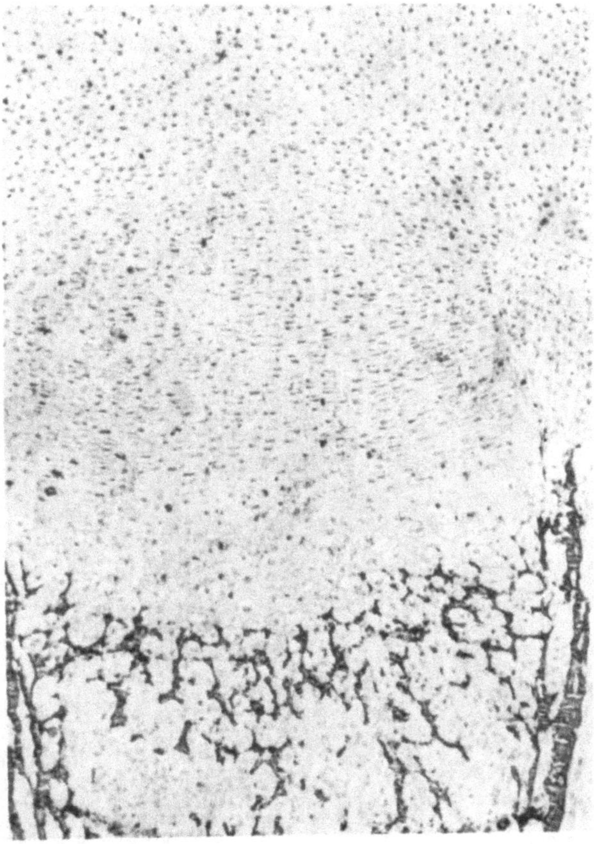

Fig. 5: Tibial epiphysis and metaphysis from a one day old experimental mouse whose mother was treated daily with 0.75 mg cortisone acetate during days 10 - 19 of gestation. Note calcification of longitudinal and transverse intercartilaginous septa at the hypertrophic zone. Methacrylate embedding, Von Kossa staining. x 90.

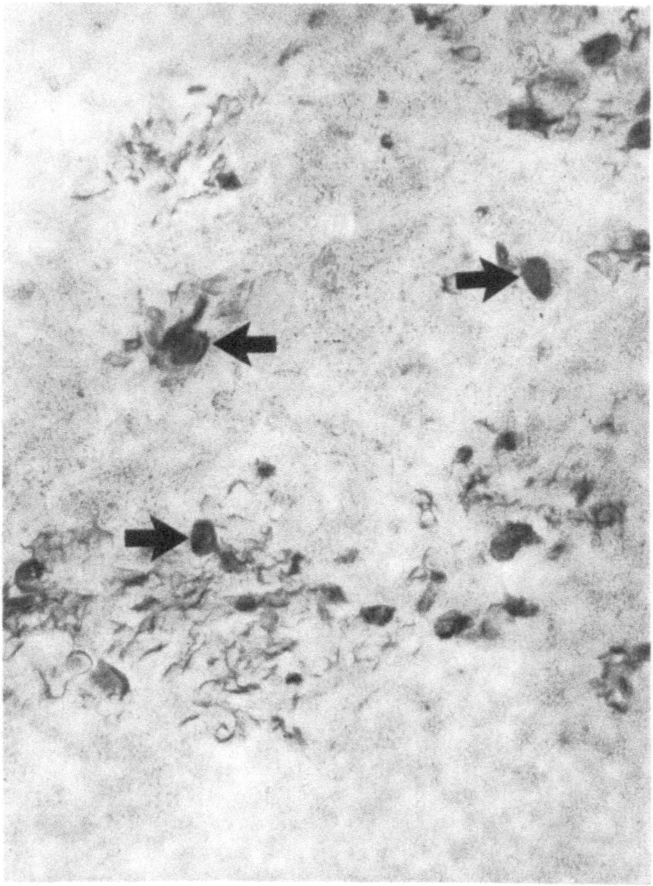

Fig. 6: TEM photograph of longitudinal intercartilaginous septum at the hypertrophic zone of a tibial epiphysis showing mineral crystals outside and inside matrix vesicles. The mother of this one day old experimental mouse was treated daily with 0.75 mg cortisone acetate during days 10 - 19 of gestation. Lead citrate and uranyl acetate staining method. x 20 520.

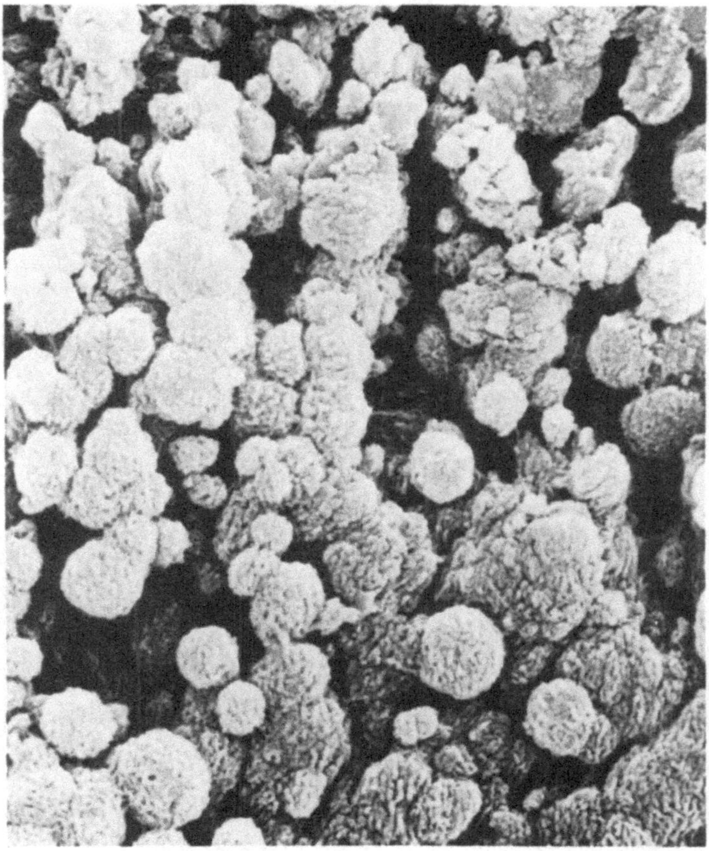

Fig. 7: SEM photograph of calcospherites at the hypertrophic zone of a tibial epiphysis in one day old experimental mouse, whose mother was treated daily with 0.75 mg cortisone acetate during days 10 - 19 of gestation. Note small and large calcospherites. NaOCl immersion for 2 hours. x 5 600.

REFERENCES

Bonucci, E., 1971, The locus of initial calcification in cartilage and bone, Clin. Orthop., 78, 108 - 139.

Dekel, S., Ornoy, A., Sekeles, E., Noff, D., Edelstein, S., 1979, Contrasting effects on bone formation and on fracture healing of cholecalciferol and of 1α hydroxycholecalciferol, Calcif. Tiss. Intl., 28, 245 - 251.

Grüneberg, H., 1963, "The Pathology of Development". A study of inherited skeletal disorders in animals, (Oxford: Blackwell Scientific Publ.)

Hurley, L.S., 1977, "Nutritional Deficiencies and Excesses", in: Handbook of Teratology, Vol. 1 (G. Wilson, H. Fraser, eds.) pp. 261 - 308, Plenum Press, New York.

Kaduri, A.J., Ornoy, A., 1974, Impaired osteogenesis in the fetus induced by administration of cortisone to pregnant mice, Isr. J. Med. Sci., 10, 476 - 481.

Nelson, M.M., Ashling, C.W., Evans, H.M., 1952, Production of multiple congenital abnormalities in young rats by maternal pteroylglutamic acid deficiency during gestation, J. Nutr., 48, 61 - 80.

Noff, D., Edelstein, S., 1978, Vitamin D and its hydroxylated metabolites in the rat. Placental and lacteal transport, subsequent metabolic pathways and tissue distribution, Horm. Res., 9, 292 - 360.

Ornoy, A., 1971, The effects of maternal hypercortisonism and hypervitaminosis D_2 on fetal osteogenesis and ossification in rats, Teratology, 4, 383 - 394.

Ornoy, A., Horowitz, A., 1972, Postnatal effects of maternal hypercortisonism on skeletal development in newborn rats, Teratology, 6, 153 - 158.

Ornoy, A., Menczel, J., Nebel, L., 1968, Alteration in the mineral composition and metabolism of rat fetuses and their placentae induced by maternal hypervitaminosis D_2, Isr. J. Med. Sci., 4, 827 - 832.

Ornoy, A., Nebel, L., Menczel, J., 1969, Impaired osteogenesis of fetal long bones induced by maternal hypervitaminosis D_2, Arch. Pathol., 87, 563 - 571.

Ornoy, A., Kaspi, T., Nebel, L., 1972, Persistent defects of bone formation in young rats following maternal hypervitaminosis D_2, Isr. J. Med. Sci., 8, 943 - 949.

Ornoy, A., Goodwin, D., Noff, D., Edelstein, S., 1978, 24,25 Dihydroxycholecalciferol is a metabolite of vitamin D essential for bone formation, Nature, 276, 517 - 519.

Ornoy, A., Levy, J., Atkin, I., Salamon, J., 1979, Scanning and transmission electron microscopic observations on the origin and structure of matrix vesicles in epiphyseal cartilage of young rats, Isr. J. Med. Sci., 15, 928 - 936.

Ornoy, A., Atkin, I., Levy, J., 1980, Ultrastructural studies on the origin and structure of matrix vesicles in bone of young rats, Acta Anat., 106, 450 - 461.

Raisz, L.G., Trummel, C.L., Holick, M.F., Deluca, H.F., 1972, 1,25 dihydroxycholecalciferol; a potent stimulation of bone resorption in tissue culture, Science, 175, 768 - 769.

Simmons, D.J., Kunin, A.S., 1967, Autoradiographic and biochemical investigations of the effects of cortisone on the bones of the rat, Clin. Orthop., 55, 201 - 215.

Sontag, L.W., Munson, P., Huff, E., 1936, Effects on the fetus of hypervitaminosis D and calcium and phosphorous deficiency during pregnancy, Am. J. Dis. Child., 51, 302 - 321.

Storey, E., 1963, The influence of adrenal cortical hormones in bone formation and resorption, Clin. Orthop., 30, 197 - 217.

Warkany, J., 1943, Effect of maternal rachitogenic diet on skeletal development of young rats, Am. J. Dis. Child., 66, 511 - 516.

The Effect of Cytosine-Arabinoside on Limb Morphogenesis in the Mouse

M. A. Rooze

Laboratoire d'Anatomie et d'Embryologie humaines de la Faculté de Médecine, Université Libre de Bruxelles, 97, rue aux Laines, B-1000 Brussels, Belgium

INTRODUCTION:

Cytosine arabinoside (C.A.) is an antimetabolic drug acting as a pyrimidine-analog which inhibits DNA synthesis. The drug is currently being used in humans for the treatment of leukemias. Various biochemical mechanisms of action of C.A. have been suggested. CHU and FISCHER (1962) have shown that C.A. is phosphorylated to a diphosphonucleotide (C.A.D.P.). C.A.D.P. inhibits the oxydation of diphosphate cytidylic acid into diphosphate deoxycytidilic acid. SILAGI (1965) suggested that C.A. is incorporated into DNA resulting in a modified DNA molecule which is unable to replicate. On the other hand, MOMPARLER (1974) provided evidence that C.A. inhibits DNA-polymerase.

The teratogenic effect of C.A. was first described by CHAUBE and MURPHY (1965) in the rat and later by KARNOFSKY and LACON (1966) in the chick. Further studies have been performed in the rat (RITTER et al., 1971, 1973; KROWKE et al., 1977; SCOTT et al., 1975); in the mouse (KOCHHAR et al., 1978). It was found that injection of C.A. was followed by a rapid decrease in DNA synthesis. The drug affected the development of both fore and hind limbs, the pattern of malformations being dependent on the dose and time of administration. The teratogenic action of C.A. could be inhibited by C.M.P. administered simultaneously or quickly after the injection of the drug. Our first results obtained in the mouse have been presented in a poster session of the XIIIth International Embryological Conference held in Berlin in 1978.

MATERIAL and METHODS:

Saline solutions (9°/₀₀ NaCl) of cytosine arabinoside at different concentrations were injected intraperitoneally in pregnant mice of different gestational ages. Two strains of mice were used, Swiss and C57BL. Lethality and teratogenicity were determined by examining fetuses collected at day 17 by Caesarian section. For macroscopic examination of the skeleton, fetuses were eviscerated and submitted either to alizarin red DAWSON'S method or to WATSON'S double staining combining alcian blue and alizarin red. For morphological purposes, pregnancies were interrupted 6, 24, 30 or 54 hours after injection of the drug. Some embryos were submitted to supravital Nile blue staining in order to demonstrate the general pattern of necrotic cells. Others were fixed in SERRA'S medium and embedded in paraffin; 10 µ thick serial sections of isolated limb buds were stained with toluidine blue or submitted to the UNNA-BRACHET'S method for demonstration of nucleic acids. In all experiments, hind and fore limbs of both sides were examined.

Teratology of the Limbs

RESULTS:

The teratogenic effects of C.A. were compared in C57BL and Swiss mice after treatment on day 9 (1, 5 or 10 mg/kg), day 10 (1, 5, 10 or 20 mg/kg) and day 11 (1, 5, 10, 25, 50 or 100 mg/kg). The following results will be considered: the general effects of the drug on the whole embryos, the structural deformities induced in the limb skeleton and the changes observed in the pattern of cell necrosis in developing limb buds at short intervals after the administration of the drug.

1. Embryolethality and teratogenicity
   Lethal doses for adult rats and mice were higher than 1 000 mg/kg. However, teratological and embryolethal doses were considerably lower and differed in both species. KOCHHAR et al. (1978) have reported that the teratogenic dose for the mouse was about 16 times lower than for the rat.

Earlier experiments had revealed that, for each gestational age, lethality increased dose-dependently. Other correlations were found between the dose of the drug and the teratogenic response of the embryos as well as between the dose and the weight of the embryos.

The comparative results in two different strains of mice obtained in this study revealed some interesting facts. C57BL embryos which received 10 mg/kg of C.A. at day 9 had a lower weight than Swiss embryos treated identically. In addition the percentage of living fetuses was lower in the C57BL strain. This indicates that C57BL fetuses are more sensitive to the action of the drug. On day 10, no statistical differences could be found between the two strains. Surprisingly, after treatment on day 11, the Swiss strain was more sensitive than the C57BL strain.

Considering these slight strain differences, it was interesting to examine and compare the structural effects of the drug on the limb skeleton in both C57BL and Swiss mice.

2. Limb skeleton deformities
   The structural defects induced by C.A. in the limb skeleton were studied macroscopically in 17-day fetuses of both strains of mice after treatment on day 9 (1, 5 or 10 mg/kg), day 10 (1, 5, 10 or 20 mg/kg), and day 11 (1, 5, 10, 25, 50 or 100 mg/kg). The results obtained under different conditions emphasize the variability of the pattern of malformations in relation to the dose and time of drug administration, the different sensitivity of both strains of mice to the teratogen and the occurrence of asymmetrical defects of variable frequency.
   a). General consideration (Tab. 1)
   No limb abnormalities were observed after the administration of 1 mg/kg on day 9, 10 and 11 as well as of 5 mg/kg on day 9 and 11. With all other drug doses the hind limbs were more selectively affected. The percentage of malformed fetuses increased with increasing dosages. As shown in Tab. 1, C.A. is more effective on days 10 and 11. It is also important to note that when one of the hind or one of the fore limbs was malformed, the contralateral limb was also abnormal. However, the pattern of malformation was not necessarily the same.

Table 1 shows that the asymmetries in the pattern of malformations were more pronounced when the drug was administrated on day 10 or day 9 (with 10 mg/kg). It is also interesting to observe that whatever the dose, the percentage of asymmetries in the hind limbs was quite constant. After treatment on day 9, a dose of 10 mg/kg C.A. induced symmetrical defects in the fore limbs and asymmetrical ones in the hind limbs. We have no interpretation for this phenomenon. However, as already suggested by MILAIRE (1978), we must bear in mind that the initial blood supply to the hind limbs is provided by the umbilical vein, which is much more developed on the left than on the right side. More detailed studies of this vascular asymmetry will perhaps reveal its importance in the genesis of asymmetrical abnormalities. Details about the asymmetrical defects induced by C.A. will be presented in the description of skeletal deformities.

Table 2 summarizes the results of a comparative analysis of the teratogenic effects of C.A. administered at 5 or 10 mg/kg on day 9, 10 or 11 in two different strains of mice. The results obtained in the fore limb revealed that the C57BL strain was more resistant to the teratogen than the Swiss strain. In addition, asymmetrical effects were less frequent in the C57BL strain. However, the differences between the two strains were smaller at high drug doses. Similar observations were made in regard to the defects induced in the hind limbs, but the differences between the two strains of mice were less obvious, particularly after the administration of 10 mg/kg on day 10 and 11. These strain differences might be related either to differences in the metabolism of the drug or to slight differences in the rate of limb development between C57BL and Swiss mice.

b) <u>Defects of the limb skeleton (Tab. 3)</u>

<u>Day 9</u>: only 10% of the fore limbs were affected by 10 mg/kg C.A. administered on day 9; the defect was a preaxial reduction of the autopod. The hind limbs remained unaffected after treatment with 5 mg/kg of C.A. The 10 mg/kg dosage, however, induced malformations in all limb segments with the exception of the girdle. Right-left asymmetries were observed in the defects induced in the same segments, the right limb being generally more severely affected than the left one. In 30% of the cases, excessive skeletal pieces were formed in the autopod, such as hyperphalangism of the 1st digit or polydactylism.

<u>Day 10</u>: all the segments of both limbs could be affected after treatment on day 10, the severity of the malformation being dose-dependent. The pectoral girdle was never absent, but all other segments of the fore limb were affected at higher dosages.

Hyperphalangism or polydactylism were rare in the fore limb. On the contrary, 33% of such defects were found in the hind limbs of the 5 mg/kg treated embryos. Surprisingly, this percentage decreased with increasing dosage. A standard pattern of malformations after treatment on day 10 was not apparent (Tab. 3). Asymmetrical defects were more frequent in the hind limbs, mainly in the autopod of which 30% were asymmetrically affected. It is interesting to note that the percentage of asymmetries increased in a proximo-distal direction. The right limb was generally more severely affected. Asymmetries appeared in the anterior stylopod and zeugopod after treatment with 20 mg/kg; they were found in the anterior autopod with any of the three doses tested. The right fore limb also seemed to be more severely affected than the left one.

<u>Day 11</u>: administration of 5 mg/kg C.A. on day 11 neither affected the fore nor the hind limbs. The stylopod was rarely affected except after treatment with 25 mg/kg. The autopod was reduced or absent, but never showed any excess material. The

asymmetries were rare and limited to the stylopod or to the zeugopod; the autopod was always symmetrically affected. The fetuses which received 50 or 100 mg/kg of C.A. were less severely affected. This was most probably due to the fact, that at these high dosages, only the more resistant fetuses survived; indeed, the number of living fetuses was much reduced. After treatment of C57BL mice on day 9, all fore limbs were normal and 20% of the hind limbs showed excessive skeletal development. After treatment on day 10, the fore limbs of the C57BL fetuses were still more resistant, except after treatment with 20 mg/kg, which induced skeletal reductions in the autopod. It is interesting to note that asymmetrical defects were less frequent in the C57BL than in the Swiss strain but also that in regard to asymmetry the left limb was more severely affected. The results obtained in the hind limbs lead to similar considerations. The autopod of the 5 mg/kg treated fetuses presented excess lesions in 70% of the cases. After treatment on day 11, the pectoral girdle remained unaffected in both strains. C57BL fetuses appeared to be particularly resistant to the administration of 10 mg/kg of the drug. A 25 mg/kg dose was too high to allow a study of strain differences.

3. Changes in the pattern of cell necrosis

The administration of C.A. was followed by typical changes in the normal pattern of physiological cell death in the developing mouse limb bud mesoderm which was described earlier by MILAIRE (1976).

As early as 6 hours after treatment, abnormal degenerative phenomena occurred in the distal mesoderm, their extent and regional density varying according to the concentration of the drug. Whatever the day of treatment, they were always found in the marginal mesoderm underlying the apical ectodermal ridge. The number of necrotic cells was generally higher on the preaxial side. In addition, the limb buds of the treated embryos were somewhat reduced with respect to those of normal embryos of the same age, particularly after the injection of 10 mg/kg of C.A. (embryos subjected to higher doses have not yet been examined in this respect).

The same distal necrotic area was still present 30 hours after treatment but apparently had moved slightly in proximal direction with respect to its initial location, a thin layer of unaffected tissue being now present between the necrotic zone and the apical ectoderm. It thus seems that a thin layer of subectodermal cells resisted the action of the drug, underwent active cell proliferation immediately after injection and forced the neighbouring necrotic cells back in proximal direction.

Similar changes occurred after treatment on day 9, 10 or 11 with 5 and 10 mg/kg of C.A. However, as shown in Tab. 1, the embryos treated on day 9 and 11 with 5 mg/kg developed normal fore and hind limbs. Either the number of affected cells was insufficient to modify the normal genesis of the limb skeleton, or the regulatory properties of the limb bud mesoderm at this stage were able to overcome the defect induced by this particular concentration of the drug.

It may thus be concluded that C.A. induces selective cell necrosis in a particular area of the subridge mesoderm, near the marginal vein. This effect is phase-specific and the resulting pattern of skeletal malformations is related to the extent and regional intensity of the degenerative phenomena. In certain cases after treatment at day 10 with 5 mg/kg, a local hyperplasia of the preaxial part of the ectodermal ridge was found to be associated with the absence of the preaxial necrotic area normally present in the deep mesoderm of the first digital presumptive area. Such changes might be similar to those observed in the genesis of hereditary or induced hyperphalangia of the first digit. Recently, MILAIRE (1978) considered the changes as a compensatory reaction of the ectoderm to the loss of mesoderm in the limb bud footplate.

The effects of C.A. on cell degeneration was examined after treatment with 50 and 100 mg/kg on day 11. The extent and intensity of the cellular damage was so prominent in these conditions that within a few hours after injection, the whole distal portion of the limb bud footplate became necrotic and was later replaced by a large necrotic cavity. This cavity was generally more extended preaxially, so that digit IV, the first one to be formed, usually remained unaffected or was slightly reduced.

Table 1: Incidence of normal and abnormal skeletal patterns in different experimental conditions (Swiss strain).

FORE LIMB

Day of Injection	9			10			11				
Dose (mg/kg)	1	5	10	5	10	20	5	10	25	50	100
Normal	100	100	90	31	21		100				
Sym. Defects			10	48	46	78		100	100	93	94
Asym. Defects				21	33	22				7	6
Asym./Sym. (%)				44	72	28				7.5	6.5
HIND LIMB											
Normal	100	100	30	14	4		100				
Sym. Defects			23	52	58	59		95	94	93	100
Asym. Defects			47	34	38	41		5	6	7	
Asym./Sym. (%)			204	65	65.5	69.5		5	6	75	
No. of Fetuses	32	34	30	29	24	37	35	44	31	27	18

Table 2: Comparison of incidence of normal and abnormal skeletal patterns in C57BL and Swiss strains.

FORE LIMB

Day of Injection	9		9		10		10		11	
Dose (mg/kg)	5		10		5		10		10	
Strain	Sw	C57	Sw	C57	Sw	C57	Sw	C57	Sw	C57
Normal	100	100	90	100	31	84	21	23		39
Sym. Defects			10		48	8	46	62	100	61
Asym. Defects					21	8	33	15		
Asym./Sym. (%)					44	100	72	24		
HIND LIMB										
Normal	100	96	30	79	14	12	4			
Sym. Defects		4	23	21	52	76	58	75	95	97
Asym. Defects			47		34	12	38	25	5	3
Asym./Sym. (%)			204	0	65	16	65.5	33.3	5	3
No. of Fetuses	34	54	30	28	29	25	24	34	44	31

Table 3: Quantitative evaluation of the skeletal pattern in different experimental conditions. (Swiss strain)

Day of injection			9		10			11				
Dose (mg/kg)			5	10	5	10	20	5	10	25	50	100
FORE LIMB	Girdle	normal	100	100	100	96	66	100	100	100	100	100
		reduced				4	34					
		absent										
		asym.					3					
	Stylo-pod	normal	100	100	66	21	8	100	98	74	97	100
		reduced			34	71	85		2	26	3	
		absent				8	7					
		asym.					3				3	
	Zeugo-pod	normal	100	100	59	21	5	100	75	49	72.5	94
		reduced			41	75	38		25	42	27.5	6
		nodules					47			6		
		absent				4	10			3		
		asym.					9				3	
	Auto-pod	normal	100	90	60	56	8.5	100			26	
		reduced		10	40	38	90		93	84	74	100
		absent							7	16		
		excess				6	1.5					
		asym.			21	34	21				3	6
Number of Fetuses			34	30	29	24	37	35	44	31	27	18
HIND LIMB	Girdle	normal	100	100	62	9	3	100	39	35	85	28
		reduced			38	91	78		56	65	15	72
		absent					19		5			
		asym.							5	3		
	Stylo-pod	normal	100	52	59		1.5	100	51	68	89	56
		reduced		32	3	28	4.5		46	29	11	44
		absent		16	38	72	94		3	3		
		asym.		17	7	13	6		3			
	Zeugo-pod	normal	100	40	55			100	36	26	78	
		reduced		50	23	55.5	10.5		37	49.5	9	94
		nodules			7	6.5	15		16	3	11	6
		absent		10	15	39	74.5		11	21.5	2	
		asym.		30	7	22	18		5	3	11	
	Auto-pod	normal	100	46	24	4	1.5	100				
		reduced		27	43	74	76		39	52	93	39
		absent					18		61	48	7	61
		excess		27	33	22	4.5					
		asym.		30	31	35	33					

REFERENCES

Chaube, S.W., Kreis, K., Uchida, Murphy, M.L., 1968, The teratogenic effect of 1 B-D-arabinofuranosylcytosine in the rat. Protection by deoxycytidine, Biochem. Pharm., 17, 1213 - 1226.

Chu, M.Y., Fischer, G.A., 1962, A proposed mechanism of action of 1 B-D-arabinofuranosylcytosine as an inhibitor of the growth of leukemic cells, Biochem. Pharm., 11, 423 - 430.

Karnovsky, D.A., Lacon, C.R., 1966, The effects of 1 B-D-arabinofuranosylcytosine on the developing chick embryo, Biochem. Pharm., 15, 1435 - 1442.

Kochhar, D.M., Penner, J.D., McDay, J.A., 1978, Limb development in mouse embryos. II. Reduction defects, cytotoxicity and inhibition of DNA sythesis produced by cytosine arabinoside, Teratology, 18, 71 - 92.

Krowke, R., Berg, P., Merker, H.-J., 1977, Effects of cytosine arabinoside, 6-amino-nicotinamide and 6-mercaptopurine riboside on ectoderm and mesoderm of mouse limb buds, Teratology, 15, 137 - 148.

Milaire, J., 1976, Rudimentation digitale au cours du développement normal de l'autopode chez les Mammifères, Colloques internationaux C.N.R.S., 266, 221 - 233.

Milaire, J., 1978, Approches morphologiques, histochimiques et expérimentales de la genèse des malformations des membres, Bull. Acad. Méd. Belg., 133, 402 - 413.

Momparler, R.L., 1974, A model for the chemotherapy of acute leukemia with 1 B-D-arabinofuranosylcytosine, Cancer Res., 34, 1775 - 1787.

Ritter, E.J., Scott, W.J., Wilson, J.G., 1971, Teratogenesis and inhibition of DNA sythesis induced in rat embryos by cytosine arabinoside, Teratology, 4, 7 - 14.

Ritter, E.J., Scott, W.J., Wilson, J.G., 1973, Relationship of normal patterns of cell death and development to malformation in the rat limb. Possible mechanisms of teratogenesis with inhibitors of DNA sythesis, Teratology, 7, 219 - 226.

Scott, W.S., Ritter, E.S., Wilson, J.G., 1975, Studies on induction of polydactyly in rats with cytosine arabinoside, Develop. Biol., 45, 103 - 111.

Silagi, S., 1965, Metabolism of 1 B-D-arabinofuranosylcytosine in L cells, Cancer Res., 25, 1446 - 1453.

Mechanisms of Limb Development Revealed by the Teratogenic Activity of Nicotinamide Analogues

John C. McLachlan

Department of Zoology, University of Oxford,
South Parks Road, Oxford OX1 3PS, U.K.

The development of the embryonic chick limb is surprisingly difficult to perturb, whether by physical damage caused by operative techniques, or by chemical treatments. Among the teratogens that have been studied for their effects on limb development, the nicotinamide analogues are notable for the attention they have received, and the profound inferences that have been drawn from their reported modes of action.

A general description of the effect of these substances has been provided by LANDAUER (1957). Most nicotinamide analogues have a teratogenic effect (LANDAUER and SALAM, 1973), but two, 3-acetylpyridine (3-AP) and 6-aminonicotinamide (6-AN), have received particular attention. The overt effects of these chemicals are rather different. 3-AP causes a condition described as "muscle hypoplasia", in which the body weight is reduced, and the limbs, particularly the legs, have a thin appearance (Fig. 1). When the amount of muscle is scored at later stages of development, it is found to be significantly reduced in animals treated with 3-AP compared to equivalent controls (TANAKA, YAMAMOTO, and HAYASHI, 1967). 6-AN is described as causing micromelia (Fig. 2), accompanied by brachycephaly, oedema, and retardation of feather germs development (LANDAUER, 1957). The teratogenic effects of both these chemicals are completely relieved if they are co-administered with nicotinamide, and it is believed that they act by competitively excluding nicotinamide. Since nicotinic acid is rather less effective than nicotinamide in alleviating the effects of these teratogens, it has been suggested that normal NAD(P) synthesis involves the direct incorporation of nicotinamide into pyridine nucleotides, rather than by a step involving de-amination to nicotinic acid (CAPLAN, 1972). Other substances (of which organophosphorus and methyl carbamate insecticides are of particular interest) also reduce NAD levels, cause malformations similar to 6-AN, and are alleviated to some extent by co-treatment with nicotinamide (PROCTOR and CASIDA, 1975), although organophosphorus compounds may have additional effects which are not relieved by nicotinamide (Meniel, 1976).

Two major hypotheses have been based on the effects of nicotinamide analogues. The first is the "phenocopy" concept advanced by LANDAUER, where it is suggested that teratogens may mimic and shed light on naturally occurring mutations (HERMAN, CLARK, and LANDAUER, 1963). The second is that proposed by CAPLAN and his co-workers (see CAPLAN, 1977, for references), which suggests that intracellular NAD plays a controlling role in muscle and cartilage differentiation. High internal pool sizes of NAD are taken to dictate muscle differentiation, while low molecular pools dictate cartilage expression. Thus the mode of action of 3-AP in causing the condition described as "muscle hypoplasia", is taken to be that the 3-AP competitively excludes nicotinamide, lowers intracellular NAD levels, and hence cuases a reduction in the amount of muscle present.

Clearly, if this theory of control of muscle and cartilage differentiation were found to be valid, it would be of the greatest importance. However,

Teratology of the Limbs

a number of criticisms can be advanced against it. First, the effect of 3-AP on the limb is rather more complex than it is often described. The thin appearance of the leg is in fact due to a reduction in all the tissues of the limb, including muscle, tendon, loose mesenchyme, and cartilage (McLACHLAN, BATEMAN, and WOLPERT, 1976). The effect on cartilage (which can be seen even from a casual glance at Fig. 1) is particularly surprising, since the theory would predict that the low levels of NAD now present would present a favourable environment for cartilage. There is a marked effect on the nerves of the limb: these are abolished within 24 hours of treatment, and this will prevent any subsequent recovery of muscle, which is dependent on nerve supply for its maintenance (EASTLICK, 1943). As the embryo's own production of NAD begins to increase (ROSENBERG and CAPLAN, 1974), some tissues may be able to recover; but muscle will seem to suffer disproportionately if the effect is scored late in development. Secondly, 3-AP is effective as late as 13 days of incubation (CAPLAN, 1970), which is long after the period during which differentiation events are taking place (generally considered to be prior to stage 25, i.e. 4 days of incubation - see for example ROSENBERG and CAPLAN, 1975). Thirdly, 6-AN treatment does not affect muscle as the theory predicts, but rather has a deleterious effect on cartilage (SEEGMILLER, OVERMAN, and MEREDITH, 1972; SEEGMILLER, 1977; McLACHLAN, 1980).

It seems therefore that the in vivo action of these teratogens does not provide support for CAPLAN's hypothesis. However, their effects can reveal some interesting clues to the mechanisms of limb development operating after the time of differentiation of the major cell types. These are mechanisms which affect the mutual interaction of these tissues, and operate in the phase of limb development which we have described as "co-ordinate growth" (McLACHLAN and WOLPERT, 1980). Clearly, any treatment that affects the normal development of a differentiated tissue, will affect these mechanisms, and the information that has been obtained is summarized below.

1. <u>The effect on feather germ formation</u>

   When the feather germs of the developing chick wing first appear at around 8 days of incubation, they have adopted a pattern which is rather constant in spacing, number, and morphology. How might this pattern respond to a treatment such as 6-AN which results in a considerable shortening of the limb? There are two possibilities:

   a). The number of feather germs could remain constant, but their spacing could decrease. This corresponds to the situation in the developing amphibian embryo, where a reduction in the number of cells of the embryo results in the formation of an embryo with the normal number of somites, each of which, however, is smaller (COOKE, 1977).

   b.) The number of feather germs could be reduced in proportion to the reduction in size of the limb.

I therefore counted the number of feather germs in proximo-distal sequence from elbow to wrist of chick wings reduced in length by treatment at various stages with 6-AN (Fig. 2, 3). It can be clearly seen that where the length of the wing is considerably reduced, the number of germs is reduced also (see McLACHLAN, 1980 for further details). This favours the theory advanced by SENGEL (1976), that development of the feather germs is controlled by a spacing mechanism such that each territory of sufficient size will initiate a feather germ when appropriately induced.

Nonetheless, it is still true that the feather germs appear slightly smaller in treated animals than in the controls, in accordance with the classic description of "down retardation". This may be because the cells of the feather germs are affected deleteriously, or because of an indirect effect on growth (Fig. 4). If the limb fails to elongate at the normal rate after 6-AN treatment, then the germs which are formed at the same density at T_2, the time of germ determination, in both treated and control wings, will be at higher density in the treated wings at a later time T_3. This may deny the developing germ enough territory to grow normally.

2. Muscle pattern

The muscle cells of the developing vertebrate limb first appear in dorsal and ventral muscle blocks, which then split up in a very striking manner to form the definitive pattern of the adult musculature (see WOLPERT, 1978). It is not known how this process is controlled, although a number of suggestions have been made.

One is that the elongation of the cartilage elements causes shearing forces which result in the splitting of the muscle block (CAREY, 1921). I have been able to eliminate this possibility by examining the muscle pattern in limbs where normal lengthening has been prevented by treatment with 6-AN. Even in grossly shortened limbs, where tension forces must have been very considerably reduced, the muscle pattern is normal (McLACHLAN, 1980).

Another suggestion has been that the nerves play a role, either directly, by a kind of "cheese cutter" effect (WORTHAM, 1948), or via shearing forces, since it has been reported that different regions of the undivided muscle blocks are capable of independent contractions (LANDMESSER and MORRIS, 1975). SHELLSWELL (1977) has been able to eliminate these possibilities by treating limbs with 3-AP before the distal muscle blocks have been innervated, and showing that the pattern of muscles was normal, even in the complete absence of nerves resulting from this treatment.

This use of nicotinamide analogues to eliminate two hypotheses that have been suggested to explain muscle splitting, has enabled attention to be focussed on a possible role for the connective tissues (WOLPERT, 1978).

3. Co-ordinate growth of the msucles

Although the pattern of the muscles in limbs shortened by 6-AN treatment is normal, their volume is not. It is reduced co-ordinately with the reduction in length of the cartilage. Their cross-sectional area, however, is quite unaffected (Tab. 1). This illustrates that the final length of the muscles is not specified in advance, but is dependent on the elongation of the cartilage, perhaps by a tension effect, while the cross-sectional area is independent of the length of the limb. This provides direct support in an embryonic system for the conclusions drawn by other authors (HAINES, 1932; GOLDSPINK, 1974) on a role for tension in controlling muscle growth in post-natal growth.

In these three areas then, it can be seen that the action of nicotinamide analogues can help to illuminate those aspects of limb morphogenesis which depend on tissue interactions, though they do not make clear the means by which cells arrive at their differentiated state in the process of giving rise to these tissues.

Table 1.

Effect of Muscles of 6-AN Treatment

Muscle	Dose (µg)	Length of Ulna (mm)	Length of Muscle (mm)	Breadth of Muscle (mm)	Area of Muscle (mm^2)
	0	4.08 (0.27)	4.47 (0.44)	0.78 (0.13)	0.28 (0.04)
FCU	10	3.47 (0.41)	3.41 (0.75)	0.81 (0.10)	0.28 (0.04)
	20	2.49 (0.57)	2.29 (0.49)	0.81 (0.11)	-
	0	4.48 (0.37)	2.95 (0.20)	0.59 (0.07)	0.11 (0.07)
FDP	10	3.47 (0.41)	2.09 (0.43)	0.63 (0.07)	0.12 (0.07)
	20	2.49 (0.57)	1.59 (0.20)	0.59 (0.07)	-

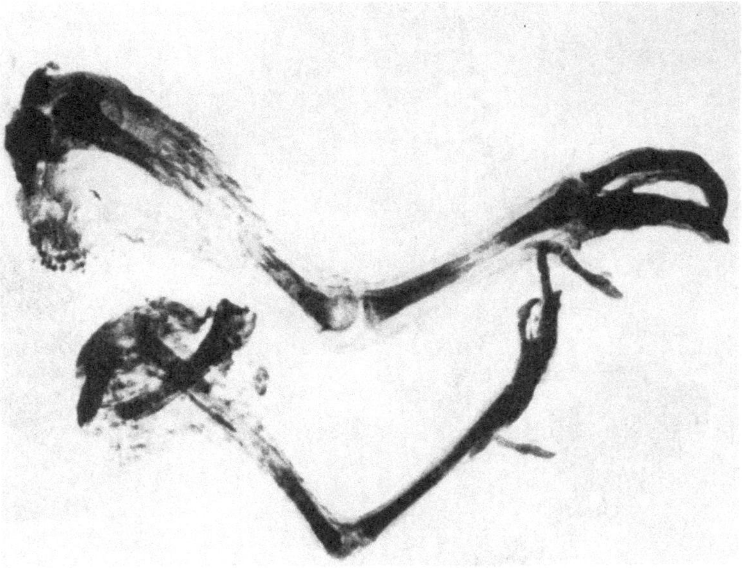

Fig. 1: Legs from (a) a normal embryo at 11 days of incubation.

(b) an embryo of same age treated at 6 days of incubation with 2 mg of 3-AP in 50 µl distilled water.

(Whole mounts stained with alcian green and cleared in methyl salicylate).

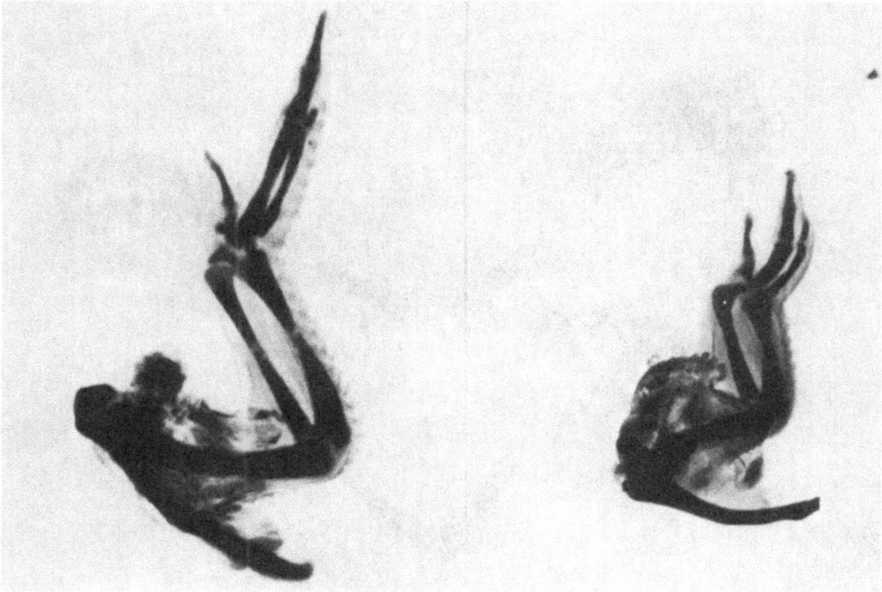

Fig. 2: Wings from (a) a normal 11 day embryo.

(b) an embryo of same age treated at 6 days of incubation with 10 µg of 6-AN.

Specimens prepared as in Fig. 1.

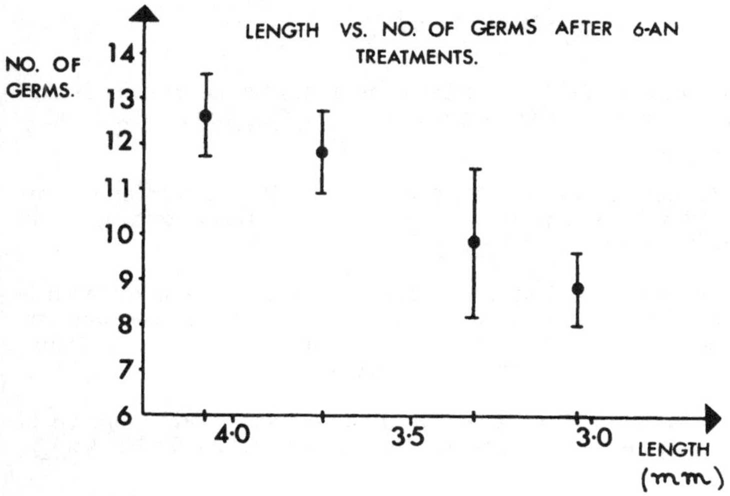

Fig. 3: Variation in number of feather germs in limbs of different lengths resulting from 6-AN treatments at different stages (for details see McLACHLAN, 1980).

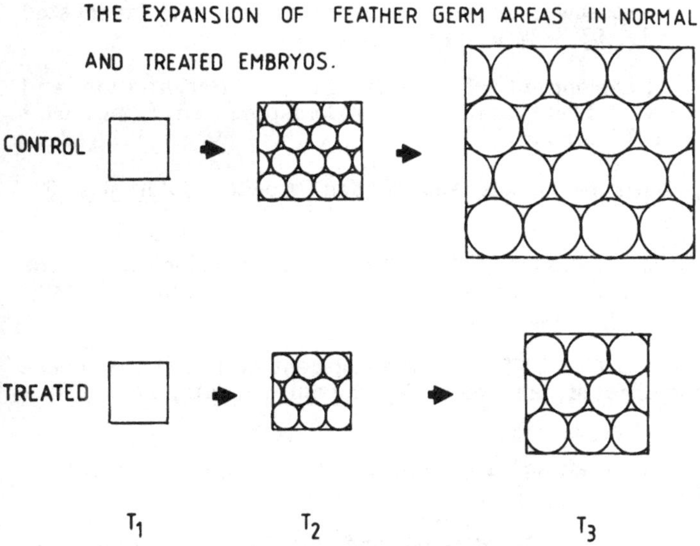

Fig. 4: The retardation of feather germs often observed after 6-AN treatment may be due to a failure of the limb to expand in the normal way. See text for discussion.

REFERENCES

Caplan, A.I., 1970, Effects of the nicotinamide sensitive teratogen 3-Acetylpyridine on chick limb cells in culture, Exp. Cell Res., 62, 341 - 345.

Caplan, A.I., 1972, Comparison of the capacity of nicotinamide and nicotinic acid to relieve the effects of muscle and cartilage teratogens in developing chick embryos, Develop. Biol., 28, 344 - 351.

Caplan A.I., 1977, Muscle, cartilage, and bone development and differentiation from chick limb mesenchymal cells, in: "Vertebrate limb and somite morphogenesis", (D.A. Ede, J.R. Hinchliffe, and M. Balls, eds.), pp. 119 - 214, Cambridge Univ. Press.

Carey, E.J., 1921, Studies in the dynamics of histogenesis IV. Tension of differential growth as a stimulus to myogenesis in the limb, Am. J. Anat., 29, 93 - 115.

Cooke, J., 1977, The control of somite number during amphibian development: models and experiments, in: "Vertebrate limb and somite morphogenesis", (D.A. Ede, J.R. Hinchliffe, and M. Balls, eds.), pp. 433 - 448, Cambridge Univ. Press.

Eastlick, H.L., 1943, Studies on transplanted embryonic limbs of the chick. 1. The development of muscle in nerveless and innervated grafts, J. Exp. Zool., 93, 27 - 45.

Goldspink, G., 1974, Development of muscle, in: "Differentiation and growth of cells in vertebrate tissues", (G. Goldspink, ed.), pp. 69 - 99, Chapman and Hall, London.

Haines, R.W., 1932, Laws of muscle and tendon growth, J. Anat., 60, 578 - 585.

Herrman, H., Clark, E.M., Landauer, W., 1963, Muscle development in the crooked neck dwarf mutant and in the 3-AP treated chick embryo, Acta. Embryol. Exp., 6, 169 - 174.

Landmesser, L., Morris, D.G., 1975, The development of functional innervation in the hind-limb of the chick, J. Physiol., Lond., 249, 301 - 326.

Landauer, W., 1957, Niacin antagonists and chick development, J. Exp. Zool., 136, 509 - 530.

Landauer, W., Salam, N., 1973, Quantitative and qualitative distinctions in developmental interference produced by various substituted pyridines. Molecular shape and teratogenicity as studied in chicken embryos, Acta. Embryol. Exp., 1973, 307 - 318.

McLachlan, J.C., Bateman, Wolpert, 1976, Effect of 3-acetylpyridine on tissue differentiation of the embryonic chick limb, Nature, 264, 267 - 269.

McLachlan, J.C., 1980, The effect of 6-aminonicotinamide on limb development, J. Embryol. exp. Morph., 55, 307 - 318.

McLachlan, J., Wolpert, L., 1980, The spatial pattern of muscle development in chick limb, in: "Development and specialization of skeletal muscle", (D. Goldspink, ed.), Cambridge Univ. Press. (In press).

Meniel, R., 1976, Pluralitie dans le determinisme des effets teratogenes des composes organophosphores, Experientia, 32, 920 - 922.

Proctor, N.H., Casida, J.E., 1975, Organophosphorus and methyl carbamate insecticide teratogenesis: diminished NAD in chicken embryos, Science, 190, 580 - 582.

Rosenberg, M.J., Caplan, A.I., 1974, Nicotinamide adenine dinucleotide levels in cells of the developing chick limbs: possible control of muscle and cartilage development, Develop. Biol., 38, 157 - 164.

Rosenberg, M.J., Caplan, A.I., 1975, Nicotinamide adenine dinucleotide levels in chick limb mesodermal cells in vitro: effects of 3-acetylpyridine and nicotinamide, J. Embryol. exp. Morph., 33, 947 - 956.

Sengel, P., 1976, in: "Morphogenesis of the skin", p. 246, Cambridge Univ. Press.

Seegmiller, R.E., 1977, Time of onset and selective response of chondrogenic core of 5-day chick limb after treatment with 6-aminonicotinamide, Develop. Biol., 58, 164 - 173.

Seegmiller, R.E., Overman, D.O., Meredith, N.R., 1972, Histological and fine structure changes in micromelia induced by 6-aminonicotinamide, Develop. Biol., 28, 555 - 572.

Shellswell, G.B., 1977, The formation of discrete muscles from the chick wing dorsal and ventral muscle masses in the absence of nerves, J. Embryol. exp. Morph., 41, 269 - 277.

Tanaka, S., Yamamoto, Y., Hayashi, Y., 1967, Effect of 3-acetylpyridine on the development of the leg muscles of the chick embryo, Embryologia, 9 306 - 332.

Wolpert, L., 1978, Pattern formation in biological development, Sci. Am., 239, 159 - 164.

Wortham, R.A., 1948, The development of the muscles and tendons in the lower leg and foot of chick embryos, J. Morph., 83, 105 - 148.

Analysis of Radiographs in Reproduction Toxicology by Means of Densitometry and Planimetry

H. Sterz, G. Hebold

Abt. MF - 2T, Medizinische Forschung, Boehringer Mannheim GmbH, Postfach 51, D-6800 Mannheim 31

INTRODUCTION:

Since the thalidomide tragedy in the early 60's, screening studies on animals to detect embryotoxic, fetotoxic, and teratogenic risk factors for humans have been an essential part of pharmaceutical research. Despite the large expenditures of time and money involved, these studies generally fail to provide a fully satisfactory answer to the question of whether or not a new drug is teratogenic in man.

This dilemma is undoubtedly due primarily to the fact that the animal species available to us are comparable to man only to a limited extent. But do we in fact utilize all the information that such a study provides?

Despite reports of intrauterine growth retardation caused by various substances (ARIYUKI et al., 1979; JAFFE and JOHNSON, 1973; KNIGHT and ROE, 1978; MERKER et al., 1975; RAPAKA et al., 1977), many investigators seem to concentrate on the discovery of malformations. More subtle effects such as supernumerary ribs or defective ossification (to name only a few) are often neglected or receive marginal attention (BRENT and JENSH, 1967).

Should a substance one day not follow the rule, that all substances capable of producing teratogenic effects in man also cause malformation, resorption and defective development in animals, and instead lead only to intrauterine growth retardation - our present standard methods of teratological screening would not suffice to recognize it.

Drug consumption during pregnancy continues to increase rather than decrease. Therefore, every item of meaningful information from our animal studies should be registered for the sake of maximum safety in the use of drugs.

Teratological screening of fetal skeletons can yield a considerable amount of information without undue extra effort, provided that:

1.) the variable number of bone anlagen in rat fetuses obtained by caesarean section is counted (ALIVERTI et al., 1979),

2.) the skeletons of fetuses of larger animal species are carefully prepared and X-rayed (NOTHDURFT and STERZ, 1977).

Our teratological screening studies are performed at a time when the fetal skeleton is in a phase of very high metabolic activity and thus an excellent yardstick for prenatal development. Exogenous disturbance of fetal development is frequently evidenced only by a slightly reduced body weight. Such underdeveloped fetuses often do not lack a single bone anlage, and are also inconspicuous in all other respects. Nonetheless, this state must be regarded as a developmental defect of the entire animal. In rat fe-

Teratology of the Limbs

tuses, this retardation is frequently associated with a smaller number of ossification centers in the phalanges and in the cervical and caudal segments of the vertebral column. These animals are, of course, readily identified, and no expensive equipment is required to detect these effects. However, there is little point in counting the bone anlagen mentioned in rabbit fetuses, because they are generally present at full term, even in cases of retarded development. It is thus all the more difficult to recognize in rabbits those transitional stages that do not present obvious skeletal anomalies or distinctly lower body weights than the controls, in spite of a retardation or even acceleration of skeletal mineralization (PALMER, 1977).

In our experience, alizarin-stained preparations are not suitable for the rapid and accurate detection of defective mineralization in rabbits. On the contrary, an abnormal degree of mineralization in an otherwise intact skeleton - be it due to retardation or to acceleration - can be totally overlooked when this method is used. More definitive methods are usually very elaborate and cannot be employed for teratological screening, although they are eminently suitable for more sophisticated studies (HEUCK, 1969).

We accordingly improved the densitometric and planimetric techniques for the evaluation of radiographs of fetal skeletons, so that all skeletons available from teratological studies can be routinely assessed with regard to the degree of mineralization. This can only be done with an image analyzer (SAACKEL, 1974).

The method we have developed allows very accurate measurement of fetotoxic effects that manifest themselves as abnormal skeletal growth in rabbit fetuses and young rats, though in principle any other animal species may be used.

The quality of X-ray pictures obtainable in teratological studies is excellent (STERZ and HEBOLD, 1978), and this was the prerequisite for successful evaluation of bone radiographs by electronic means (Figs. 1 and 2). The significance of our work thus lies in the fact that this method makes it possible to register the complete informational content of radiographs, if necessary (Figs. 3 and 4).

This method was described in detail three years ago (STERZ and SAACKEL, 1977). The bone anlage under analysis is placed under a microscope and the magnified image viewed on a television monitor. The resolution of the image into dots allows the digitization of the video signal corresponding to the brightness of each individual dot. The entire image can thus be converted into an array of numerical values from which a computer can then derive the structure, area, and total density of the bone.

It is of course essential to include a reference wedge in every radiograph.

To assess the information yield of this method, we needed answers to the following two questions:

1. Which bones of the fetal skeleton are suitable for measurement?

2. Does the litter size affect the comparability of the results?

With regard to question 1:

Many bone anlagen are suitable as regards the technique of measurement, the exception being those that appear at widely varying times, such as the 5th sternal center.

It is easiest to measure small bones - such as sternal centers, metatarsal and metacarpal bones, phalanges, and vertebral centers that give sharply defined shadow images. However, a sharply defined image is not absolutely essential since any desired rectangular segment of a large bone may be measured.

Our experience has shown the phalanges to be suitable, although mineralization is relatively weak at 30 days p.c., when we obtain the fetuses by caesarean section. The metatarsals are better suited than the metacarpals on account of their more advanced mineralization. We have obtained very good results with measurements of the mineralized epiphysis of the tibia. Presumably, the other epiphyses of the long bones are also suitable, as are the sternal centers and several cervical vertebrae.

With regard to question 2:

Litter size is important when extremely small or extremely large litters are produced. The former usually exhibit better mineralization than average, and the latter poorer mineralization. We accordingly decided to exclude litters of less than four or more than ten from evaluation.

METHODOLOGY:

In order to establish the usefulness of our method, we examined substances that affect mineralization. As retardation of mineralization is far more frequent than acceleration, we selected two ß-stimulators, since these drugs are known to retard mineralization. We further investigated the effects of thalidomide on the rabbit and of vitamin-A acid on the rat. The ß-stimulators and vitamin-A acid were administered orally to pregnant rabbits and rats during organogenesis, just as in teratological screening studies, whereas thalidomide was administered from the 9th to 12th day p.c. (also by gavage). The 4th sternal center, 4th metatarsal bones, the proximal phalanges of the toes of the 4th hindpaw, and the proximal ends of both tibias were selected for measurement.

RESULTS:

1. ß-Stimulators

a.) Our method enabled us to determine a distinct, dose-dependent decrease of mineralization by 17 - 67% in the 4th metatarsal bone of the fetus (Tab. 1). This effect was evident not only at high, maternally toxic doses, but also at a lower dose equivalent to 10 times the pharmacologically effective dose. It is important to note that the fetal skeletons of all animal groups had passed through a normal, routine examination and generally appeared to be entirely normally mineralized to the naked eye, except for the group that had been treated with the high, maternally toxic dose. The fetuses of this group exhibited a poorly visible retardation of the development of the os basioccipitale and an abnormal shape of the sternal centers. The mean fetal weights of the proband groups were not distinctly different from those of the control groups.

b.) If ß-stimulation was preeceded by ß-blockade, the retardation induced by ß-stimulation was distinctly less (Tab. 2).

c.) Not all bones were affected to the same extent: small bone anlagen, such as the phalanges, proved to be more sensitive than larger ones. However, we assume on the basis of studies to date that changes in the larger bone anlagen (such as the metatarsals and the epiphyseal ends of long bones) are more significant, since anomalous mineralization in these bones is less readily corrected later on.

d.) We did not observe any difference between left and right limbs in the ß-stimulator study.

e.) It was interesting to note that the defective mineralization visible in other bones was masked in the case of the sternum.
At high drug levels, there is apparently a competitive effect between the deforming and retarding actions of the drug, with the retardant action predominating as the dose is increased. Only further increase of the dosage produced defective mineralization. For this reason, the sternum can be used for such measurements only when it is not the target organ. Accordingly, we prefer using the limb skeleton and measure the phalanges, metatarsals, and mineralized epiphyseal ends of long bones.

2. Thalidomide

Although administration of 200 mg of thalidomide produced a high percentage of malformed limbs, none of the bones we examined showed signs of defective ossification (Tab. 2).

3. Vitamin-A acid

There was no difference in ossification between the controls and the weanlings of rats that had received 6 or 18 mg of vitamin-A acid per kg of body weight from the 7th to 16th day of gestation, whereas the doses under investigation produced a clear-cut teratogenic effect in a parallel experiment.

DISCUSSION:

Our method makes it possible to detect fetotoxic effects even when the drug does not produce anomalies or a lower fetal weight. We thus have a highly useful supplement to the general screening program for the resolution of suspect or borderline cases that turn up in the radiographs and that cannot be classified on the basis of visual inspection alone. For the first time, suspected radiographic evidence of defective ossification can be quickly and easily verified or refuted.

The "no-effect" level of a drug with regard to the fetus can be determined more accurately.

These measurements also reveal the significance of defective ossification in the postnatal period. Radiographs of animals raised for an arbitrary length of time can be evaluated and we can then determine whether or not the defect has been corrected, or terminated in a pathologic state that is known as osteogenesis imperfecta or osteopetrosis when it occurs in man - to name only the two most important syndromes (WARKANY, 1971).

The distinct retardation of mineralization produced by ß-stimulators, which is not accompanied by obvious deformation of the bones under investigation, is scarcely considered relevant with regard to man since other animal experiments have shown that such defective mineralization of bone is corrected within a few weeks after birth. Even pronounced rib deformation - so-called "wavy ribs" - in newborn rats disappears after 8 - 10 days (STERZ and HEBOLD, 1980).

ACKNOWLEDGEMENTS

This project received financial support from the Bundesministerium für Forschung und Technologie (Federal Ministry of Research and Technology) of the Federal Republic of Germany (Project No. CMT 12).

We would like to thank Mrs. GERTRUD OLESZEK for her excellent preparations of the skeletons, and Miss ANNETTE HÖFER for performing the measurements so assiduously.

Table 1: Influence of two ß-receptor stimulants on the mineralization of the rabbit fetus. (30 d.p.c.[1])

Drug	mg/kg day	Os Metatarsale IV: bone density (%)	Os Metatarsale IV: bone area (%)
Control		100	100
Doxaminol[2]	10	83	88
Doxaminol	40	67	74
Doxaminol	160	33	42
Buphenine	3 x 250	78	81

Table 2: Influence of different substances on the mineralization of the rabbit fetus. (30 d.p.c.[1])

Drug	mg/kg day	Bone Density (%): tibia	Bone Density (%): sternal center No. IV	Bone Density (%): prox. phalanx IV hind paw
Control		100	100	100
Doxaminol[2]	80	77	79	72
Carazolol[3] + Doxaminol	50 + 80	90	91	99
Buphenine	3 x 250	78	96	85
Thalidomide	200	100	100	100

[1]d.p.c. = dies post conceptionem
[2]WHO-registration as a generic name has been applied for.
[3]ß-receptor blocker

Pharmacologic threshold dosis in our rabbit strain:
Doxaminol = ~ 1 mg/kg; Buphenine = ~ 20 mg/kg

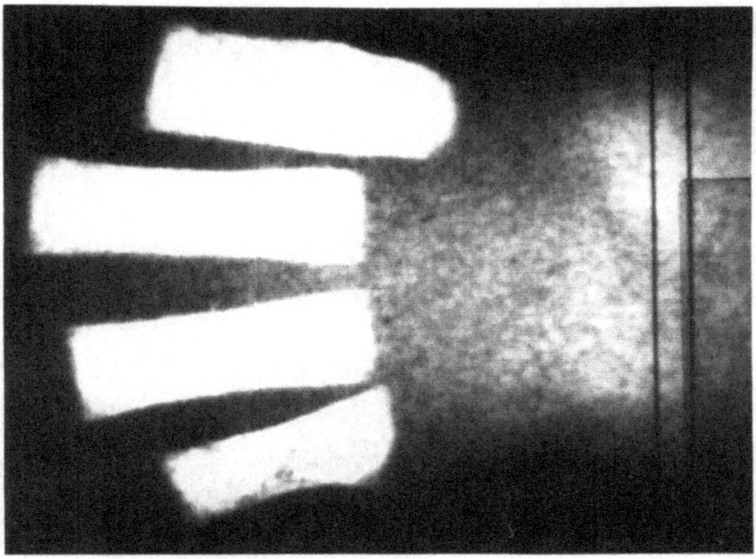

Fig. 1: Radiograph showing the mineralization of the metatarsal bones. Rabbit fetus, 30th day post conceptionem.

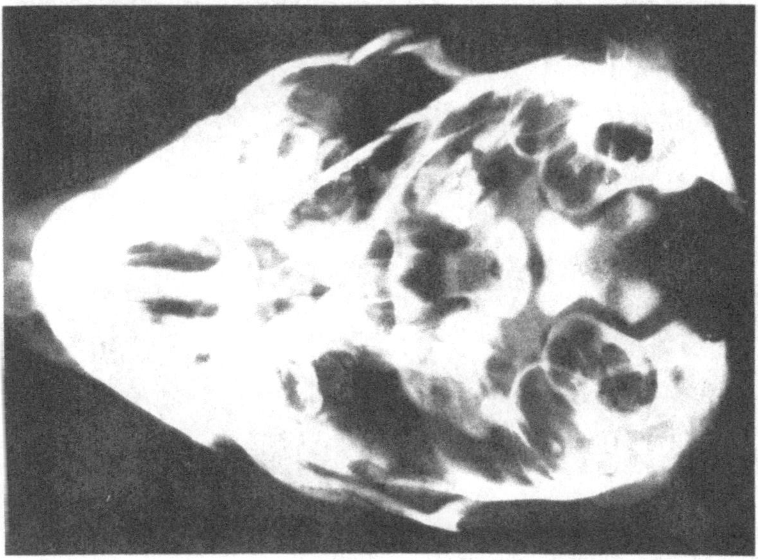

Fig. 2: Radiograph showing the mineralization of the cranial bones after removal of skin, calotte, brain, mandibula with tongue, and hyoid bone. Rabbit fetus, 30th day p.c.

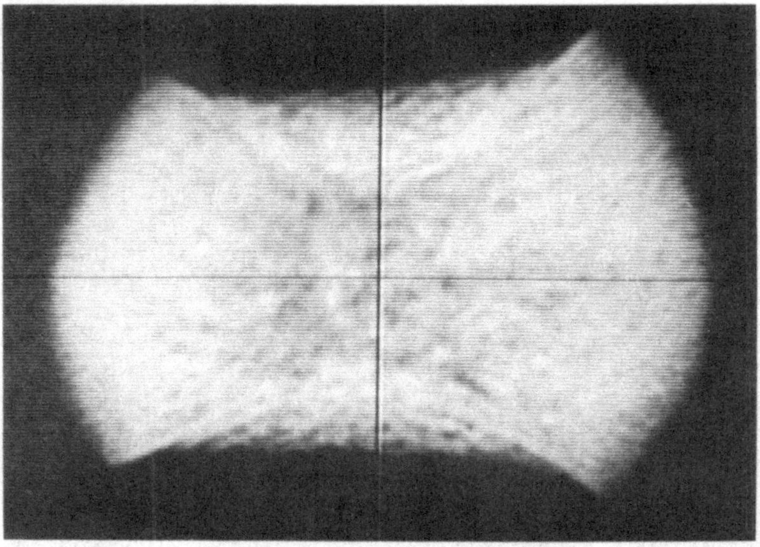

Fig. 3: TV-monitor image of well ossified sternal center III. Rabbit fetus, 30th day p.c.

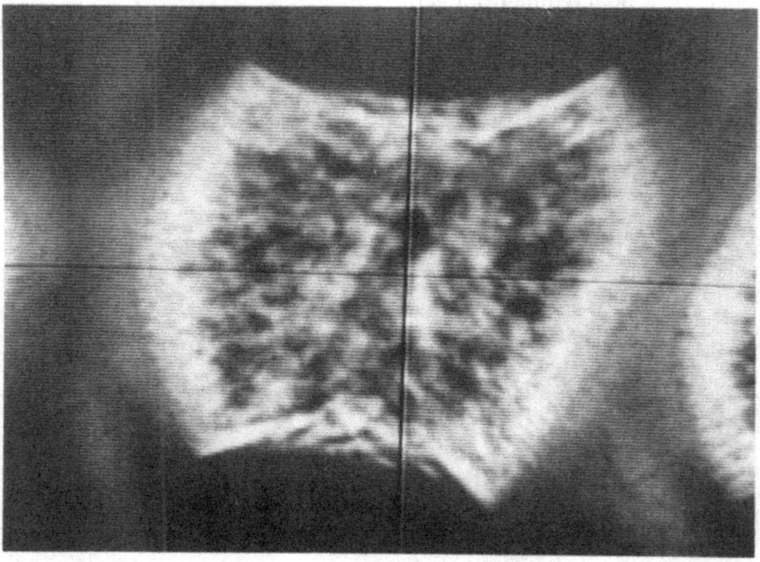

Fig. 4: TV-monitor image of poorly ossified sternal center III. Rabbit fetus, 30th day p.c. A higher incidence of such weakly ossified bones in drug-treated animal groups should be sufficient reason for evaluation of mineralization by a reliable method such as the one presented here.

REFERENCES

Aliverti, V., Bonanomi, L., Giavini, E., Leone, V.G., Mariani, L., 1979, The extent of fetal ossification as an index of delayed development in teratogenic studies on the rat, Teratology, 20, 237 - 242.

Ariyuki, F., Higaki, K., Yasuda, M., 1979, Relationship between low body weight and retardation of ossification of the skeleton in rat fetuses: Analysis of SFD induced by maternal fasting and hypervitaminosis D_2, Teratology, 20, 150 - 151.

Brent, R.L., Jensh, R.P., 1967, Intrauterine growth retardation, in: "Advances in Teratology", (D.H.M. Woollam, ed.), Vol. 2, pp. 139 - 227, Academic Press, New York and London.

Heuck, F., 1969, Mikroradiographische Untersuchungen der Mineralisation des gesunden und kranken Knochengewebes, Der Radiologe, 9, 142 - 154.

Jaffe, N.R., Johnson, E.M., 1973, Alterations in the ontogeny and specific activity of phosphomonoesterases associated with abnormal chondrogenesis and osteogenesis in the limbs of fetuses from folic acid-deficient pregnant rats, Teratology, 8, 33 - 50.

Knight, E., Roe, D.A., 1978, Effects of salicylamide and protein restriction on the skeletal development of the rat fetus, Teratology, 18, 17 - 22.

Merker, H.-J., Franke, L., Günther, Th., 1975, The effect of D-Penicillamine of (sic) the skeletal development of rat foetuses, Naunyn-Schmied. Arch. Pharmacol., 287, 359 - 376.

Nothdurft, H., Sterz, H., 1977, Routine radiography of the skeletons of 31-day-old rabbit fetuses, in: "Methods in Prenatal Toxicology", (D. Neubert, H.-J. Merker, T.E. Kwasigroch, eds.), pp. 155 - 164, Georg Thieme Publ., Stuttgart.

Palmer, A.K., 1977, Incidence of sporadic malformations, anomalies and variations in random bred laboratory animals, in: "Methods in Prenatal Toxicology", (D. Neubert, H.-J. Merker, T.E. Kwasigroch, eds.), pp. 52 - 71, Georg Thieme Publ., Stuttgart.

Rapaka, R.S., Parr, R.W., Liu, T.-Z., Bhatnagar, R.S., 1977, Biochemical basis of skeletal defects induced by hydralazine: inhibition of collagen synthesis and secretion in embryonic chicken cartilage in vitro, Teratology, 15, 185 - 194.

Saackel, L.R., 1974, Elektronische Auswertung von Mikroradiogrammen, Biomed. Technik, 19, 10 - 14.

Sterz, H., Hebold, G., 1978, Der Wert röntgenologischer Untersuchungen in der Fetotoxizität, in: "Embryotoxikologische Probleme in der Arzneimittelforschung, (B. Schnieders, G. Stille, P. Grosdanoff, eds.), pp. 61 - 63, Dietrich Reimer Verlag, Berlin.

Sterz, H., Hebold, G., 1980, Increased incidence of wavy ribs in rat fetuses due to vasoactive substances, Poster Presentation, 8th Confer. Europ. Teratology Soc., Münster (FRG), Sept. 1 - 4, 1980, Teratology, in press.

Sterz, H., Saackel, L.R., 1977, Automated television scanning technique for the quantitative evaluation of X-ray shadows of individual bones, in: "Methods in Prenatal Toxicology", (D. Neubert, H.-J. Merker, T.E. Kwasigroch, eds.), pp. 362 - 370, Georg Thieme Publ., Stuttgart.

Warkany, J., 1971, in: "Congenital Malformations", pp. 134 - 151, 824 - 836, 863 - 869, Year Book Medical Publishers, Chicago.

Limb Malformations Induced in the Rat by Amniotic Puncture

Jean-Jacques Houben

Laboratoire d'Anatomie et d'Embryologie humaines de la Faculté de Médecine, Université Libre de Bruxelles, 97, rue aux Laines, B-1000 Brussels, Belgium

The frequent occurrence of annular constrictions in pediatric surgery has drawn the attention to the mechanisms involved in the pathogenesis of the well known Congenital Constriction Band Syndrome (C.C.B.S.).

CLAVERT (1979) established some interesting correlations between clinical aspects of C.C.B.S. and experimentally induced malformations in the rabbit.

TRASLER et al. (1956) accomplished amniotic sac puncture in mouse embryos on day 13 of gestation. A no. 26 hypodermic needle was inserted into the amniotic sac without injection; abortion and foetal resorption were noticed; the examination of surviving foetuses revealed a high incidence of cleft palate.

Uterine vascular clamping performed in the rat (BRENT and FRANKLIN, 1960) as well as intra-uterine hypoxia resulted in growth retardation and limb anomalies. Some investigators (GULIENETTI et al., 1962; KENDRICK and FEILD, 1967; KENNEDY and PERSAUD, 1977) have studied different aspects of malformations induced by amniocentesis. The putative involvement of the maternal adrenal gland was excluded. Limb deficiencies (KINO, 1975) and associated defects were described in detail.

A few hours after amniotic puncture and oligohydramnios (KINO, 1972; PERSAUD, 1973), hemorrhages involving the limbs appeared. The same phenomenon could be induced by hypertonic glucose injected into the amniotic sac of rabbit embryos (CLAVERT, 1979). Contractions of the uterine muscle were thought to be responsible for circulatory disturbances (KINO, 1972; SINGH and SINGH, 1974). Uterine muscle relaxant administered before amniotic puncture significantly reduced the incidence of hemorrhages and limb malformations.

In the present study the effects of amniotic puncture on limb morphogenesis have been examined in the rat following treatment on gestational days 9 to 17.

MATERIAL and METHODS:

Fourty-nine pregnant C.O.B.S. rats (Charles River) were used in this study. Surgical procedures were performed under deep ether anesthesia. The morning when sperm was detected in vaginal smears was designated as day 0 of gestation. Amniotic sac punctures were performed between day 9 and day 17 with a glass micropipette (ϕ 0.3mm). After laparotomy by midline incision, the uterine horn was pulled out of the abdominal cavity, and the pipette was carefully introduced through the antimesometrial part of the uterine wall; the horns were constantly moistened by sterile HANKS solution to prevent dehydration. Groups of untreated embryos were used as controls.

Teratology of the Limbs

The following experiments were performed:

1.) 262 amniotic punctures were made and 128 embryos were left untreated (controls). The amount of amniotic fluid lost varied between 0.01 ml and 0.40 ml. Control and treated foetuses were collected on day 20 of gestation; the number of implantation sites were counted and malformations were detected by WATSON'S method (Alcian blue/ alizarin skeletal staining).

2.) Several treated pregnant rats were sacrificed, one, two or three days after surgery and the embryos were removed for standard histological studies.

3.) In order to confirm the site of puncture and the absence of direct trauma of the embryo, methyl green or indian ink were injected into the amniotic cavities of 15 embryos which were then immediately examined by microscopy.

4.) Some embryos were submitted to hypertonic glucose injection (1M osmolarity) into the amnion. 39 foetuses were treated between days 12 and 15 of gestation.

RESULTS:

1.) General effects of amniotic puncture:
Correlation was found between limb deficiencies and associated anomalies induced by amniotic puncture (without any compensatory injection) and the stage of development at the time of treatment. The quantity of amniotic fluid lost could not be evaluated precisely because of spontaneous and variable drainage through the site of puncture; this volume was estimated to be between 0.001 ml and 0.010 ml. The results are summarized in Table 1.

a.) Treatment on day 9, 10, and 11:
A micropipette was rapidly inserted and removed in order to take care of severe oligohydramnios. No abnormality was observed in the treated embryos and the incidence of mortality was 20%. The of resorption in the control group was 10%.

b.) Treatment on day 12:
Amniocentesis was performed with an empty micropipette which was slowly introduced. The amniotic fluid rose gradually and spontaneously in the capillary tube. Oligohydramnios occurred with a loss of fluid estimated to range from 1/10 to 1/3 of the total amniotic volume.

Amniocentesis on day 12 resulted in 22.6% mortality. Two embryos were severely growth retarded. One showed a hematoma in the tail, the other a left ulnar club-hand; no anomaly was detected in the osseous skeleton.

c.) Treatment on day 13:
The incidence of foetal death following 42 amniocentesis experiments was 38.1%. Brachy metatarsy and complete adactyly of the forelimbs were observed in two embryos (4.8%); vestigial nails were found implanted on the malformed extremities.

d.) Treatment on day 14:
It was possible to insert the micropipette into the space between the abdominal wall and the prominent four limb buds. Only five anterior limbs were affected (7.1%) in four embryos. Seventeen treated foetuses (30.4%) died and were resorbed. All five affected extremities were fore limbs (Fig. 1 a).

More than 0.25 ml of amniotic fluid were drained in 20 cases. The risidual amount of amniotic fluid was reduced to less than 10% of its normal value. The corresponding embryos, however, did not show any limb defects.

e.) Treatment on day 15:
Sixty-three amniocenteses were performed which induced limb malformations in 27 (42.8%) embryos. The observed rate of mortality (23%) was lower than that obtained at earlier stages.

This lower incidence of mortality cannot be considered as a sign of resistance, since the number of normal surviving foetuses was also the lowest of the series. It thus seems that day 15 can be considered as a stage of greatest sensitivity to experimental oligohydramnios. Anterior limbs were found affected 17 times and posterior limbs 28 times. This difference is of high statistical significance ($X^2 < 0.005$). The digital rays, including metacarpi and metatarsi were most frequently affected (Fig. 1 c and d). The carpus (tarsus) was found malformed in two cases and the elbow in one case. One club-hand and four club-feet were observed. The other abnormalities were: syndactyly of soft tissues (1 case), constrictive band (1 case), hematoma of trunk and tail (2 cases), complete amelia (1 case) and short umbilical cord (1 case). Complete amelia can only be explained by proximal constrictive band applied to a preexistent normal limb.

2.) Damages induced in the developing limb buds:

At the 14 day stage, the distal part of the forelimb bud acquired the characteristic shape of a foot plate which was clearly distinguishable from the more proximal zeugopod segment; digital outgrowths appeared along the marginal border of the footplate.

One day after amniotic puncture, vascular disruption and interstitial hemorrhage were found localized under the apical ectoderm. Two days later the affected areas were replaced by large cavities bordered by a cellular envelope and filled with large amounts of blood. A great number of macrophages could be seen around the cavities. These kinds of "cysts" were frequently separated from the ectoderm by a thin layer of healthy mesoderm (Fig. 1 b). The marginal vein probably was the original site of the hemorrhage. At the 15 day stage all digital rays were distinctly present and vascular damage, after amniocentesis was now localized between the digital condensations.

3.) Site of puncture and possible direct injuries to the embryos:

As revealed after injection of methyl green or indian ink, puncture of the amniotic cavity was effectively accomplished in 12 out of 15 injections. In two cases, hemorrhage appeared in the placenta with coloured marks, an injury which was most probably responsible for foetal death. In only one case were the embryo and extra embryonic membranes found unstained. A larger series of experiments was not performed because extensive data are available in the literature (CLAVERT, 1979).

4.) The influence of hypertonic glucose:

The injection of hypertonic glucose caused a high percentage of mortality in the foetuses treated on days 12, 13 and 14, but the number of malformed embryos was much lower than expected (Table 2). As a matter of fact, oligohydramnios and hypertonic glucose injection induced a similar amount of limb malformations.

DISCUSSION and CONCLUSIONS:

The results confirm the teratogenic influence of amniotic puncture performed on different developmental stages in the rat. This treatment resulted in severe malformations of the limbs with occasional associated defects, as other experiments have suggested (LOVE and VICKERS, 1972; LEIST and GRAUWILER, 1974; DEMYER and BAIRD, 1979).

Some particular aspects of the present study should be pointed out. One case of obvious constrictive band was observed with severe malposition of the hindlimb buds; this foetus was alive and was immediately examined at the opening of its annexes.

Histological studies of affected limb buds have confirmed the structural aspects of the damages already described in other reports. The topographical distribution of hemorrhages appeared particularly selectively: in the embryos treated before day 14, the hematoma were localized along the marginal vein; they appeared in the interdigital spaces in the embryos treated at later stages.

In contrast to uterine vascular clamping and hypoxia (PETTER et al., 1971), amniocentesis induced specific hemorrhages; when the uterine horns were isolated from maternal circulation for more than 5 minutes before the foetuses were sacrificed, dissemination and superficial hemorrhages occurred.

Hypertonic glucose injected into the amniotic cavity of the rat increased the rate of mortality but did not change the frequency of limb malformations induced by amniotic puncture performed without any injection.

Although day 15 was a stage of particularly great sensitivity, the amount of amniotic fluid removed did not affect the mortality rate.

KENNEDY and PERSAUD (1979) recently proposed a hypothesis on the present syndrome. The loss of amniotic fluid caused by puncture combined with uterine contractions was thought to disturb the foeto-maternal circulation.

Ischemia followed by repairing processes was responsible for the defects. The high sensitivity on day 15, the etiology of the constriction band as well as the clinical implications of the syndrome described, should be studied by further experiments.

Table 1:

Incidence of death and malformations induced by amniocentesis on different days of gestation:

Gestational day	Total number of treated embryos	Normal foetuses nr	Normal foetuses %	Resorption sites nr	Resorption sites %	Malformed foetuses nr	Malformed foetuses %
9, 10, 11	25	20	80.0	5	20.0	0	0.0
12	62	44	71.0	16	25.8	2	3.2
13	42	24	57.1	16	38.1	2	4.8
14	56	35	62.5	17	30.4	4	7.1
15	63	21	33.4	15	23.8	27	42.8
16, 17	14	13	92.8	1	7.2	0	0.0
	262	157	59.9	70	26.7	35	13.4

Table 2:

Comparison between oligohydramnios and hypertonic glucose injection on days 12, 13, and 14 of gestation in rat fetuses.

Experiment	Nr. of treated foetuses	Normal surviving foetuses		Resorption sites		Malformed foetuses	
		nr.	%	nr.	%	nr.	%
Amniocentesis with oligohydramnios	160	103°	64.3	47°	30.7	8	5.0
Hypertonic glucose injection	39	17°	43.6	20°	51.3	2	5.1

°X^2 significant < 0.01

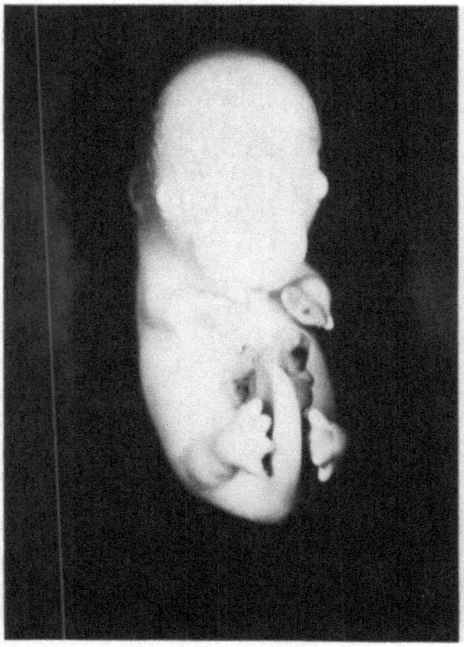

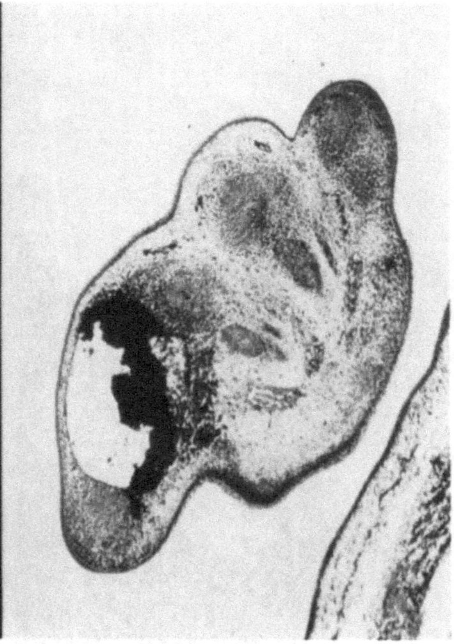

Fig. 1 a: Amniocentesis performed on day 14; distal hematoma and necrosis of anterior extremities.

Fig. 1 b: Hemorrhage in the interdigital area with intact ectoderm. Trichrome de Masson. x 60.

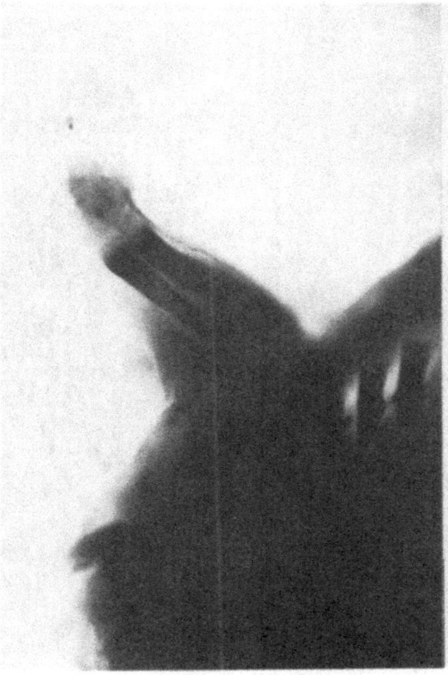

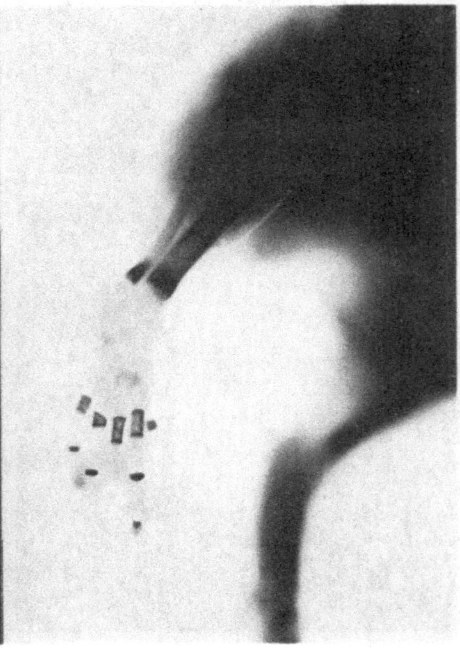

Fig. 1 c: Important dysplasia of the forelimb. Radius and ulna are normal. Carpus, metacarpus and digits are absent. Presence of a distal phalanx at the extremity. Watson's staining.

Fig. 1 d: Metacarpal defects with absence of phalanges causing brachydactyly. Watson's staining.

REFERENCES

Brent and Franklin, 1960, Uterine vascular clamping: new procedure for the study of congenital malformations, Science, 132, 89 - 91.

Clavert, J.M., 1979, Contribution expérimentale à l' étude de la pathogénie de la maladie amniotique, Thèse 148, Faculté de Médecine, Univ. Louis Pasteur, Strasbourg, France.

Demyer, W., Baird, I., 1979, Mortality and Skeletal Malformations from Amniocentesis and Oligohydramnios in Rats: Cleft Palate, Clubfoot, Microstomia and Adactyly, Teratology, 2, 33 - 38.

Gulienetti, R., Kalter, H., Davis, N.C., 1962, Amniotic fluid volume and experimentally-induced congenital malformations, Biol. Neonat., 4, 300 - 309.

Kendrick, F., Feild, L., 1967, Congenital anomalies induced in normal and adrenalectomized rats by amniocentesis, Anat. Rec., 159, 353 - 356.

Kennedy, A., Persaud, T.V.N., 1977, Pathogenesis of developmental defects induced in the rat by amniotic sac puncture, Acta Anat., 97, 23 - 35.

Kennedy, L.A., Persaud, T.V.N., 1979, Experimental amniocentesis and teratogenesis: clinical implications, in: "Advances in the Study of Birth Defects", Vol. 1, Teratologic Mechanisms. (T.V.N. Persaud, ed.), pp. 163 - 175, MTP Press Limited.

Kino, Y., 1972, Reductive malformation of the limbs in the rat fetus following amniocentesis, Congen. Anom. (Japan), 12, 35 - 44.

Kino, Y., 1975, Clinical and experimental studies of the congenital constriction band syndrome with an emphasis on its etiology, J. Bone Jt. Surg., 57A, No. 5, 636 - 643.

Leist, K.H., Grauwiler, J., 1974, Fetal pathology in rats following uterine vessel clamping on day 14 of gestation, Teratology, 10, 55 - 68.

Love, A.M., Vickers, T.H., 1972, Amniocentesis dysmelia in rats, Br. J. Exp. Pathol., 53, 435 - 444.

Persaud, T.V.N., 1973, Meromelia and other developmental abnormalities in experimental oligohydramnios, Anat. Anz. Bd., 133, 499 - 502.

Petter, C., Bourbon, J., Maltier, J.P., et Jost, A., 1971, Production d'hémorragies des extrémités chez le foetus de rat soumis à une hypoxie in utero, C.R. Acad. Sci., Paris, 272, 2488 - 2490.

Singh, S., Singh, G., 1974, Role of uterine contraction in producing hemorrhages in rat fetuses after amniocentesis, Teratology, 10, 145 - 148.

Trasler, D.G., Walker, B.E., Fraser, F.C., 1956, Congenital malformations produced by amniotic sac puncture, Science, 124, 439.

The Effect of Sodium Salicylate on Limb Development

F. Beck and A. P. Gulamhusein

Dept. of Anatomy, University of Leicester,
University Road, Leicester LE1 7RH, U.K.

Salicylates have a long therapeutic history as antipyretics, antirheumatics, pain killers and placebos. Congenital malformations in man have an even longer history (WARKANY, 1977) and show no sign of diminishing in number. Could the first be causally related (even to a small degree) with the second?

It is well known that salicylates are embryotoxic in rats (WARKANY and TAKASC, 1959; KIMMEL et al., 1971), but apart from isolated experiments in monkeys, for example, (WILSON et al., 1975) which also showed embryotoxicity, very little work has been done on alternative species. In the present study the effect of sodium salicylate on ferrets has been investigated and compared with that on the rat. A measure of the possible danger to man has been adduced by comparing human maternal serum levels after treatment with teratogenic levels in rats and ferrets.

Ferrets were paired when the vulva and testicles indicated that both partners were fertile (BECK et al., 1976). Mating was determined by direct observation and checked by the presence of sperm in the vaginal smear immediately after coitus. Pregnancy was timed from the moment of mating. At 13.0 or 18.0 days of gestation the animals were injected with one of 3 doses of sodium salicylate and subsequently were killed at 35 days (gestation is 42 days). The presence of resorption sites was noted and surviving embryos were examined for external malformation, 1/3 of the survivors were eviscerated, stained with alizarin and their skeletons were subsequently examined for abnormalities. The remainder were examined by Wilson's freehand razor sectioning technique (WILSON, 1965). Rats were mated in the usual way, pregnancy was timed from midnight of the night preceding the finding of a plug or positive vaginal smear. At 8.5 or 11.5 days the rats were injected subcutaneously with 400 mg/kg of sodium salicylate. This dose was equivalent to the highest possible dose, compatible with significant fetal survival at term in ferrets; pilot experiments showed that it was also the minimal reasonably effective dose in our particular rat strain. Rats were killed at 20.5 days and the uterine contents examined in a similar way to that of the ferrets. Results are shown in Table 1. Eight and a half days of gestation in the rat is roughly equivalent to 13.0 days in the ferret; 11.5 days in the rat (circa 25 somites) is in some respects a similar age to 18 days in the ferret but in other parameters it is a little behind in development, for instance, in the ferret there are circa 31 somites and the neural tube is closed (BECK, 1975). The blood salicylate levels were determined 1, 2,3, and 24 hours after subcutaneous injection of rats and ferrets at 8.5 or 13 and 11.5 or 18 days after injection using TRINDER'S (1954) method. Using six animals of each species a conversion factor to serum levels was calculated. It was found that after a subcutaneous injection of 125 or 400 mg/kg serum levels were virtually identical in the ferret and rat. At 125 mg the concentration was 37 - 39 mg% after 1 hr, 33.6 - 35 mg% after 2 hrs and 28.5 - 30.5 mg% after 3 hrs. After 24 hrs levels were indistinguishable from background. Similarly at 400 mg/kg levels were 70 - 71 mg% after 1 hr, 68 - 69 mg% after 2 hrs, 51 - 54 mg% after 3 hrs and unmeasurable after 24 hrs.

Teratology of the Limbs

KNOBEN et al. (1978) have reported that in man anti inflammatory doses of aspirin produce plasma levels of 20 - 30 mg%. At these levels LEVY et al. (1972) have shown that conjugating mechanisms are saturated and the half life of a given dose increases to 22 hours. Clearly, therefore, doses sometimes therapeutically administered (and often taken in suicide bids) give human serum levels well below those found to be embryotoxic in the rat and equivalent to those described as embryotoxic in ferrets. Many factors must be operative in determining the fact that salicylates are more embryotoxic in the ferret than in the rat. Maternal pharmacokinetic factors and detoxifying mechanisms have hardly been studied in the ferret but since factors other than serum levels are operative it is possible that embryo salicylate levels are higher in the ferret for a given serum level than they are in the rat. It has been shown by JACKSON (1948) that salicylates cross 'the placenta' and WILSON et al. (1975) have shown that salicylate levels were more easily maintained in their strain of rats than in the monkey (in which the drug was also demonstrated to be less teratogenic).

Numerous malformations (Fig. 4 - 6) involving the eyes, lips, palate, cardiovascular system and urogenital system were found in both species (see GULAMHUSEIN et al.,) and there was evidence of critical periods in so far as some malformations were found at the earlier stages of gestation only and some at the later stages. Limb defects were an example of this phenomenon for they were found only in ferrets at 18.0 days of gestation and not at 13.0 days. None were seen in the rat possibly because at 11.5 days the rat is a little less mature than the ferret from the point of view of limb development (see above). Only the forelimbs were affected in the ferret at 18 days of gestation (Fig. 1 - 3). It is interesting that forelimb defects were only present if the animals also had tail defects (Fig. 6); furthermore, the left forelimb was consistently more affected than the right (Fig. 1 - 3).

One might speculate that the left seventh intersegmental artery from which the left subclavian artery develops arises in the early stages from the descending aorta <u>below</u> the level at which the ductus arteriosus is responsible for mixing deoxygenated blood with the oxygenated blood in the aorta. On the other hand, the right seventh intersegmental artery arises from the right horn of the aortic bulb well <u>before</u> the entry of the ductus (Fig. 7). It is likely therefore, that the right limb bud is developing at a higher oxygen tension than the left and <u>possibly</u> this may make it less susceptible to the teratogenic action of salicylate (Fig. 7).

ZIMMERMANN and we (in preparation) have explanted mouse forelimb buds in Trowell type culture on days 11, 12, or 13 of gestation in the presence of 100, 300 and 1 000 µg sodium salicylate/ml of culture medium (see this symposium for method). We obtained dose dependent inhibition of cartilage formation which was most marked at 11.0 days of gestation (43 somites). This correlates well with preliminary in vitro results in the ferret where the very few limb buds so far explanted have been shown to be maximally sensitive to salicylate at 22 days of gestation (40 - 47 somites). Electron microscopic studies on the mouse embryos showed changes of the proteoglycan matrix in the cartilage as well as changes in the cartilage cells themselves. At 1 000 µg/ml necrosis of cartilage cells was widespread but adjacent blastema remained unaffected. Clearly, therefore, salicylate has a direct action on embryonic tissue. Its' precise nature is unknown but a number of possibilities exist including inhibition of glycosaminoglycan or collagen synthesis, disturbance of prostaglandin synthesis and a direct effect on cell differentiation.

Finally, the nature of salicylate action on embryonic rat tissues has been further examined by our group (McGARRITY et al., in press) by means of the technique of NEW et al. (1976). The optimum teratogenic dose in vivo of subcutaneously injected sodium salicylate in our strain of rats at 9.5 days was found to be 450 mg/kg. Three hours after injection serum levels (TRINDER, 1954) were found to be 65 mg%. Eighteen hours after injection serum levels were 20 mg/100 ml. 9.5 day embryo rat egg cylinders were then cultured in vitro.

(a) For 24 hrs in normal serum to which 65 mg% sodium salicylate had been added followed by 24 hrs in normal serum.
(b) For 24 hrs in rat serum obtained 3 hrs after subcutaneous injection of sodium salicylate (containing 65% sodium salicylate) followed by 24 hrs in normal serum.
(c) For 24 hrs in rat serum to which 30 mg% of sodium salicylate was added followed by 24 hrs in normal serum.
(d) For 24 hrs in rat serum from rats injected 18 hrs previously with 450 mg/100 ml of sodium salicylate (containing 25 mg% sodium salicylate) followed by 24 hrs in normal serum.
(e) Controls cultured in normal serum for 48 hrs.

The types of malformation seen after salicylate exposure at 9 1/2 days do not (as may be expected) include limb defects. The embryo has just 3 - 5 somites at 9 1/2 days and only about 25 somites at 11 1/2 days. The purpose of the whole embryo in vitro culture experiment was to see whether the same level and types of abnormality were obtained after culture in serum to which salicylate was added as was found after culture in serum for salicylate treated animals. Hence, the culture technique was used to determine whether any teratogenic effect was due to the effect of the drug on the mother. Table 2 illustrates some of the anomalies seen in culture and shows quite clearly that no maternal effect was demonstrable. It allows one to confirm the conclusion assumed in the results of the in vivo experiment and partially predictable from the limb bud culture experiment, that during the phase of histiotrophic nutrition sodium salicylate, rather than one of its metabolites, is the effective teratogen acting directly on the embryonic tissues.

ACKNOWLEDGEMENTS

We are grateful for a grant in aid of research from the Medical Research Council Drs. Zimmermann, Al-Alousi and Harrison-Sage as well as Messrs. McGarrity and Samani participated in the experimental work. We are also grateful to the technical staff of the Anatomy Department for excellent technical assistance.

Table 1:

The Effect of Sodium Salicylates on Rats and Ferrets

(1) Day of injection + dose	(2) No. of animals	(3) No. of implantations	(4) Resorptions (%)	(5) No. of fetuses showing external or internal malformations (% 3)	(6) Mean fetal weight
(F 13.0 (400 mg/kg)	8	75	68 (91 %)	6 (8 %)	3.13
(R 8.5 (400 mg/kg)	10	91	21 (23 %)	13 (14 %)	3.11
(F 18.0 (400 mg/kg)	8	70	46 (66 %)	23 (33 %)	2.17
(R 11.5 (400 mg/kg)	10	98	9 (9 %)	10 (10 %)	3.21
F 13.0 (250 mg/kg)	7	55	17 (31 %)	9 *	3.74
F 18.0 (250 mg/kg)	6	57	21 (37 %)	12 (21 %)	3.59
F 13.0 (125 mg/kg)	8	67	22 (33 %)	5 (8 %)	3.66
F 18.0 (125 mg/kg)	8	76	33 (43 %)	3 (4 %)	3.68
F 13/18 (control)	8	73	6 (8 %)	1 (1 %)	4.04
R 8.5 (control)	7	57	0	0	3.65
R 11.5 (control)	5	51	0	0	3.78

* Hydramnios

R = Rat; F = Ferret; Control = 1 ml saline (R) 5 ml saline (F)

Table 2:

The Effect of Sodium Salicylate on Development of Rat Embryos In Vitro

Serum	Total No. of embryos	Vitelline circulation	Normal body shape	Normal closure of neural tube	Mean somite No.
Control	41	100 % (41)	83 % (34)	88 % (36)	24.0 ± 2.38
Removed 3 hrs after injection. Salicylate level 60 mg %	36	22 % (8)	0 % (0)	5.5 % (2)	7.9 ± 0.56
Removed 18 hrs after salicylate injection. Salicylate level 20 mg %	23	82 % (19)	69 % (16)	65 % (15)	20.9 ± 1.22
Salicylate added 65 mg %	26	42 % (1)	0 % (0)	0 % (0)	8.8 ± 0.24
Salicylate added 30 mg %	31	84 % (26)	35 % (11)	13 % (4)	18.0 ± 0.55

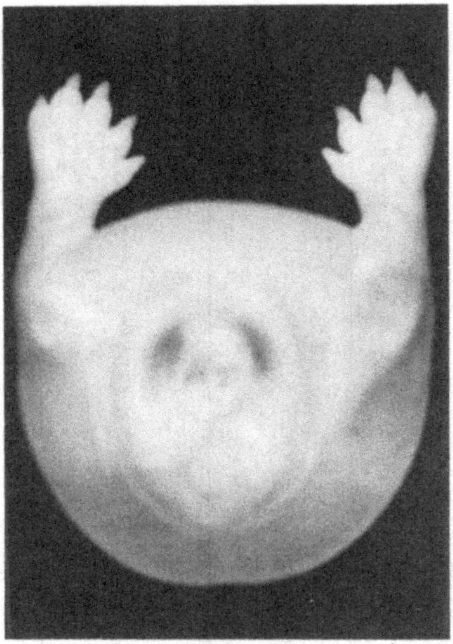

Fig. 1: 35 day normal ferret fetal forelimbs seen from below. x 3.6

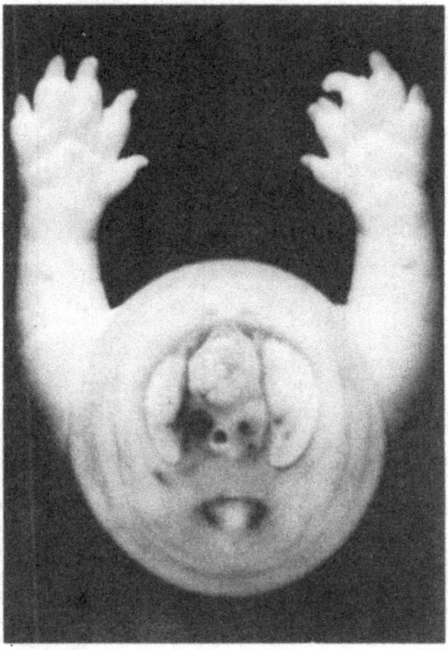

Fig. 2: 35 day ferret fetal forelimbs from a mother treated with sodium salicylate - seen from below. The left forelimb is abnormal; the right is normal. x 3.6

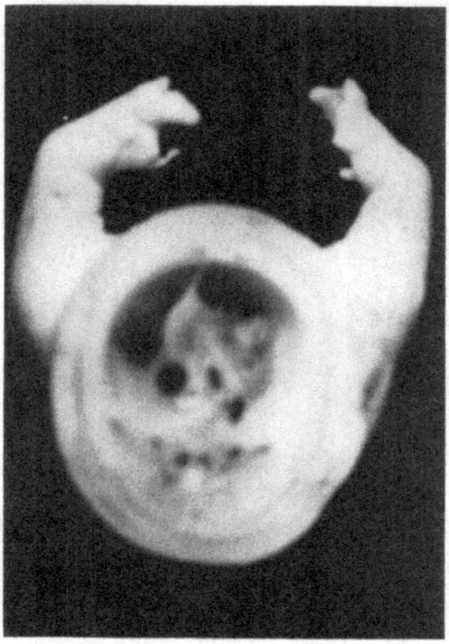

Fig. 3: 35 day ferret fetal forelimbs from a mother treated with sodium salicylate. Seen from below. Both limbs are abnormal - the left more so than the right. x 3.6

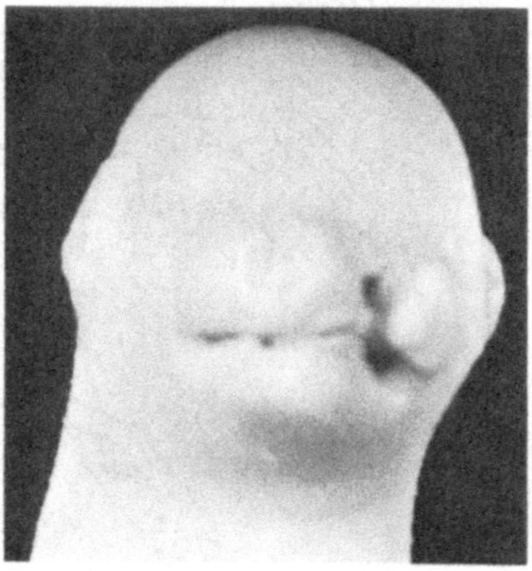

Fig. 4: Cleft lip in a 35 day fetal ferret from a mother treated with sodium salicylate. x 4

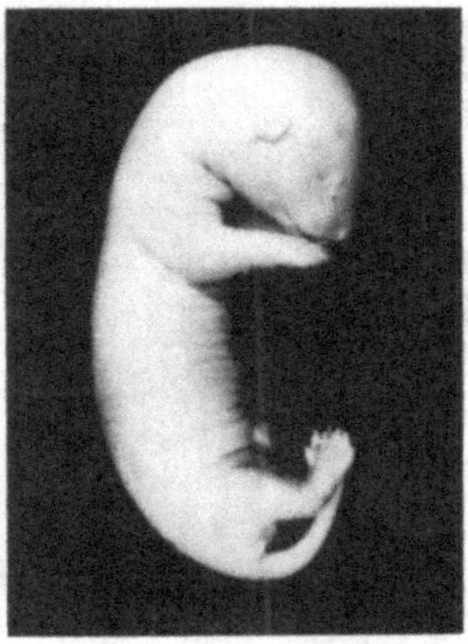

Fig. 5: Normal 35 day fetal ferret. x 1

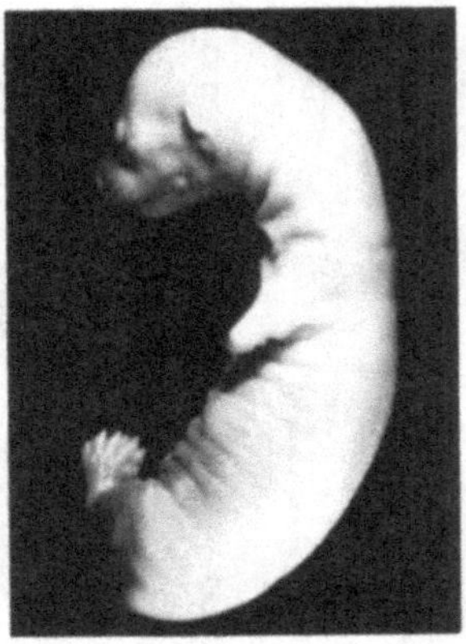

Fig. 6: 35 day fetal ferret from mother treated with sodium salicylate. Note absence of tail. x 1.1

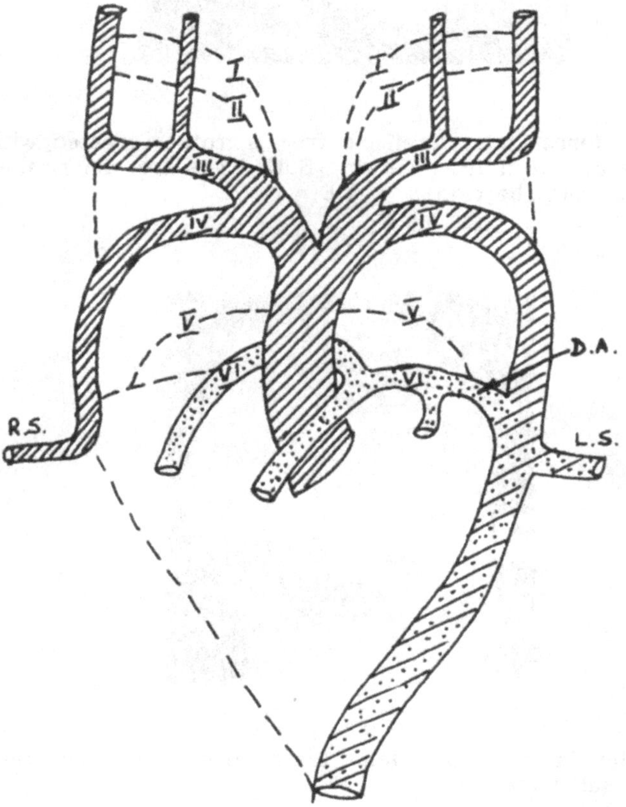

Fig. 7: To show the relative paucity of oxygenated blood passing to the left subclavian artery (LS) when compared with the right (RS).

DA = Ductus arteriosus. I - VI branchial arch arteries. For explanation see text.

REFERENCES

Beck, F., 1975, The ferret as a teratological model, in: "New approaches to the evaluation of abnormal embryonic development", (D. Neubert, H.-J. Merker, eds.), pp. 8 - 20, Georg Thieme, Publ., Stuttgart.

Beck, F., Schön, H., Mould, G., Swidzinska, P., Curry, S., Grauwiler, J., 1976, Comparison of the teratogenic effects of mustine hydrochloride in rats and ferrets. The value of the ferret as an experimental animal in teratology, Teratology, 13, 151 - 166.

Gulamhusein, A.P., Harrison-Sage, C., Beck, F., Al-Alousi, A., 1980, Salicylate-induced teratogenesis in the ferret, Life Sci., 27, 1799 - 1805.

Jackson, A.V., 1948, Toxic effects of salicylate on the foetus and the mother, J. Pathol. Bact. 60, 587 - 593.

Kimmel, C.A., Wilson, J.G., Schumacher, H.J., 1971, Studies on the metabolism and identification of the causative agent in aspirin teratogenesis in rats, Teratology, 4, 15 - 24.

Knoben, J.E., Anderson, P.O., Watanabe, A.S., 1978, Clinical drug data, in: Drug Intelligence Publications, pp. 318 - 319, Illinois.

Levy, G., Tsuchiya, T., Lewis, P.A., 1972, Limited capacity for salicyl phenolic glucuronide formation and its effects on the kinetics of salicylate elimination in man, Clin. Pharmacol. Ther. 13, 258 - 268.

McGarrity, C., Samani, N., Beck, F., Gulamhusein, A.P., The effect of sodium salicylate on the rat embryo in culture : An in vitro model for the morphological assessment of teratogenicity, J. Anat. (London), (in press).

New, D.A.T., Coppola, P.T., Cockcroft, D., 1976, Improved development of rat head fold embryos in culture resulting from low oxygen and modification of culture serum, J. Reprod. Fert. 48, 219 - 222.

Trinder, P., 1954, Rapid determination of salicylate in biological fluids. Biochem. J. 57, 301 - 303.

Warkany, J., Takasc, E., 1959, Experimental production of congenital malformation in rats by salicylate poisoning, Amer. J. Pathol. 35, 315 - 331.

Warkany, J., 1977, History of Teratology, in: "Handbook of Teratology," Vol. 1, (J.G. Wilson, F.C. Fraser, eds.), pp. 3 - 46, Plenum Press, New York.

Wilson, J.G., 1965, Methods of examining rat fetuses for malformations, in: "Teratology, Principles and Techniques", (J.G. Wilson, J. Warkany, eds.), pp. 262 - 277, Univ. of Chicago Press.

Wilson, J.G., Ritter, E.J., Scott, W.J., Fradkin, R., 1975, Comparative distribution and embryotoxicity of acetylsalicylic acid in pregnant rats and rhesus monkeys, Toxicol. Appl. Pharmacol. 41, 67 - 78.

α,α'-Dipyridyl Teratogenicity in the Rat

S. Lilja

Institut für Toxikologie und Embryonal-Pharmakologie, Freie Universität Berlin, Garystraße 9, D-1000 Berlin 33

INTRODUCTION:

The mesenchyme and its extracellular components play an important role in limb development. Therefore, a disturbance of mesenchyme development may induce embryotoxic or teratogenic effects. When lathyrogenic substances, such as D-penicillamine or ß-aminopropionitrile, are given at critical stages of gestation, malformations are produced (HALL, 1972; BARROW and STEFFEK, 1974; MERKER et al., 1975; WILEY and JONEJA, 1976). α,α'-Dipyridyl (α,α'-DIP) seems to have similar effects (OOHIRA and NOGAMI, 1978). α,α'-DIP is a chelator for ferrous iron, which is involved in enzyme reactions, such as electron transport in mitochondria. Ferrous iron is also necessary in the biosynthesis of collagen. Some proline residues in the precursor chains of collagen, pro-α 1 and pro-α 2, are converted to hydroxyproline by protocollagen hydroxylase, an enzyme that requires ferrous iron for activity. It has been shown that α,α'-DIP inhibits the hydroxylation of proline and accumulates procollagen intracellularly (JUVA et al., 1966). MÜLLER et al. (1971) found that this substance impairs the conversion of procollagen to collagen. However, considering the role of ferrous iron in enzyme reactions, in oxygen transport and in the biosynthesis of collagen, it can be assumed that these modes of action lead to a number of other effects. This was confirmed by OOHIRA and NOGAMI (1978), who reported on limb anomalies produced by α,α'-DIP in rats. These teratogenic effects could not be explained by an inhibition of collagen synthesis alone. In order to analyse the effects of α,α'-DIP on limb development more precisely, we morphologically examined rat embryos exposed to this substance in vivo.

MATERIALS and METHODS:

Pregnant Wistar rats (Winkelmann; Borchen, W. Germany) (day of conception = day 0), weighing about 250 g were used. 68 mg/kg α,α'-DIP (Sigma Chemical Co., St. Louis Mo., USA) in 8 ml 15% ethanol were injected intraperitoneally to pregnant rats on day 12.5 of gestation. Control animals received a corresponding amount of 15% ethanol.

To examine external and skeletal malformations, the rats were sacrificed on day 21 of pregnancy. The fetuses were removed and weighed. For the determination of the cartilaginous and bony parts the fetuses were fixed in 10% formaldehyde, stained with alcian blue, cleared with KOH and stained with alizarin red.

For light and electron microscopic investigations limb buds were removed at various stages after administration of α,α'-DIP. Removal was performed every 2 hours starting with 2 hours after injection until 16 hours after injection and then again after 24 h, 48 h, 72 h and 98 h. For light microscopy the limb buds were fixed in Bouin's solution and embedded in paraffin. 5 µm thick sections were cut and stained with hematoxylin and eosine. For electron microscopy the limb buds were fixed in 0.1 M phos-

Teratology of the Limbs

phate buffer (pH 7.2) containing 1% glutaraldehyde and 1% tannic acid. Postfixation was performed in 2% OsO_4 in 0.2 M phosphate buffer (pH 7.2). The samples were dehydrated in an acetone series and embedded in Mikropal. Sectioning was carried out in a LKB-microtome and contrasting was performed with uranyl acetate/lead citrate. The sections were examined with a SIEMENS Elmiskop 101. For light microscopic investigations sections were cut at 1 µm and stained with alkaline GIEMSA solution (60° C, 1 min).

RESULTS:

Administration of α,α'-DIP to rats on day 12.5 of pregnancy caused a rather high resorption rate (44%). The weights of live fetuses decreased compared to control experiments (Table 1). External malformations of the digits of the forelimb were found in 83%. Separately counted hindlimb malformations amounted to 44%. A fusion of the 3rd and 4th digits (Fig. 1 a) was the most frequent digital anomaly observed in alcian blue and alizarin red stained forelimbs on day 21. After staining the cartilaginous skeleton with alcian blue, this phenomenon was established as early as on day 16. This fusion may affect all regions of the rays (metacarpalia and phalanges) or only parts of them. The distal bone anlagen of the phalanges frequently remain separated and the metacarpalia are fused (Fig. 1 b).

There was another striking feature in the forelimb. 22 hours after treatment with α,α'-DIP a bleb was noticed (Fig. 1 c).

A characteristic morphological finding of the limb buds only a few hours after injection of α,α'-DIP, was the appearance of necroses (Fig. 2 a). Electron microscopic examination demonstrated shrinking necroses which first appeared 4 hours after treatment (Fig. 2 b). This type of necroses is characterized by a condensation of the cytoplasm, pyknosis of the nuclei and shrinkage of the cell volume. In the endphase of necroses the cell is deformed by deep invaginations and finally breaks up. The fragments are phagocytized by normal neighbouring cells. The necroses are evenly distributed in the distal parts of the limb buds. The necroses lead to formation of cell depleted zones and wide intercellular spaces. This phenomenon is particulary pronounced below the apical ectodermal ridge (AER) (Fig. 3). Compared to controls with numerous mesenchymal cells directly under the basal lamina and long finger-like processes reaching the basement membrane, the treated limb buds often exhibit areas with no cellular processes. In many limbs the marginal sinus is enlarged and filled with numerous blood cells. Frequently, only a small amount of cellular material is seen between this vessel and the epithelial basal lamina. In a few cases the endothelium expands to the basal lamina below the apical ridge (AER). Necroses are seldom seen in the epithelium and endothelium of the vessels. However, the epithelial cells apparently form only a very loose structure (Fig. 2, b). 45 hours after treatment necroses are no longer demonstrable.
From light microscopic observations the first blastemata appear after 45 hours. The pattern of the blastema already indicates the fusion of the 3rd and 4th digits (Fig. 4, a). A characteristic feature is the increase of enlarged vessels in the surrounding of the newly formed blastema (Fig. 4, a). 72 hours after exposure to α,α'-DIP the formation of new vessels can be observed in the electron microscope (Fig. 4, b).

DISCUSSION:

It seems reasonable to attribute these malformations observed after application of α,α'-DIP to a cytotoxic effect of the substance. There are many teratogenic substances, such as DNA- and RNA-synthesis inhibitors, which induce necroses (RITTER et al., 1971, 1973; SCOTT et al., 1971; MERKER, 1977). However, the malformation pattern of α,α'-DIP is different from that of other necroses producing substances. Therefore, other mechanisms have to be considered: the blebs observed in the forelimb (Fig. 1 c) suggest a disturbance in the epithelio-mesenchymal interaction. This in fact is seen electron microscopically in the area of the apical ectodermal ridge (AER) (Fig. 3). The region between the epithelium and the mesenchyme shows large intercellular spaces and a lack of cellular processes compared to limb buds from control experiments. However, the contact between epithelium and mesenchyme seems to play an important role in the regulation of proliferation, differentiation and pattern formation in this area (SEARL and ZWILLING, 1964; ZWILLING, 1961). Thus, the formation of new blastema might be disturbed and this might lead to a wrong pattern. In fact, light microscopic data show a fusion of the blastemata probably as a result of the presence of an insufficient amount of vital cells. On the other hand, an additional finding has to be discussed in this respect. In the surroundings of the mis-developed blastema, numerous vessels are seen (Fig. 4, a). The morphological findings indicate the formation of additional vessels (Fig. 4, b) compared to the control. It would therefore be tempting to correlate the wrong distribution and localization of the blastema to the formation of new vessels according to the hypothesis of CAPLAN and KOUTROUPAS, (1973). We can speculate that formation of a ferrous chelate complex may cause oxygen deficiency which then acts as an impulse for the development of new vessels. However, this model of malformation requires further investigation.

ACKNOWLEDGEMENTS

I wish to thank Mrs. U. KRÜGER and Mrs. H. STÜRJE for their expert technical assistance.

This work was supported by grants from the Deutsche Forschungsgemeinschaft awarded to Sonderforschungsbereich 29 - Embryonale Entwicklung und Differenzierung - "Embryonal-Pharmakologie".

Table 1:

EFFECTS OF α,α'-DIPYRIDYL ON RAT EMBRYOS EXPOSED TO SINGLE I.P. INJECTIONS ON DAY 12.5 AND EXAMINED ON DAY 21.

Dose mg/kg	Litters (n)	Resorption (%)	Live Fetuses (n)	Wet Weight g ± S.D.	Digital Malformations *	
					Forelimb %	Hindlimb %
68	15	44	95	3.77 ± 0.51	83	44
0	3	15	23	4.94 ± 0.37	0	0

* External malformations in fore- and hindlimbs were separately counted.

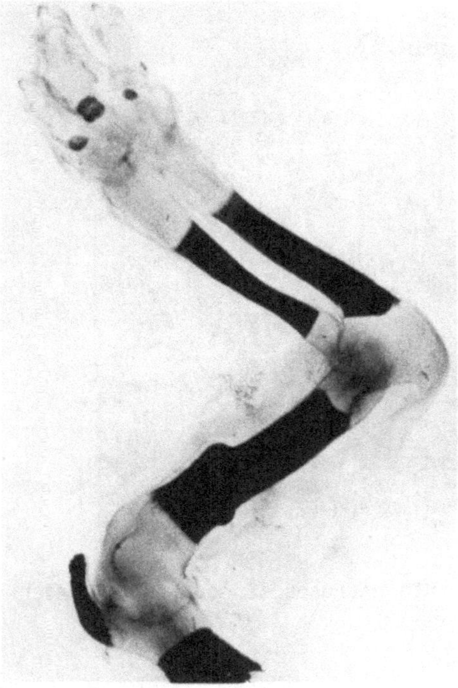

Fig. 1 a: Alcian blue and alizarin red stained rat forelimb on day 21. Maternal treatment with 68 mg/kg α,α'-DIP on day 12.5 of gestation. Note the fusion of the 3rd and 4th digits.

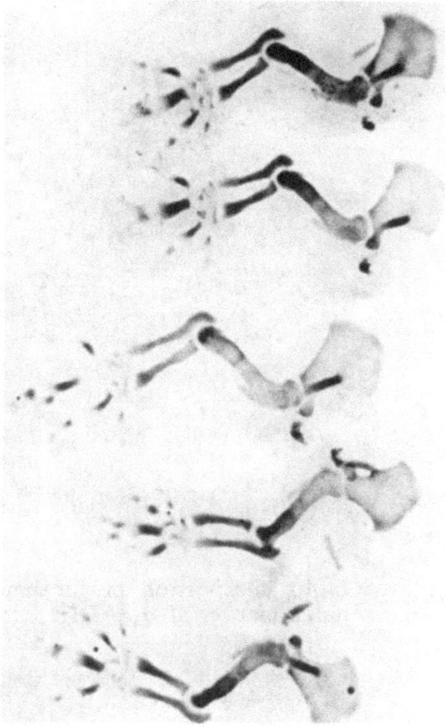

Fig. 1 b: Digital abnormalities in the forelimbs of 16 day old rat fetuses after maternal injection of α,α'-DIP. Variations of the digital defect with 3rd and 4th digits fused.

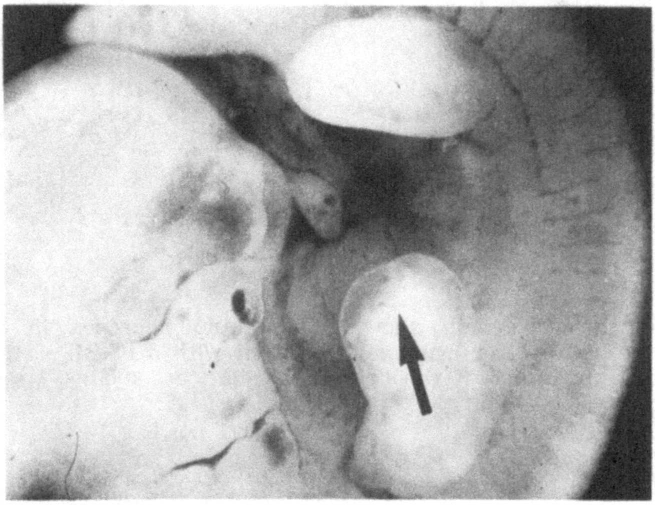

Fig. 1 c: Rat fetus with bleb in forelimb (→) 22 hours after maternal treatment with α,α'-DIP.

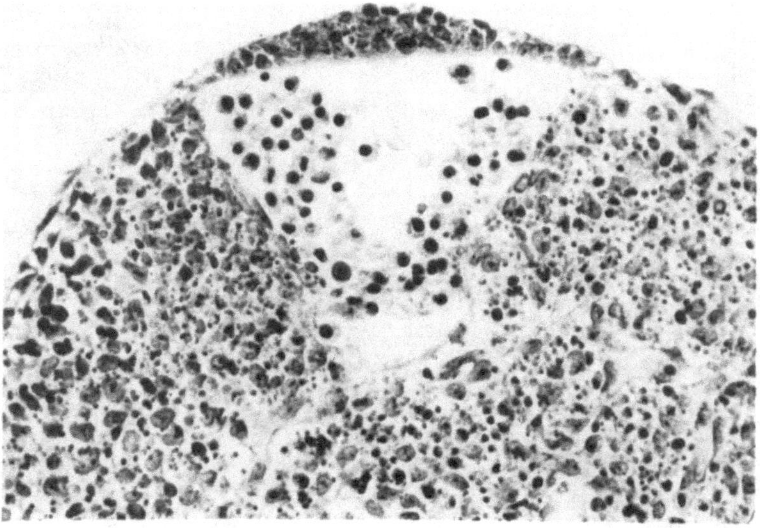

Fig. 2 a: Light micrograph of forelimb with necroses 12 hours after maternal injection of α,α'-DIP. x 300.

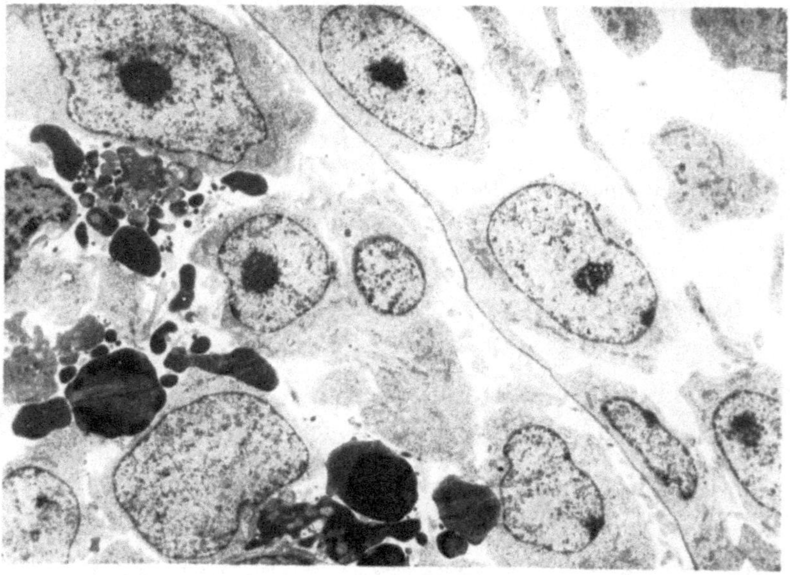

Fig. 2 b: Electron micrograph showing shrinking necroses in a forelimb bud 4 hours after maternal treatment with α,α'-DIP. Note also the loose appearance of the epithelial cells. x 4000.

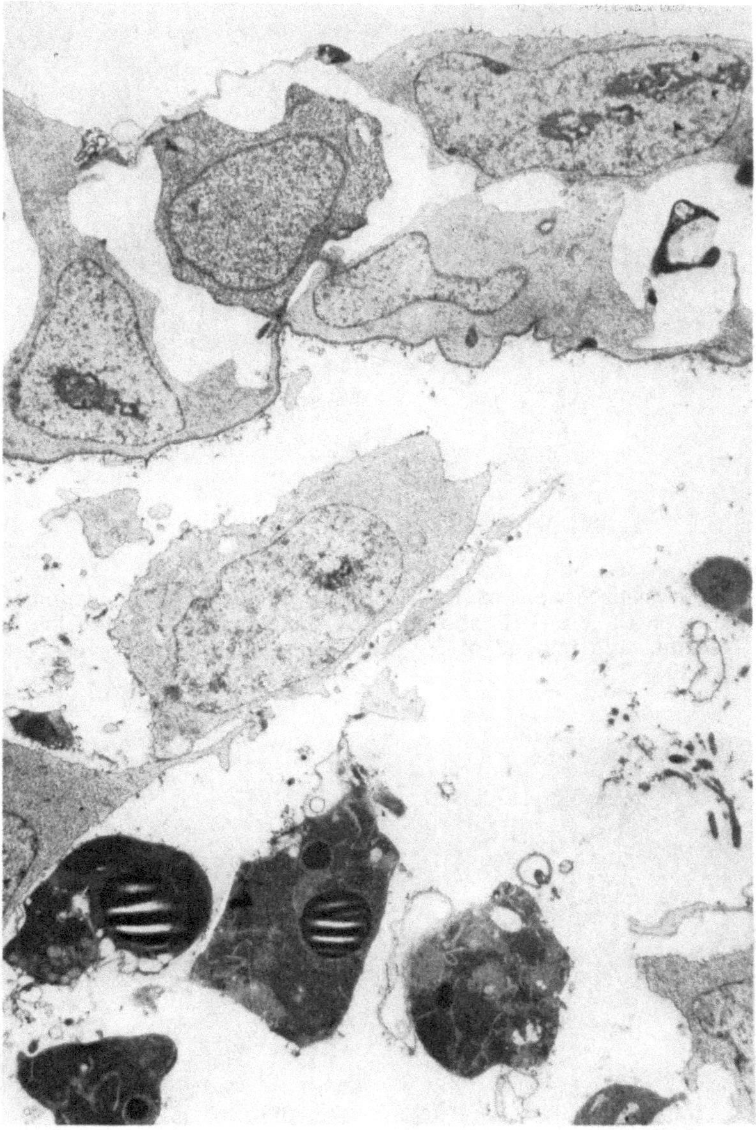

Fig. 3 Electron micrograph demonstrating the area of the apical ectodermal ridge (AER) of the rat forelimb 6 hours after maternal injection of α,α'-DIP. The region between the epithelium and the mesenchyme has a rather empty appearance. Compared to limb buds from control experiments there are only a few cellular processes. x 5400.

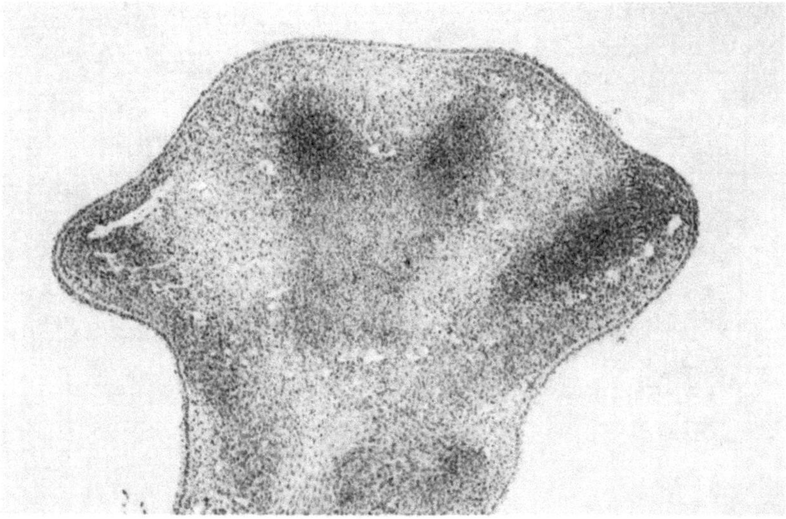

Fig. 4 a: Light micrograph of rat forelimb 72 hours after maternal treatment with α,α'-DIP showing the development of the blastema in 4 digital rays instead of 5. Note also the numerous vessels. x 100.

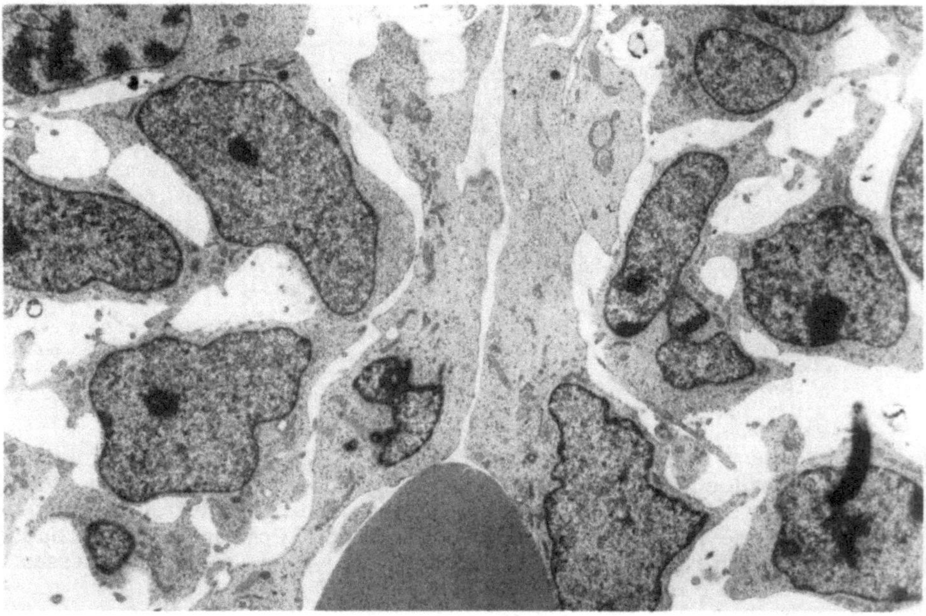

Fig. 4 b: Electron micrograph showing the formation of additional vessels in a rat forelimb 72 hours after maternal injection of α,α'-DIP. x 5000.

REFERENCES

Barrow, M.V., Steffek, A.J., 1974, Teratologic and other embryo-toxic effects of ß-aminopropionitrile in rats, Teratology, 10, 165 - 172.

Caplan, A.J., Koutroupas, S., 1973, The control of muscle and cartilage development in the chick limb: The role of differential vascularization, J. Embryol. exp. Morph., 29, 571 - 583.

Hall, B.V., 1972, Skeletal defects in embryonic chicks induced by administration of beta-aminopropionitrile, Teratology, 5, 81 - 88.

Juva, K., Prockop, D.J., Cooper, G.W., Lash, J.W., 1966, Hydroxylation of proline and the intracellular accumulation of a polypeptide precursor of collagen, Science, 152, 92 - 94.

Merker, H.-J., 1977, Considerations on the problem of critical period during the development of limb skeleton, in: Morphogenesis and malformation of the limb, (D. Bergsma, W. Lenz, eds.), 2nd International Conference on morphogenesis and malformation, Titisee, W. Germany, Alan R. Liss, Inc., New York.

Merker, H.-J., Franke, L., Günther, Th., 1975, The effect of D-penicillamine on the skeletal development of rat foetuses, Naunyn Schmied. Arch. Pharmacol., 287, 359 - 376.

Müller, P., McGoodwin, E.B., Martin, G.R., 1971, Studies on protocollagen: Identification of a precursor of proto α1, Biochem. Biophys. Res. Commun., 44, 110 - 117.

Oohira, A., Nogami, H., 1978, Limb anomalies produced by 2,2'-dipyridyl in rats, Teratology, 18, 63 - 70.

Ritter, E.J., Scott, W.J., Wilson, J.G., 1971, Teratogenesis and inhibition of DNA synthesis induced in rat embryos by cytosine arabinoside, Teratology, 4, 7 - 14.

Ritter, E.J., Scott, W.J., Wilson, J.G., 1973, Relationship of temporal patterns of cell death and development to malformations in the rat limb. Possible mechanisms of teratogenesis with inhibitors of DNA synthesis, Teratology, 7, 219 - 226.

Scott, W.J., Ritter, E.J., Wilson, J.G., 1971, DNA synthesis inhibition and cell death associated with hydroxyurea teratogenesis in rat embryos, Develop. Biol., 26, 306 - 315.

Searl, R.L., Zwilling, E., 1964, Regeneration of the apical ectodermal ridge of the chick limb bud, Develop. Biol., 9, 38 - 55.

Wiley, M., Joneja, M.G., 1976, The teratogenic effects of ß-aminopropionitrile in hamsters, Teratology, 14, 43 - 52.

Zwilling, E., 1961, Limb morphogenesis, Adv. Morphog., 1, 301 - 330.

D. Limb Defects in Man

Approaches to Classification of Limb Defects

W. Lenz

Westfälische Wilhelms-Universität, Institut für Humangenetik,
Vesaliusweg 12/14, D-4400 Münster

The first principle of classification is morphology. In some malformation types, classification by morphology is entirely satisfactory, i.e. there is no overlap between types, and there is a perfect correlation between morphology and genetic cause, as in the APERT syndrome, in cleidocranial dysostosis, in the thrombocytopenia radius aplasia syndrome, in some types of hereditary brachydactyly or splithand-splitfoot.

In many other malformation types, however, no such close correlation exists. The phenotype is highly variable in some families with autosomal dominant splithand-splitfoot, type C brachydactyly, or the HOLT-ORAM syndrome, or in the autosomal recessive Fanconi anemia. The hand malformations shown by some HOLT-ORAM cases are virtually identical to those seen in thalidomide embryopathy or in a variety of chromosomal aberrations and autosomal dominant as well as recessive syndromes. Aplasia of radius or triphalangy of thumb are good morphological descriptions but these are heterogenous groups. On the other hand, in one etiologically homogenous group one may find cases of aplasia, hypoplasia, triphalangy, and duplication of the thumb. Only extensive family studies will show the total range of manifestations due to one gene.

In a monogenic type of malformation virtually no problem arises from purely coincidental presence of two different malformations in the same family. While such coincidental familial cases do occur by pure chance, their frequency depends on the incidence of the respective malformations which is generally low, i.e., below 0.1 per cent or even 0.01 per cent, for most types of limb defects. The recurrence risk for monogenic malformations in sibs, on the other hand, is 25 per cent or 50 per cent, i.e., 250 to 500 times higher than the risk due to chance. This, however, is what happens in populations. In the medical literature there is an unfortunate tendency to publish rare coincidences.

Sometimes unwarranted conclusions have been based on such highly selected reports, such as the idea, that all types of limb malformations are basically interrelated as various forms of one very general category of dysmelia or ectromelia.

The majority of limb defects do not follow simple mendelian patterns. Most cases are sporadic. Morphological classification is possible, but has severe limitations. We may put two similar cases, which etiologically may be different, into the same category for morphological reasons. On the other hand we may put two cases in distinct categories, though they have the same etiology. We really do not know, how similar two cases have to be, to invoke the same name. There is one approach, however, which may help us to get out of this dilemma, i.e., comparison of left arm or leg, with the right counterpart, and comparison of arms with legs. Many limb defects are more or less asymmetrical. We may find a certain malformation on the one side associated with strikingly variable malformations on the opposite side. The most simple hypothesis is, that the malformations on both sides

Teratology of the Limbs

of the same person are due to the same cause. Again, chance associations of etiologically different malformations on the right and on the left side are so extremely unlikely to occur, that we may neglect them. Thus, the comparison of malformations on opposite sides shows, that morphological categories like total amelia, distal defect of the humerus and the forearm, humeroradial synostosis, ulnar defects, sometimes in combination with thumb defects, may belong to one broad category.

If we extend this type of reasoning to a comparison of arm and leg malformations, we will again find a characteristic spectrum of defects of the femur and the fibula associated with the spectrum of arm malformations. Originally, we called this spectrum the femur-fibula-ulna syndrome. I now prefer, however, to call it the femur-fibula-ulna complex, since a syndrome, in my opinion, should have a minimum of signs present in every case. This is not true for the FFU-complex. A similar situation, i.e. an etiological uniform or supposedly uniform entity, comprising cases which have not one single symptom in common, is probably not exceptional. Let me quote three examples. In thalidomide embryopathy, one child may have no ears, paralysis of the rectus muscles and renal dystopia, a second child may have no arms, but normal ears, eye muscles and kidneys, and a third may have triphalangeal thumbs, inguinal hernia and anorectal stenosis, but none of the malformations shown by the other two. In the autosomal dominant HOLT-ORAM-syndrome, the mother may have triphalangeal thumbs and no cardiac defect, her child may have partial proximal humerus defect, radioulnar synostosis, aplasia of the first and of the second ray, and a defect of the atrial septum. In one type of autosomal dominant splithand-splitfoot malformation, aplasia of the ulna with only the thumb present, defect of the tibiae, syndactyly and various forms of splithand and splitfoot do occur in different members of the family in various combinations. If this can happen in entities with known environmental or genetic cause, we can expect it also in complex malformations of unknown etiology.

The next approach is basically similar to the study of associations of limb defects: the study of associations of limb defects with malformations affecting other organs. I will give three examples of this. In focal dermal hypoplasia, a dermatological condition with a characteristic pattern of cutaneous defects, pigmentation and papillomas of the mucous membranes, various defects of fingers, toes and long bones may be seen, which certainly do not fit into any narrow morphological category. By the common link of the dermatological symptoms, we are able to define the limb malformation complex of focal dermal hypoplasia. Focal dermal hypoplasia occurs almost exclusively in females, it is probably due to an X-linked gene lethal in the male sex. The irregular limb defects in females as well as the osteopathia striata of focal dermal hypoplasia may be explained as an effect of the functional Lyon mosaic of cells in which either the normal or the abnormal X-linked gene is inactivated.

Another complex of distal limb defects is associated with microglossia (aglossia, ankyloglosson). There is some overlap of the hand defects of the microglossia-adactyly complex with those seen in the pectoralis aplasia-hand malformation complex, but as a group both are certainly distinct. Cases of pectoralis aplasia as a rule show only defects of the homolateral hand, whereas in the microglossia complex more severe arm defects as well as distal defects of the feet are seen. The spectrum of limb defects associated with microglossia is strikingly similar to that associated with splenogonadal fusion. Therefore, both may in fact represent different aspects of one basically identical condition.

Etiological classification would be a rather simple business, if most or even a substantial proportion of all malformations were due to definite single causes, which can be traced by a questionnaire as most cases of dysmelia in the years 1960 to 1962 were due to thalidomide. Thalidomide, however, was rather exceptional in human teratology and should not, as the public and even some teratologists are inclined to believe, be accepted as a generally valid paradigma. Several attempts have been made to link malformations with the intake of drugs, notably mellizine, bendectin, duogenon and other steroid hormones. As no distinctive pattern can be discerned in the type of malformations observed following intake of any of these substances, and the malformations appear to be samples of those expected to occur in any population, all such studies confute rather than confirm the idea of an etiological connection.

APPROACHES TO CLASSIFICATION

1. MORPHOLOGY
2. FAMILIAL AGGREGATION
3. ASSOCIATION
   a) limb defects
   b) other defects
4. FACTORS IN PREGNANCY

REFERENCES

Lenz, W., Majewski, F., Fehlbildungen der Gliedmaßen, in: "Lehrbuch der Röntgendiagnostik" Bd. 2, Teil 2, 6. Auflage, (Schinz, ed.), pp. 261 - 349, Georg Thieme Verlag, Stuttgart, in press.

Formal Genesis of Syndactyly

G. M. Lösch

Medizinische Hochschule Lübeck, Klinik für Plastische Chirurgie,
Ratzeburger Allee 160, D-2400 Lübeck 1

In an effort to classify the malformations of the hand with regard to morphogenetic criteria demonstrated by us on the 5th European Anatomical Congress in Prague, 1979 (LÖSCH, et al., 1979, 1981), the syndactylies (D.C.) are divided in Group I "FAILURE OF DIFFERENTIATION OF PARTS", into osseous and cutaneous forms, based on the classification of the International Confederation of Societies of Hand Surgery (SWANSON, 1976).

In the past (LÖSCH, 1970) the osseous and cutaneous syndactylies were designated by us as primary forms according to the morphogenesis and placed in contrast to the Acro- and bridge-syndactylies (GRUBER, 1937). The latter occur as a symptom within the malformation syndrome with ring constrictions, pseudoligaments, acral defects and syndactylism (LÖSCH, DUNCKER, 1971; LÖSCH, SCHRADER, 1981; TEMTAMY, McKUSICK, 1969, 1978; WEHR, 1981).

Special anatomy and formal genesis of the cutaneous syndactyly:

In this paper we will confine ourselves to reflections on the formal development of primary osseous and cutaneous syndactylies on the basis of special anatomical investigations. In the case of a primary cutaneous syndactyly, two or more fingers may be webbed more or less towards the distal end. In the complete syndactyly the nails may be united to one common nail plate, the adjoining nail walls being completely absent. In the area where the vagina fibrosa inserts to the skeleton of the finger rays (Fig. 1), we find strongly developed fibrous septa originating from the syndactylous finger areas facing each other. These are the non-separated "CLEELAND's Ligaments". The ligamentum metacarpeum transversum superficialis may be shifted distally. The longitudinal fibres of the palmar aponeurosis spread out and extend very far distally to the rim of the syndactyly.

The thumb may be kept in adduction and slight opposition by transverse fibres originating from the fasciculi transversi of the palmar aponeurosis (LÖSCH, 1970). The tendons of the flexor digitorum profundus, otherwise normal, may broaden in a fan-shape at the distal phalanx in syndactylous fingers and web with the neighbouring tendons so that insertions can be observed also in the neighbouring distal phalanx. The division point of vessels and nerves in the syndactylous interdigital space may be shifted distally. In the case of cutaneous syndactyly the skeleton and joints may be developed normally. However, the syndactyly may be complicated by clinodactyly, camptodactyly and arthrogryposis. In the case of a primary cutaneous syndactyly we find the axial differentiation and segmentation of the skeleton of the finger rays to be normal.

The crucial phase in the development of syndactylism in triphalangeal fingers is supposed to be between the 32nd and 33rd day of development (stage 16 and 17) at a crown-rump length of 10.0 to 13.0 mm (DEGEN-

Teratology of the Limbs

HARDT, 1950). At the beginning of this phase the axial ray and soft-part segmentation between the thumb and second finger is definitely defined. It can be supposed that in the case of cutaneous syndactyly a separation of the marginal sinus has not taken place. Nevertheless, an axial formation and segmentation of the skeleton into phalanges can be observed. KELLEY (1973) speculates that interdigital zones prior to their demise may serve as areas of proliferation for mesenchymal cells contributing to digital formation and that mesenchymal cells from proliferation centers in interdigital zones may play a role in the development of digits. Our investigations showed that special structures, such as "CLEELAND's ligaments" (CLEELAND, 1878) are differentiated from the mesenchyma of the interdigital spaces. It can be assumed that if the relation between ectoderm and mesoderm remains intact, bones, joints and tendons can develop to normal shape and the fingers grow to normal length (LÖSCH, SCHRADER, 1981). Cutaneous syndactyly can be complicated by bone deformity, clinodactyly, camptodactyly and arthrogryposis. These deformations can be attributed to disturbances in the morphogenetic processes of the interdigital mesenchymes, and the disturbance in the process of necrosis with its distal-to-proximal progression may play a role here (SAUNDERS, 1948; MILAIRE, 1969). It may be possible that disturbances in the process of cell death have an effect on the growth in digital length and on the correct alignment of the fingers. The distal shift of the vessel and nerve separation may be attributable to disturbances in the formation of the fine fibrous structures of the interdigital spaces.

Special anatomy and formal development of osseous syndactylism:

The "classical form" of osseous syndactyly is found in the Apert syndrome. APERT (1906) recognized the biological regularity of a well definable type of malformation which is characterized by an excessively high, narrow and flattened skull with a bulging forehead, hypoplasia of the zygoma, antimongoloid palpebral fissures, saddle nose, high-arched palate and syndactylism of the four extremities. He proposed the name ACROCEPHALOSYNDACTYLY. According to BLANK (1960) 150 cases of APERT syndrome have been described in the literature. According to BLAUTH and SCHNEIDER-SICKERT (1976) most cases of osseous syndactyly can be associated to the APERT syndrome in the closer sense, corresponding to type I of the Acrocephalosyndactyly according to TEMTAMY (1966) and McKUSICK (1971). PFEIFFER (1964), TEMTAMY (1966) and McKUSICK (1971) classified three further form variations of Acrocephalosyndactyly showing pure cutaneous syndactylies. In regard to the APERT syndrome, BLAUTH and SCHNEIDER-SICKERT (1976) distinguished three types of form and therapy of malformed hands depending on the degree of severity. We have been able to dissect both hands of a female stillborn child with Acrocephalosyndactyly, and two further spoon-shaped hands with osseous syndactyly which were available as isolated specimens together with both feet (LÖSCH, 1970).

SKELETON

Due to a primary disorder in the skeleton blastema of the hand, normal segmentation of the individual finger rays (Fig. 2) fails to develop at the distal end of the 2nd to 4th finger, seldom from the thumb to the 4th finger. Proximally, the axial condensation and differentiation of the mesenchyma is usually still unimpaired. In one hand (case 5, right hand, LÖSCH, 1970) we found a basal fusion of the 4th and 5th metacarpals. In the medial part there was no separation into rays and no segmentation into phalanges. The distal phalanx was formed by a single mesenchymal condensation not segmented in rays and indented only at the distal rim between

the 2nd and 3rd ray. The common basal element and the distal phalanx are separated by more or less distinct interarticular spaces. In regard to the developmental factors, the coordination between ectoderm and mesoderm for the growth in length remains available, but there is no segmentation of the ectodermal ridge at the distal end and consequently no division of the mesodermal maintenance factor (SAUNDERS, 1948) which is quite a controversial question today. So the cell death between the finger rays does not take place and consequently the individual fingers, which are growing independently, are not separated during growth. The impairment of the mesenchyma anlagen in the thumb in most cases implies abnormally short and wide phalanges. The joints are correspondingly malformed. If there exists a distal osseous syndactyly between the thumb and the common distal phalanx of the 2nd and 4th finger, this is of some importance to the subsequent formation of the thumb which is abnormally long and pointed (Fig. 2). In the 5th finger there will be no segmentation of the anlage in the proximal and middle phalanges in any case. While cutaneous syndactylies with a normal number of phalanges exhibit fine fibrous structures such as the "CLEELAND's ligaments", the osseous syndactylies show, in the space between the common basal skeleton elements of the 2nd to 4th finger, ample fibrous tissue and numerous transverse fibres running from one bone surface to another. According to KELLEY (1970) this condition may be due to deep-seated disorder in the proliferation centres of the interdigital zones. KELLEY (1970) speculated that prior to their demise interdigital zones may serve as areas of proliferation for mesenchymal cells contributing to digit formation. In this connection it seems to be interesting to refer to KELLEY (1973) who wrote as follows:
"It is interesting to speculate that an increase in collagen-like fibrils is associated with increased cell death, decreased maintenance activity and associated epithelial thinning".

In comparing this with normal development one could conclude that the crucial phase for the determination of osseous syndactyly in spoon-shaped hands is probably between the 30th and 32nd day of development (7.5 to 10.0 mm) according to BARDEEN and LEWIS (1901), KEIBEL, MALL (1910), PETERSEN (1930). It can be concluded from the existing but still limited range of variations of this osseous syndactylism that not only normal development has been disturbed but that the final anatomy of malformation is also defined to a certain extent by the regulative mechanisms which control the development of the normal form and have also a regulating effect towards normality if normal development is impaired (LÖSCH, 1970). The differentiation of the anlagen in the individual phalanges takes place at a later time; according to GRAY, GARDNER, O'RAHILLY (1957) at 30 to 50 mm. Therefore, the lack of segmentation in proximal and middle phalanges of the skeleton element of the 2nd to 4th finger which is separated axially at the base and syndactylous at the distal end, may possibly be regarded as a consequence of the primary disturbance.

TENDONS

The missing segmentation in the proximal and middle phalanges and the absence of the proximal interphalangeal joint in all hands examined implies the lack of the characteristic insertion of the superficialis tendon (Fig. 3). In all specimens, the tendons of the M. flexor digitorum profundus et superficialis end on the distal phalanx which they have in common, and also in the distal joint. They radiate fan-shaped and web with their inserting bundles of fibres (Fig. 3). If the osseous syndactyly extends from the 1st to the 4th finger, this fan-shaped connection and webbing with the neighbouring tendons occurs also at the tendon of the M. flexor pollicis longus. The individual tendon which is normally meant for one finger ray, therefore inserts in the whole region of the common distal phalanx. This is a consequence of the individual finger rays having no lateral limitation. The assignment of the mesenchyma anlagen of the dorsal aponeuroses to the syndactylous finger rays is disturbed. The absence of lateral limitation of the skeleton causes the fusion. The distal osseous syndactyly of the thumb and 2nd finger in the right hand of case 4 (LÖSCH, 1970) and the fibrous connection between the heads of the corresponding metacarpals will entail an extreme syndactyly. Abnormal ligamentous or fibrous webbing is also found in malformations with narrowness of the 1st interdigital space (I.D.d.(1), (a) LÖSCH et al., 1980/81; LÖSCH, SCHRADER, 1978). It is supposed that the extreme syndactyly causes the abnormal differentiation of juncturae tendinum between the tendons of M. extensor pollicis longus. The insertion of M. lumbricalis II may be shifted to the syndactylous skeleton plate, its tendon extending fan-shaped distally (case 5, both hands, LÖSCH, 1970) (Fig. 4), the tendon in one hand (case 5, right hand, LÖSCH, 1970) being strengthened by the tendon of M. interosseus dorsalis II. Since we know that the tendons at the palmar and dorsal sides differentiate in situ in the mesenchyma at a crown-rump length between 13.5 and 25 mm, it must be assumed that the impairment of their insertion behaviour at the palmar and dorsal sides is a consequence of the disturbed distal skeleton differentiation. The final anlage of the crura of the superficialis tendon develops at a crown-rump length of 22 mm (DYLEVSKY, 1967; CIHAK, 1963; DYLEVSKY, MRAZKOVA, 1970). The separation of the superficialis and profundus tendons is not completed until a crown-rump length of 25 mm is reached (DYLEVSKY, 1968).

VESSELS and NERVES

Quite frequently the division point of N. and A. digitalis palmaris proprii from their common trunk is shifted more or less distally. The cases are rare where only one nerve or only one vessel (Fig. 5) is present in the interdigital spaces of the spoon-shaped hand, branching off bilaterally and dorsally. It may happen that the end branches of the strong vessels and nerves do not run palmarly, but dorsally to the syndactylous end plate. Normally the soft part separation of the finger rays is accomplished at a crown-rump length of 18 mm (BLECHSCHMIDT, PETERSEN, 1967), and the separation of the A. digitalis communis into Aa. digitales palmares propriae is then defined. (It is remarkable and encouraging to carry out further examinations, that in spite of the varying mode of genesis of nerves and arteries there is an identical deviation of their definite form in most cases).

PALMAR APONEUROSIS, PALMAR SKIN and NAIL

While the osseous and chondral syndactyly primarily determines the shape of the hands, the palmar aponeurosis develops later on according to the existing malformation. The palmar aponeurosis extends further distally than normal and frequently ends with bow-shaped bands which keep the syndactylous fingers. The tight bands of the palmar aponeurosis are particularly noticeable. They embrace the thenar, extending into the phalanges not only ulnarly but also radially, thus making its abduction impossible. In addition, a widely distalized ligamentum palmare transversum subcutaneum acts in the same way (Fig. 6).

The malformations of the palmar aponeurosis and its derivates must be regarded as tertiary, because their development does not start until a fetus has a crown-rump length of 30 mm (CIHAK, 1967, DYLEVSKY, 1968, 1969, a, b). Furthermore, we find strong disordered fibrous tissue bundles between the fingers in the tela subcutanea which fix the fingers to each other additionally. The palmar skin of the spoon-shaped hand is characterized by a complete system of papillary ridges in the finger region. The finger nails are differentiated according to the shape of the distal phalanx and the lateral fusion of the skeleton blastema.

CONCLUSION:

In conclusion it can be assumed in regard to primary cutaneous syndactyly that the division of the marginal sinus with subsequent cell death in the interdigital space has not taken place whereas the relation between ectoderm and mesoderm has remained intact, allowing bone development and growth in length of the fingers. From this point of view it can be assumed that the primary osseous syndactylism is a stronger disturbance with further-reaching effects, while the primary cutaneous syndactylism represents weaker disturbance, although it is in close relation with the primary osseous syndactylism. Also, in regard to the cutaneous syndactylism it can be assumed that morphogenetic mechanisms act upon the development of malformation to a varying extent and consequently play an essential role in the much different degrees of finger separation. There exists a difference in the length-growth velocity between the radial and ulnar parts of the extremities in general (SEICHERT, 1966) and also an ulnoradial gradient of the growth velocity of the hand plate in all mammals (MILAIRE, 1965). The question whether or not this could explain the most frequent occurrence of cutaneous syndactylism between the ulnar fingers, remains open.

REFERENCES

Apert, H.E., 1906, De l'acrocéphalosyndactylie, Bull. Mèm. Soc. Méd. Hôp., Paris, 23, 1310 - 1330.

Bardeen, R., Lewis, W.H., 1901, Development of the limbs, body-wall and back in man, Am. J. Anat., 1, 1 - 35.

Blank, C.E., 1960, Apert's syndrome. A type of acrocephalosyndactyly - observations on a British series of 39 cases, Ann. hum. Genet., 24, 141.

Blauth, W., Schneider-Sickert, F., 1976, Handfehlbildungen, Springer, Berlin-Heidelberg-New York.

Blechschmidt, E., Petersen, D., 1967, Die frühembryonalen Entwicklungsbewegungen des menschlichen Armes als Faktor möglicher Mißbildungen, Ergeb. Chir. Orthop., 49, 62 - 111.

Degenhardt, K.H., 1950, Zum entwicklungsmechanischen Problem der Akrocephalosyndaktylie, Z. menschl. Vererb. u. Konstit. Lehre, 29, 791 - 819.

Dylevský, I., 1967, Contribution to the ontogenesis of the flexor digitorum superficialis and the flexor digitorum profundus in man, Folia Morph., Praha, 15, 330 - 335.

Dylevský, I., 1968, Tendons of the M. flexor digitorum superficialis et profundus in the ontogenesis of the human hand, Folia Morph., Praha, 16, 124 - 130.

Dylevský, I., 1969 a, Ontogenesis of the M. palmaris longus in man, Folia Morph., Praha, 17, 23 - 28.

Dylevský, I., 1969 b, Critical comments on the so-called development theory of Dupuytren's contracture, Sborn lék, 71, 289 - 296.

Dylevský, I., Mŕazková, O., 1970, Phylogenetic differences in pattern and composition of dorsal finger aponeurosis, Folia Morph., Praha, 18, 161 - 167.

Cihák, R., 1963, The development of the dorsal interossei in the human hand, Cs. Morfol., 11, 199 - 208.

Cihák, R., 1967, The occurence of mm. contrahentes and their changes during the development of the human hand, Folia Morph., Praha, 15, 197 - 205.

Cleeland, I., 1878, On the cutaneous ligaments of the phalanges, J. Anat. Physiol., London, 12, 526.

Gray, D.J., Gardner, E., O'Rahilly, R., 1957, The prenatal development of the skeleton and joints of the human hand, Am. J. Anat., 101, 169 - 223.

Gruber, G.B., 1937, Die Entwicklungsstörungen der menschlichen Gliedmaßen, in: Die Morphologie der Mißbildungen des Menschen und der Tiere, (E. Schwalbe, G.B. Gruber, eds.), Tl. III., Gustav Fischer, Jena.

Keibel, F., Mall, F., 1910, Handbuch der Entwicklungsgeschichte des Menschen, Bd. 1, Hirzl, Leipzig.

Kelley, R.O., 1970, An alectron microscopic study of mesenchyme during development of interdigital spaces in man, Anat. Rec., 168, 43 - 53.

Kelley, R.O., 1973, Fine structure of the apical rim-mesenchyme complex during limb morphogenesis in man, J. Embryol. exp. Morph., 29/1, 117 - 131.

McKusick, V.A., 1971, Mendelian inheritance in man, 3rd edition, Johns Hopkins University Press, Baltimore, London.

Milaire, J., 1965, Aspects of limb morphogenesis in mammals, in: Organogenesis, (R.L. De Haan, H. Ursprung, eds.), pp. 283 - 300, Holt, Rinehart and Winston, New York.

Milaire, J., 1969, Étude Morphogénétique de la Syndactylie postaxiale provoquée chez le rat par l'hadacine. I. Analyse des anomalies chez l'adulte, le foetus a Terme et les Embryons de 15, 16 et 17 jours, Arch. Biol., Liége, 80, 167 - 253.

Lösch, G.M., 1970, Syndaktylien - Anatomie, Entwicklung, therapeutische Aspekte - Normale und Pathologische Anatomie, Monographien in zwangloser Folge, W. Bargmann, W. Dörr, eds.) Heft 23, Georg Thieme, Stuttgart.

Lösch, G.M., Duncker, H.R., 1971, Acrosyndactylism - Transactions 5th World Congress of Plastic and Reconstructive Surgery, Melbourne, 22 - 26 February, 1971, pp. 671 - 676, Butterworth.

Lösch, G.M., Buck-Gramcko, D., Schrader, M., Cihák, R., 1979, Versuch einer Klassifikation der Extremitätenfehlbildungen unter Berücksichtigung von morphogenetischen Faktoren, 5th European Anatomical Congress, 22nd Scientific Conference of the Faculty of Medicine, Charles University Prague, 10 - 14 September, 1979, Vortrag, Summary p. 246.

Lösch, G.M., Buck-Gramcko, D., Schrader, M., Cihák, R., Seichert, V., Versuch einer Klassifikation der Fehlbildungen der Hand unter Berücksichtigung morphogenetischer Kriterien, Handchirurgie, im Druck.

Lösch, G.M., Schrader, M., 1978, Connective tissue structures in the first intermetacarpal space in cases of malformations of the hand with and without syndactyly, Chir. plastica, Berlin, 4, 145 - 159.

Lösch, G.M., Schrader, M., Fehlbildungen der Hand, in: Spezielle Chirurgie für die Praxis, Bd. III, Teil 3, (F. Baumgard, K. Kremer, H.W. Schreiber, eds.), Georg Thieme, Stuttgart, (im Druck).

Petersen, H., 1930, Die Organe des Skelettsystems, in: Handbuch der mikroskopischen Anatomie des Menschen, Bd. II/2, (W. von Möllendorf, ed.), Springer, Berlin.

Pfeiffer, R.A., 1964, Dominante erbliche Akrocephalosyndaktylie, Z. Kinderheilk., 90, 301 - 320.

Saunders, J.W., Jr., 1948, The proximo-distal sequence of origin of the parts of the chick wing and the role of the ectoderm, J. exp. Zool., 108, 363 - 403.

Seichert, V., 1966, Differential growth pattern in the chick embryo wingbud between the 3rd, 5th, and 7th day of incubation, Folia Morph., Praha, 14/4, 325 - 334.

Swanson, A.B., 1976, A classification for congenital limb malformations, J. Hand Surg., 1, 8 - 22.

Temtamy, S.A., 1966, Genetic factors in hand malformations, Ph.D. Thesis, Johns Hopkins University, Baltimore.

Temtamy, S., McKusick, V.A., 1969, Synopsis of hand malformations with particular emphasis on genetic factors, Birth Defects, Original article series, New York, National Foundation - March of Dimes III, 125 - 184.

Temtamy, S.A., McKusick, V.A., 1978, The genetics of hand malformations, Birth Defects, Original article series, New York, National Foundation -March of Dimes XIV, No. 3.

Wehr, Ch., 1981, Fehlbildungen mit Schnürfurchen, Pseudoligamenten, akralen Defekten und Syndaktylien, Diss., Lübeck.

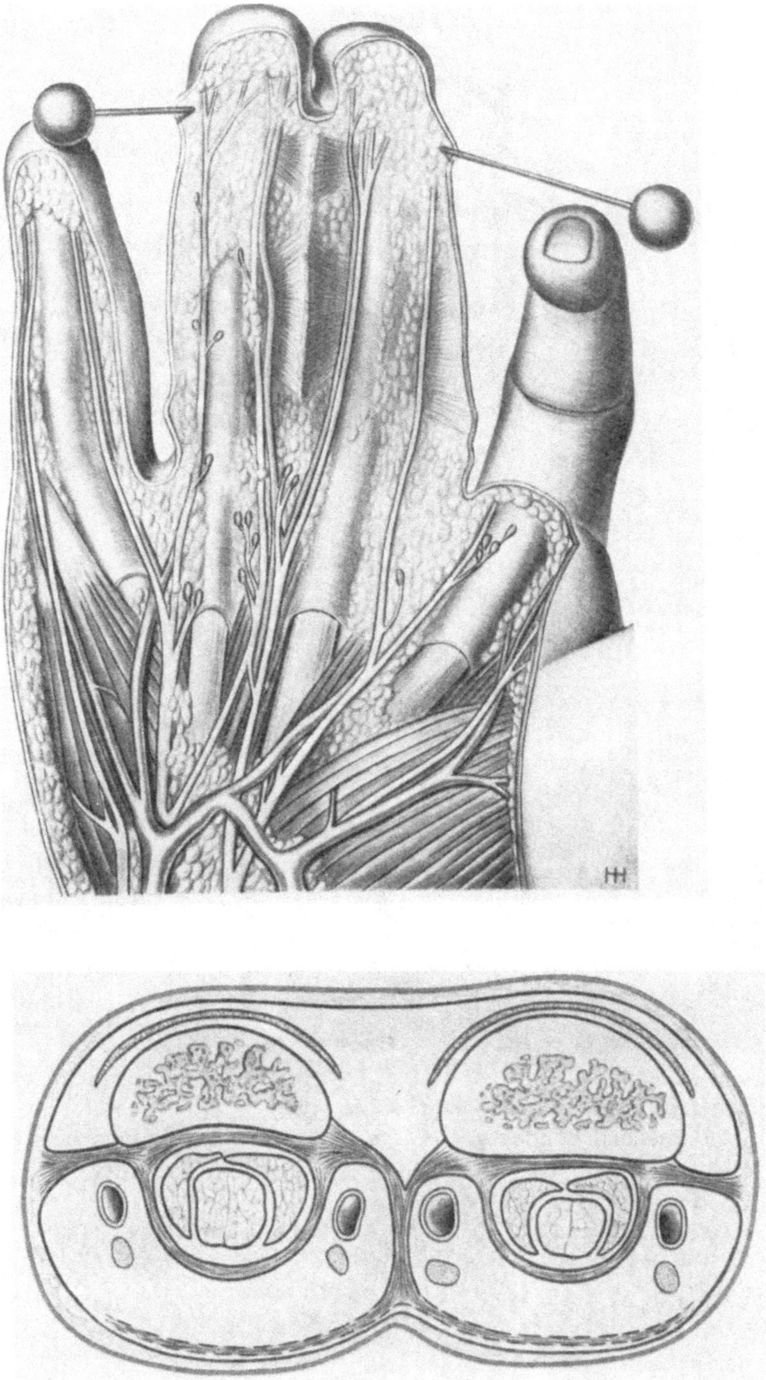

Fig. 1: Case 2, right hand (LÖSCH, 1970).
Cutaneous syndactyly of the 3rd and 4th finger. Fusion of the Cleeland's ligaments in the syndactylous interdigital space.

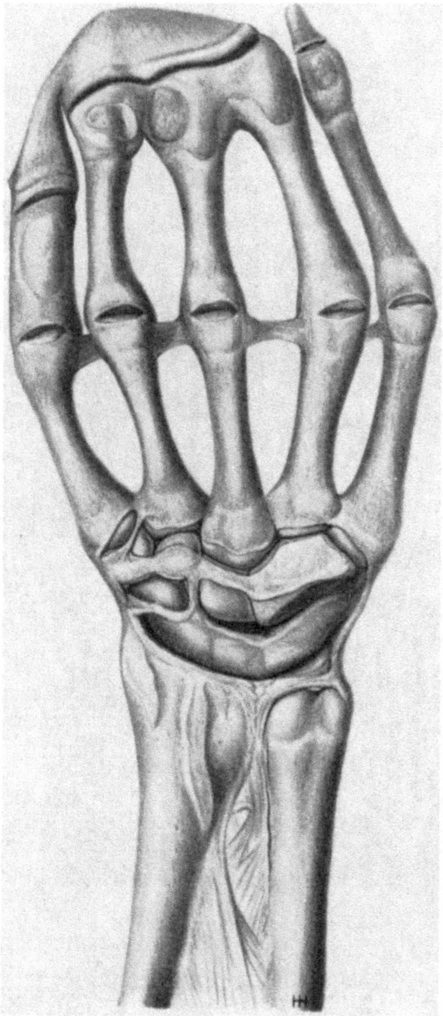

Fig. 2: Case 4, right hand (LÖSCH, 1970).
Osseous syndactyly of the 1st to the 4th finger.

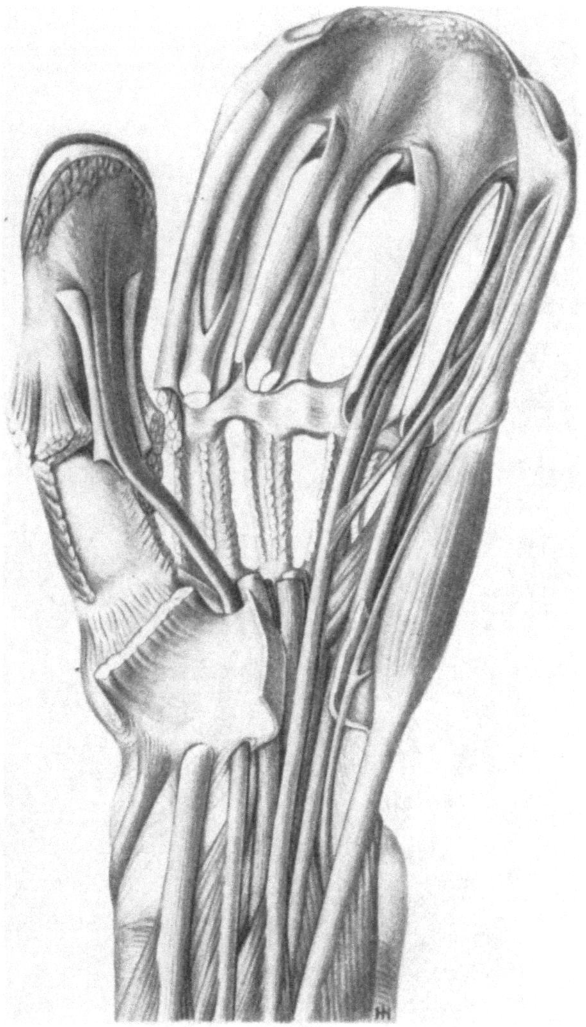

Fig. 3 Case 4, left hand (LÖSCH, 1970).
Osseous syndactyly of the 2nd to 5th finger. Layer of tendons. Note the mutual embracing of the superficialis and profundus tendon in the 3rd finger.

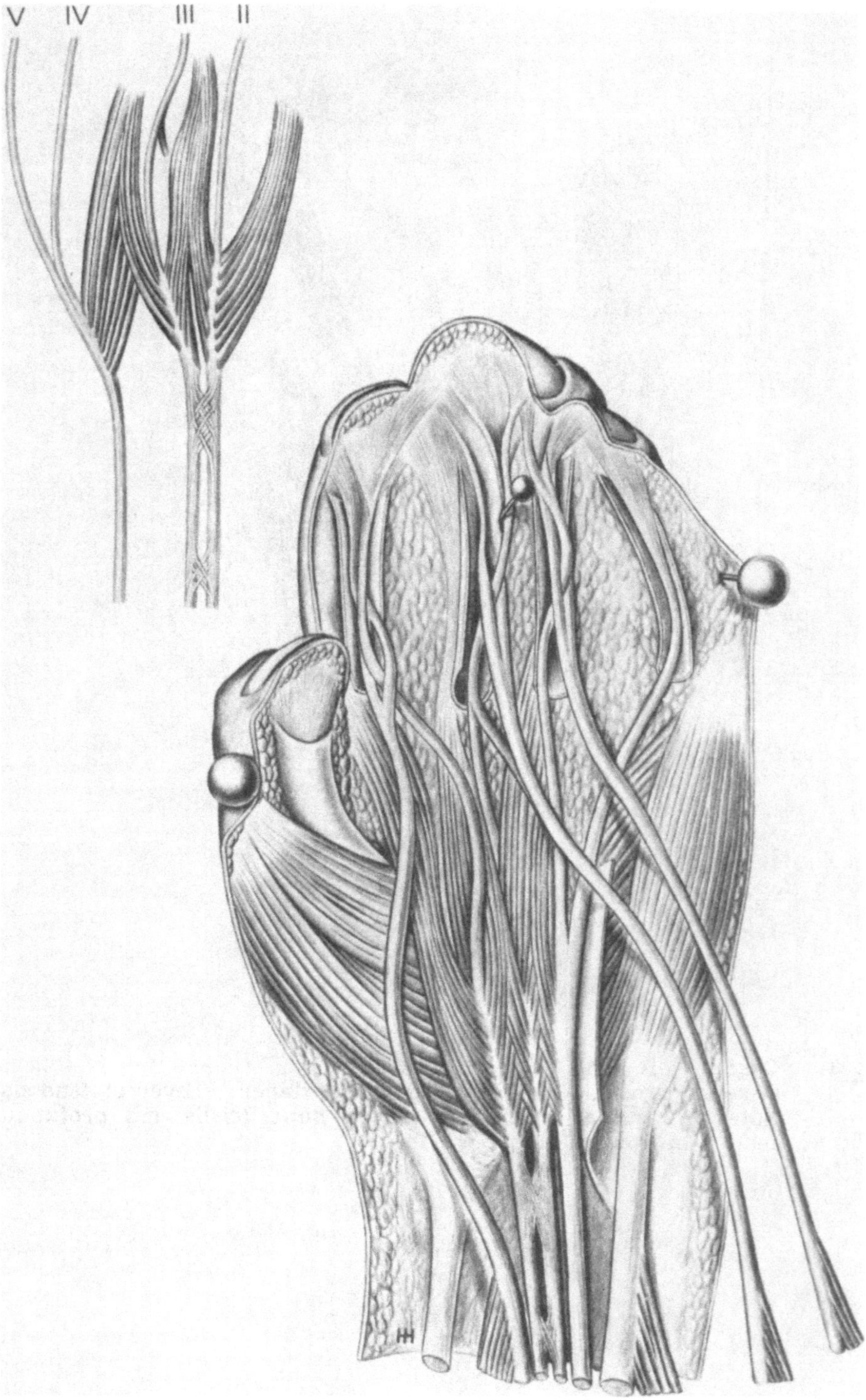

Fig. 4: Case 5, left hand (LÖSCH, 1970).
Preparation of the tendons and muscles.

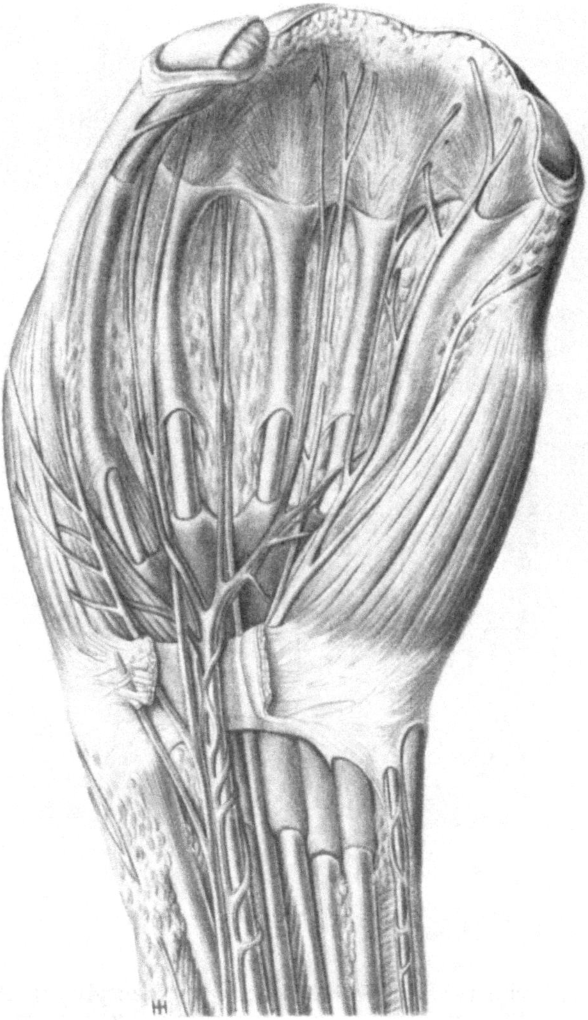

Fig. 5: Case 5, right hand (LÖSCH, 1970).
Distally shifted or missing division point of the Nn. digitales proprii and Aa.digitaes propriae.

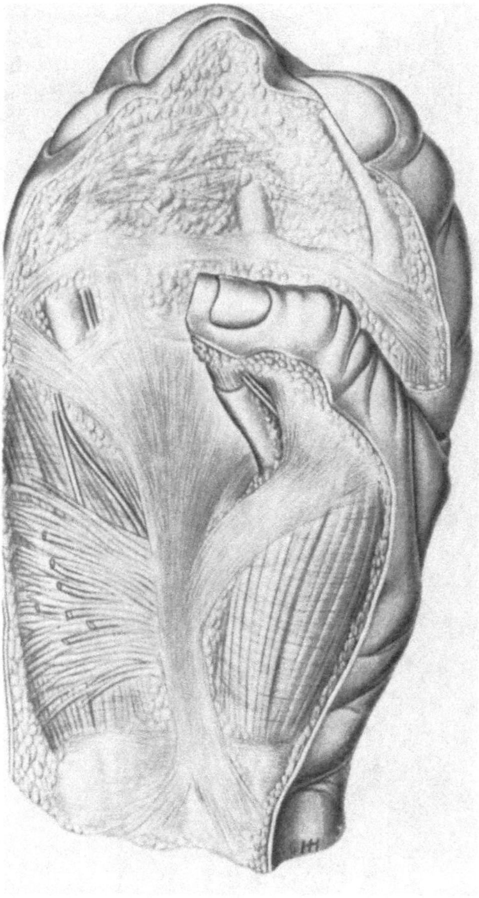

Fig. 6: Case 5, right hand with osseous syndactyly of the 2nd to 5th finger. Strong linkage of the thumb by the radial and ulnar bands of the palmar aponeurosis. Ligamentum palmare transversum subcutaneum shifted distally.

Thalidomide and the Neural Crest

Janet McCredie

Department of Surgery, The University of Sydney,
Sydney, N.S.W. 2006, Australia

The spectrum of congenital malformations caused by thalidomide is well-known to German medical scientists, but a brief summary is pertinent, since some members of this symposium may not have had any personal experience of the thalidomide problem.

The hall-mark of thalidomide embryopathy was dysmelia, or reduction deformity of the limbs. This ranged from amelia (absence of a limb) to minor digital defects. Between these two extremes, various degrees of phocomelia were seen, the majority being bilateral and symmetrical, with upper limbs more frequently involved than lower limbs (LENZ and KNAPP, 1962; PFEIFFER and KOSENOW, 1962; HENKEL and WILLERT, 1969). Absence or hypoplasia of the radius and thumb was the most frequent upper limb defect.

Whilst dysmelia was the most striking feature of the disease, many defects of cranio-facial structures and internal organs were also part of the spectrum (McBRIDE, 1961; LENZ, 1962; SPIERS, 1962; PLEISS, 1962; SMITHELLS, 1962). Major abnormalities of the viscera were responsible for considerable perinatal wastage, so that the less severely affected children survived. Internal defects were generally associated with limb defects, e.g. congenital heart disease and upper limb malformation (British Ministry of Health, 1964), but some cases were recorded with internal defects and normal limbs (SMITHELLS, 1962).

During 1970 and 1971, I was consulted over radiographs of children seeking medico-legal compensation. Claims had been received on behalf of deformed children who were born before thalidomide was released onto the Australian market. Differentiation of thalidomide victims from these others was clinically difficult. Was there any specific radiological feature of thalidomide embryopathy? A review of the radiological literature and an assessment of the available radiographs did not provide any answer to this question.

Another question of a more basic nature captured my attention. What was the pathology underlying these deformities? How did thalidomide act to produce these grotesque bones and joints? That radiology mirrors pathology is an accepted fact. Yet there was no record of what tissue was involved in this condition. It had been assumed for a decade that thalidomide acted upon mesoderm, since the systems involved were all of mesodermal origin (McBRIDE, 1961; PLEISS, 1962; WOOLLAM, 1965). Yet histopathology had not been established (TUCHMANN-DUPLEISSIS, 1975).

Dysmorphology is a radiologist's trade. The task of a radiologist in any diagnostic dilemma is to analyse the pattern of an illness as depicted in radiographs, and to deduce the nature of the disease from the radiological evidence. What is it? Where is it? These are standard questions in the process of pattern analysis which is the basis of diagnostic radiology.

Teratology of the Limbs

My initial analysis of the radiographs of 5 Australian thalidomide victims in 1970-71, plus a study of 100 thalidomide cases in U.K. in 1972, yielded evidence that a sensory peripheral neuropathic process had occurred in the embryo (McCREDIE, 1973; McCREDIE and McBRIDE, 1973). The disease pattern in the skeleton matched that of adults with sensory peripheral neuropathy of long-standing. Such patients suffer slow destruction of bones and joints in the neuropathic zones. Diabetes, tabes dorsalis, leprosy and syringamyelia are four causes of sensory neuropathy with secondary skeletal dystrophy such as CHARCOT'S joints. In this condition, bones and joints undergo gradual destruction, with tapering, fusion or disappearance of bones, and destruction and dislocation of joints. Equivalent signs were obvious in the radiographs of thalidomide children (McCREDIE, 1973; McCREDIE and McBRIDE, 1973).

The comparison was supported by the fact that thalidomide was itself a strong sensory neurotoxin. When the drug was first released, it became a popular sedative in convalescent hospitals and homes for the aged, until reports of the serious side effect of sensory peripheral neuropathy curtailed its widespread use (LE QUESNE, 1978). Neurological follow-up studies on adults with the sensory neuropathy demonstrated its particularly intractable character (FULLERTON and O'SULLIVAN, 1968). Most drug-induced sensory neuropathies recover when the drug is withdrawn. This was not the case with thalidomide. Symptoms persisted, with little change, many years later (LE QUESNE, 1978).

The distribution of the congenital defects caused by thalidomide had intrigued other researchers. LENZ and KNAPP (1962), LENZ (1965), and NOWACK (1965), established the sensitive period (21 to 42 days gestation) and a relationship between the date of ingestion of the drug and the site and type of resultant deformity. Within the sensitive period, there was a cranio-caudal sequence in time. Early in the sensitive period, head and neck defects resulted, then arm defects, and later still, deformities in the lower limbs. This parallelled the normal cranio-caudal sequence of embryonic development.

HENKEL and WILLERT (1969) studied the pattern of disease from an anatomic viewpoint. In their series of cases, mainly due to thalidomide, they demonstrated the peculiar order of disappearance of bones from the skeleton. HENKEL and WILLERT established that the pattern of dysmelia was one of elimination of longitudinal segments of the skeleton. In the upper limb, radius disappeared first, often accompanied by the thumb. Then the disease shifted to the proximal end of the humerus, whittling it away in a proximo-distal direction. Ulna and ulnar digits were the last to disappear. In the lower limb, loss of bone began in the distal tibia, leaving a residual triangular block at its proximal end. The proximal end of the femur was involved next, with progressive elimination of its shaft leaving a distal triangular block before it disappeared entirely. Finally fibula and foot disappeared (Fig. 1).

My own study in 1970-1972, was a quest for a mechanism underlying this pattern. The radiological study led me to formulate a hypothesis of "embryonic neuropathy" or neural crest injury (McCREDIE, 1973, 1974, 1975, 1976). This in turn led to a series of biological experiments in Sydney, commencing in 1973 (McCREDIE and McLEOD, 1974; McCREDIE, 1975; McBRIDE, 1974, 1976). The main observations and deductions from which the neural crest hypothesis was constructed, are presented below.

Recurrence of radial aplasia with absent or abnormal thumb (over 60% in my series) was a phenomenon which was too focal and too frequent to be a coincidence. It implied an underlying organisation, and this organisation was not typical of any primary bone disease (McCREDIE, 1973). Longitudinal segmental ablation of tissues could fit an arterial or a neural distribution. Anastomoses between embryonic blood vessels would mediate against arterial infarction as the cause. Maintenence of the end-organ relationship between nerve and periphery favoured a neural basis for this disease. Using the dermatome maps of the arm, hypothetical subtraction of the 6th cervical dermatome and its underlying bones should achieve the morphology of absence of radius and thumb (Fig. 2).

What, then, is the segmental sensory nerve supply of bone? This question had been answered in 1943 by INMAN and SAUNDERS, who had drafted the "sclerotome maps" on the basis of combined clinical and experimental studies. They defined a sclerotome as "a longitudinal band of skeletal structures supplied by one spinal segmental sensory nerve". They observed that the sclerotome not only lay beneath, but also extended beyond the myotome and dermotome of the same nerve supply. They noted that there was up to one segment of overlapping innervation from adjacent sclerotomes.

Application of the sclerotome maps to the radiographs of dysmelia provides a logical interpretation of the dysmorphology, where no explanation was previously available. Figures 3 - 6 illustrate the "sclerotome subtraction" method of interpretation (McCREDIE, 1975, 1977). Subtraction of C6 achieves variants of radial aplasia, subtraction of C7 would theoretically result in a lobster-claw defect, and subtraction of C8 would be consistent with ulnar aplasia. In the humerus, the parallel sclerotomes are difficult to read. However, it is evident that the more sclerotomes subtracted, the smaller the mass of the humerus, and the shorter the arm becomes. Hypoplasia of the scapula can be explained by sclerotome loss within the shoulder girdle.

In the leg, the sclerotomes show a spiral twist which brings the L4 and L5 sclerotomes from the lateral aspect of proximal femur to the medial aspect of distal tibia and tarsus. This reflects the normal rotation of the hind limb during embryonic development. Subtraction of sclerotomes may be single or multiple, total or partial, proximal or distal. The final skeletal morphology can be calculated by subtraction of one sclerotome or complexes of sclerotomes (McCREDIE, 1975, 1977).

The sclerotome subtraction method of interpretation implies that thalidomide acts upon embryonic sensory nerves, and that the skeletal defects are secondary to sensorineural disturbance. This raises a number of vital biological questions. For instance, what is the timing of the development of the neural crest and its derivatives, which include sensory peripheral and autonomic nerves? The crest is visible from day 18 of gestation in the human embryo (HAMILTON and MOSSMAN, 1972). It is a rapidly dividing and widely migrating tissue in early embryogenesis (HORSTADIUS, 1950; JOHNSTON, 1966; WESTON, 1970). The stage at which it migrates and divides coincides with the thalidomide sensitive period of 21 - 42 days gestation in humans. Besides the sensory peripheral and autonomic nervous systems, the neural crest gives rise to a proportion of the cells which form facial and spinal cartilages, to Schwann cells, meninges, odontoblasts and melanocytes. The transformation of the two strips of neural crest cells into the ganglia of the sensory nervous system takes place in cranio-caudal progression from day 18. Thus this tissue evolves during the thalidomide-sensitive phase of embryonic development (21 - 42 days gestation). At any one stage during this period, the development of limb buds is comparatively primitive, compared with the precocious maturation of neural crest. It is reasonable to propose that thalidomide might seek the same target tissue in the embryo as in the adult, since that tissue is developing rapidly during the period in which the drug has been shown to assert its teratogenic action.

The presence of nerves in limb buds has been denied for many years, on the basis of the histological studies of BARDEEN and LEWIS in 1901 (GARDNER, 1950; GARDNER and O'RAHILLY, 1976; WOLPERT, 1976). The technology of 1901 is no longer acceptable in the neuropathology laboratories of 1980. CAMERON studied mammalian limb buds in 1977, using rabbit embryos of 260 to 290 hours gestation, which is the peak period of thalidomide sensitivity. Light and electron microscopic examination of forelimb buds showed nerve trunks (Fig. 7) passing through the proximal third of the limb bud and surrounded by undifferentiated mesenchyme, 30 hours before chondrification was due to commence in the bud (McCREDIE, CAMERON and SHOOBRIDGE, 1978). Thus axons are present in the mammalian limb bud during the sensitive period.

The question of whether a biological relationship exists between sensory neurons and limb growth has been explored at length by MARCUS SINGER and his colleagues (SINGER, 1943, 1964, 1974). Regeneration of the limb of the newt has been shown to be sensory nerve dependant at an early stage. All nerves possess some trophic activity, but SINGER'S experiments have shown that sensory neurons possesses a quantitatively greater neurotrophism than other nerve cells. EGAR, YNTEMA and SINGER repeated YNTEMA'S early experiments with "aneurigenic limbs" in amphibian larvae, and showed by electron microscopy that 62% of such nerveless limbs did, in fact, contain nerve fibres. BAZZOLI, MANSON, SCOTT and WILSON (1977) induced phocomelia in the limb regenerates of amphibia by feeding the animals with thalidomide during the nerve dependant phase.

Although extrapolation from adult newt to human embryo is generally unacceptable, most scientists acknowledge DARWIN'S theory of evolution, whereby man and newt share common prehistoric ancestors. It is not unlikely that modern man shares a number of basic physiologic and anatomic functions with the newts of today. There has been no revolution in the structure of limbs in man or newt in the past 150 million years. Contrary to criticism on this question (GARDNER and O'RAHILLY, 1976), it is not irrational to suppose that a neurotrophic function similar to that of newt regeneration pertains in the human embryo.

From the foregoing, it can be concluded that neural crest is present, rapidly developing, and potentially vulnerable during the period when the embryo is sensitive to thalidomide. The pharmacology of the drug itself needs to be taken into account. Three particular properties of this drug deserve consideration. Firstly, its target organ in adults was the sensory nervous system. Secondly, its method of breakdown in vivo and in vitro was by simple hydrolysis. Thirdly, the 12 products of hydrolysis were non-teratogenic (SCHUMACHER, BLAKE and GILLETTE, 1968). The intact molecule was the teratogen, and thus the period of teratogenic activity was limited to a short period between ingestion and hydrolysis in plasma, with maximum plasma concentration at 1 hour after ingestion in rabbit. Such a pulsed insult to a chronologically synchronised embryo should hypothetically inflict a short, sharp injury. Taking into account the cranio-caudal progression of embryonic development, this injury should hypothetically take place at the site of maximum sensitivity within that cranio-caudal gradient. This prediction is borne out by the sclerotomes. Because of its pharmacokinetics, thalidomide can produce precise ablations at single neural levels. Embryos which develop asymmetrically, would show asymmetry of defects. Multiple doses would induce neural damage at separated levels, and would result in a scatter of deformities in the newborn child.

The autonomic nervous system is also derived from the neural crest, although its segmental arrangement is less obvious than that of the sensory nervous system (Fig. 8). Nevertheless, it is possible to correlate some multiple malformation syndromes on the basis of their embryonic nerve supply (McCREDIE, 1976). The association of congenital heart disease with upper limb malformations, as recorded in thalidomide embryopathy (British Ministry of Health, 1964), can be interpreted as resulting from a single injury to the neural crest in the lower cervical region. Similarly, complexes of leg deformities with ano-rectal or uro-genital malformations can be interpreted as lumbo-sacral neural crest injury.

In order to test whether or not neural crest causes limb malformations, SHOOBRIDGE performed diathermy ablations upon chick embryos of 48 hours incubation (stage 11 - 13 of HAMBURGER and HAMILTON). Segments were ablated from the left crest in the region of presumptive somite levels 26 - 30, which is the area of presumptive sciatic innervation. Seven of the seventeen survivors had absence of the left foot. Residual spinal cord and dorsal root ganglion mass was measured. No significant reduction in the spinal cord was found, but dorsal root ganglion mass was significantly depleted on the operated side when compared with the unoperated side, and with controls. The diathermy technique lacks sufficient precision to provide a conclusive answer to this particular question, but the results suggest that a relationship may exist between neural crest injury and limb malformation (McCREDIE, CAMERON and SHOOBRIDGE, 1978).

The arguments presented here may be summarised as the hypothesis of neural crest injury (McCREDIE, 1973). This hypothesis (Fig. 9, 10, 11) proposes the following pathogenetic mechanism:

(i) that an embryo may suffer an injury to a segment of developing neural crest, as a result of exposure to a sensory neurotoxic agent,

(ii) that such injury impedes the trophic function of sensory neurons at the injured level,

(iii) that this causes failure of formation of the sensory peripheral field of skeletal structures supplied by that segment. This results in absence or hypoplasia of bones, joints, and soft tissues within the zone of supply. The distribution tends to be bilateral and symmetrical, because the majority of embryos develop in a symmetrical fashion,

(iv) that the autonomic field of visceral structures supplied by that neural crest segment fails to form in some degree, which results in aplasia, hypoplasia, atresia or stenosis of internal organs,

(v) that the final expression of neural crest injury is dysmelia, and/or associated internal malformations in the newborn baby.

REFERENCES

Bardeen, R.B., Lewis, W.H.,1901, Am. J. Anat., 1, 1.

Bazzoli, A.S., Manson, J., Scott, W.J., Wilson, J.G., 1977, J. Embryol. exp. Morph., 41, 125.

Egar, M., Yntema, C.L., Singer, M., 1973, J. exp. Zool., 186, 91.

Fullerton, P.M., O'Sullivan, D.J., 1968, J. Neurol. Neurosurg. Psychiatry, 31, 543.

Gardner, E., O'Rahilly, R., 1976, Lancet, 1, 635.

Gardner, E., 1950, Physiol. Rev., 30, 127.

Hamburger, V., Hamilton, H.L., 1951, J. Morphol., 88, 49.

Henkel, H.L., Willert, H.G., 1969, J. Bone Joint Surg., 51-B, 399.

Horstadius, S.S., 1950, in: The Neural Crest, O.U.P., London.

Hamilton, W.J., Mossman, H.W., 1972, in: Human Embryology, Heffer and Sons, Cambridge.

Inman, V., Saunders, J.B., 1944, J. Nerv. Ment. Dis., 99, 660.

Johnston, M.C., 1966, Anat. Rec., 156, 143.

Knapp, K., Lenz, W., Nowack, E., 1962, Lancet, 2, 725.

Lenz, W., Knapp, K., 1962, Deutsch. med. Wschr., 87, 1232.

Lenz, W., 1962, Lancet, 1, 271.

Lenz, W., 1965, Ann. N.Y. Acad. Sci., 123, 228.

Le Quesne, P.M., 1975, in: Peripheral Neuropathy, (P.J. Dyck, P.K. Thomas, E. Lambert, W.B. Saunders, eds.) Philadelphia.

McBride, W.G., 1961, Lancet, 2, 1358.

McBride, W.G., 1974, Teratology, 10, 283.

McBride, W.G., 1976, Teratology, 14, 71.

Ministry of Health Reports on Public Health and Medical Subjects No. 112: Deformities caused by thalidomide. H.M. Stationary Office, 1964.

McCredie, J., McBride, W., 1973, Clin. Radiol., 24, 204.

McCredie, J., 1973, Lancet, 2, 1058.

McCredie, J., 1974, Med. J. Aust., 1, 159.

McCredie, J., 1975, Clin. Radiol., 26, 47.

McCredie, J., McLeod, J., 1974, Lancet, 1, 1111.

McCredie, J., 1975, Proc. Aust. Assoc. Neurol., 12, 135.

McCredie, J., 1975, Paediatr. Radiol., 3, 162.

McCredie, J., 1976, Med. Hypotheses, 2, 63.

McCredie, J., 1976, J. Neurol. Sci., 28, 373.

McCredie, J., Loewenthal, J., 1978, Am. J. Surg., 135, 293.

McCredie, J., Reid, I.S., 1978, J. Pediat., 92, 5, 62.

McCredie, J., 1977, Birth Defects, Orig. Art. Series, 13, 3D, 65.

McCredie, J., Cameron, J., Shoobridge, R., 1978, Lancet, 2, 761.

Nowack, E., 1965, Humangenetik, 1, 516.

Pfeiffer, R.A., Kosenow, W., 1962, Lancet, 1, 45.

Pleiss, G., 1962, Lancet, 1, 1128.

Schumacher, H., Blake, D.A., Gillette, J.R., 1968, J. Pharm. exp. Ther., 160, 201.

Smithells, R.W., 1962, Lancet, 1, 1270.

Singer, M., 1943, J. exp. Zool., 92, 297.

Singer, M., 1964, in: Progress in Brain Research, (Singer and Schade, eds.) 13, 228.

Singer, M., 1974, Ann. N.Y. Acad. Sci., 228, 308.

Tuchmann-Duplessis, H., 1975, in: Drug Effects on the Fetus, Adis Press, Hong Kong.

Woollam, D.H.M., 1965, Proc. Roy. Soc. Med., 58, 497.

Wolpert, L., 1976, Brit. Med. Bull., 32, 1, 65.

Weston, J.A., 1970, Adv. Morphogenesis, 8, 41.

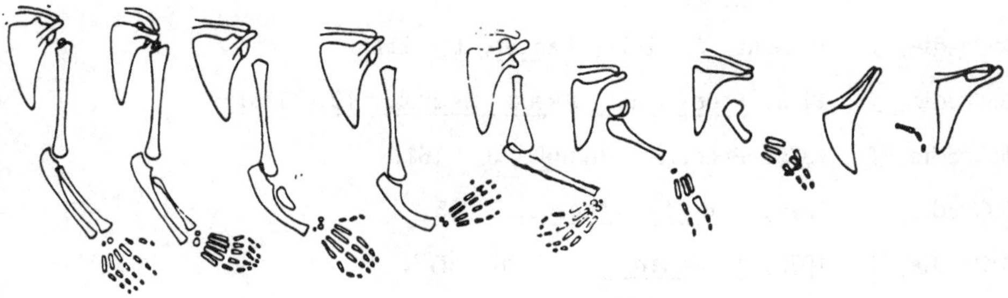

Fig. 1
Teratological sequence of dysmelia of the upper extremities.

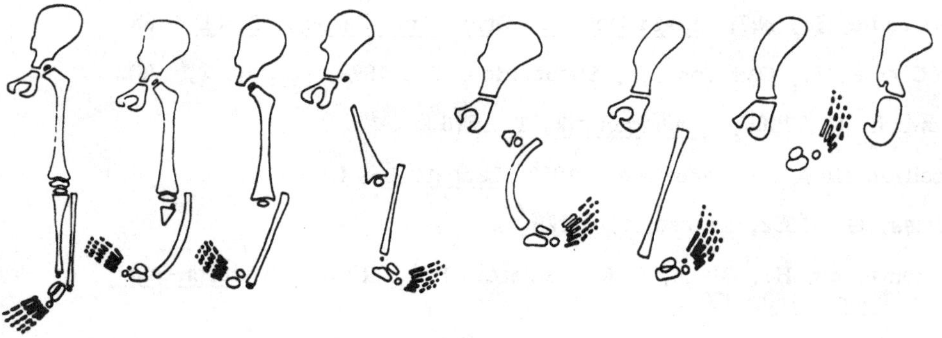

Fig. 2
Teratological sequence of dysmelia of the lower extremities.

Henkel, L. and Willert, H-G.: J. Bone Joint Surg., (1969), 51-B, 3: 399

Fig. 1: The pattern of dysmelia. Reprinted with permission of H.L. HENKEL and H.G. WILLERT, and of the J. Bone Joint Surg.

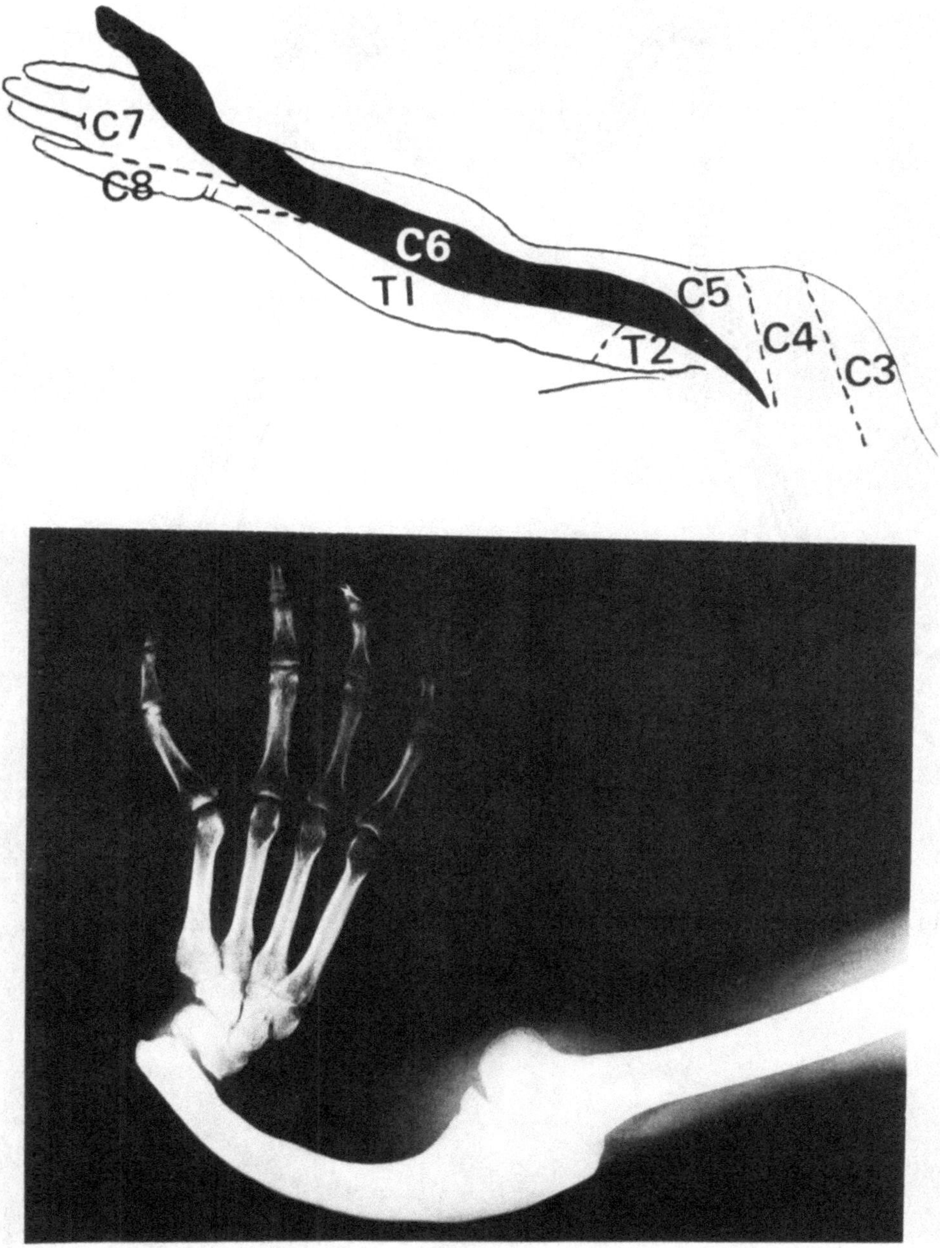

Fig. 2: "Dermatome subtraction". A hypothetical mechanism by which radial aplasia and absent thumb might be explained. (Reprinted by courtesy of Med. Hypotheses).

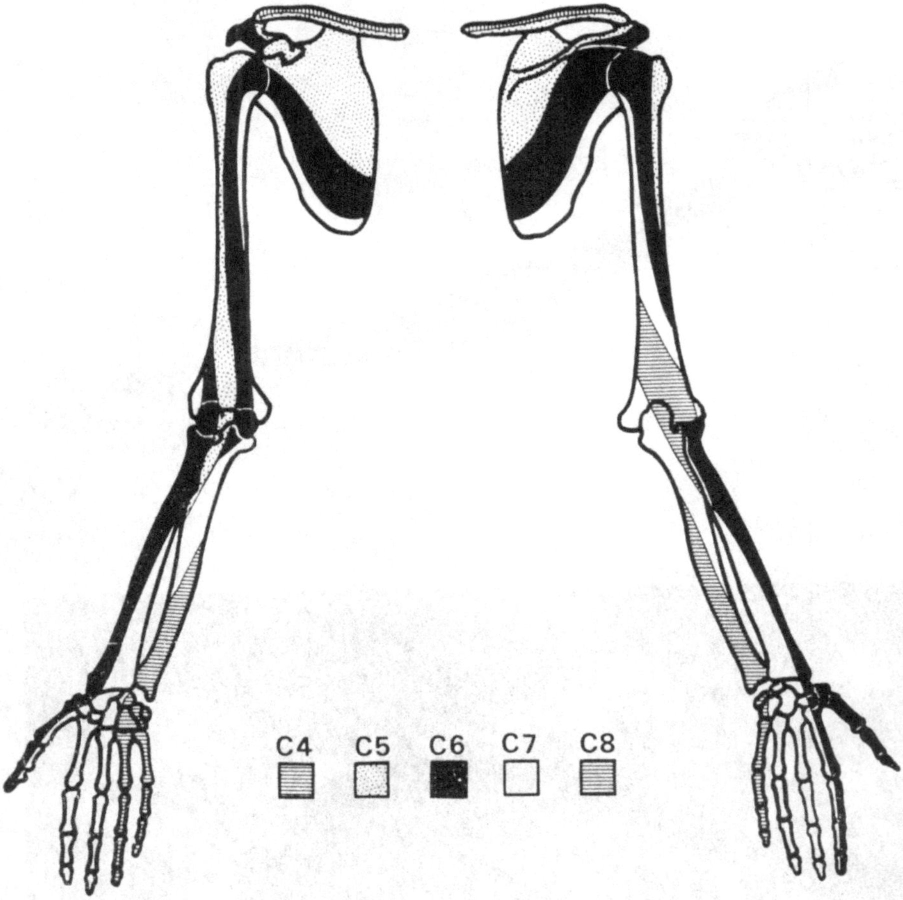

Fig. 3: Sclerotome map of the upper limbs, anterior and posterior views. (after INMAN and SAUNDERS, J. Nerv. Ment. Dis., 1944).

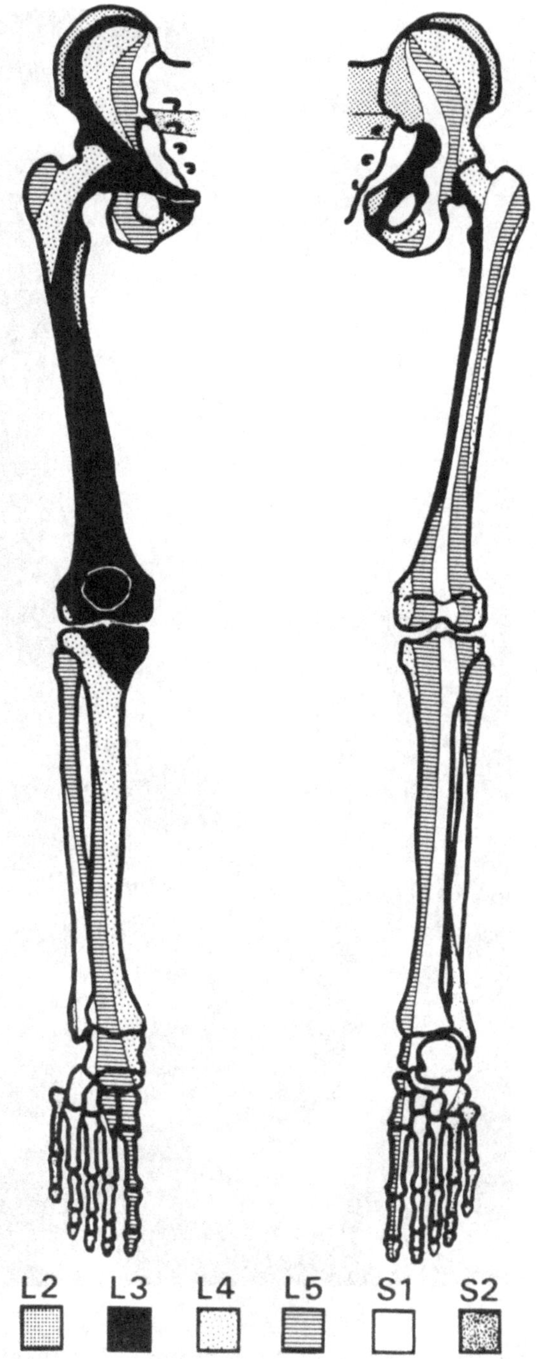

Fig. 4: Sclerotome maps of the lower limbs, anterior and posterior views (after INMAN and SAUNDERS).

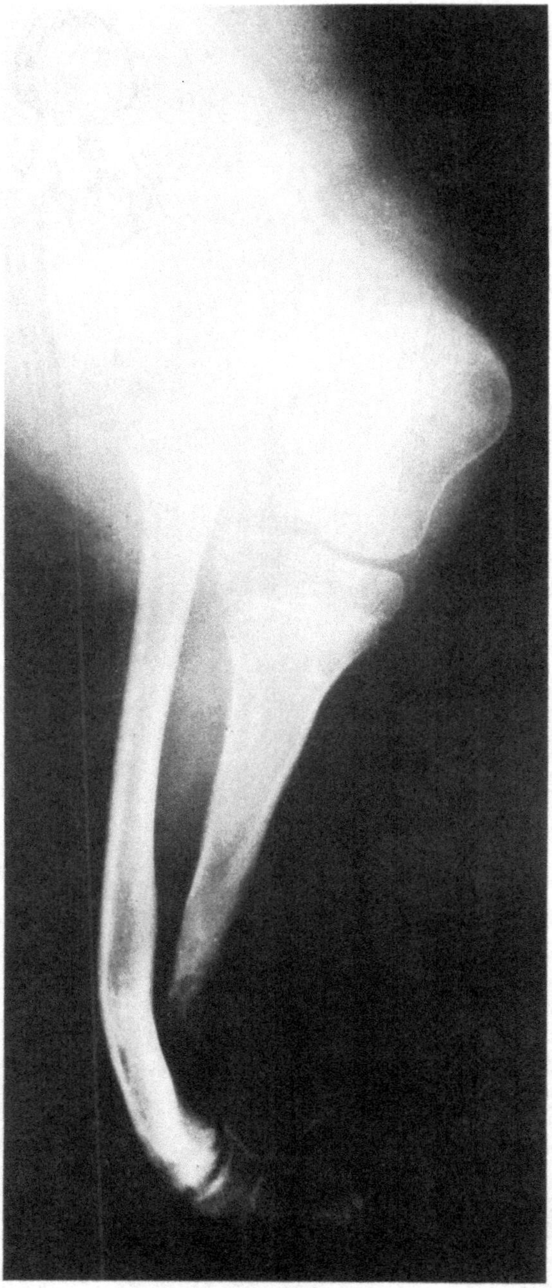

Fig. 5: Subtraction of L4 sclerotome around the knee joint produces one of the typical defects of thalidomide embryopathy.

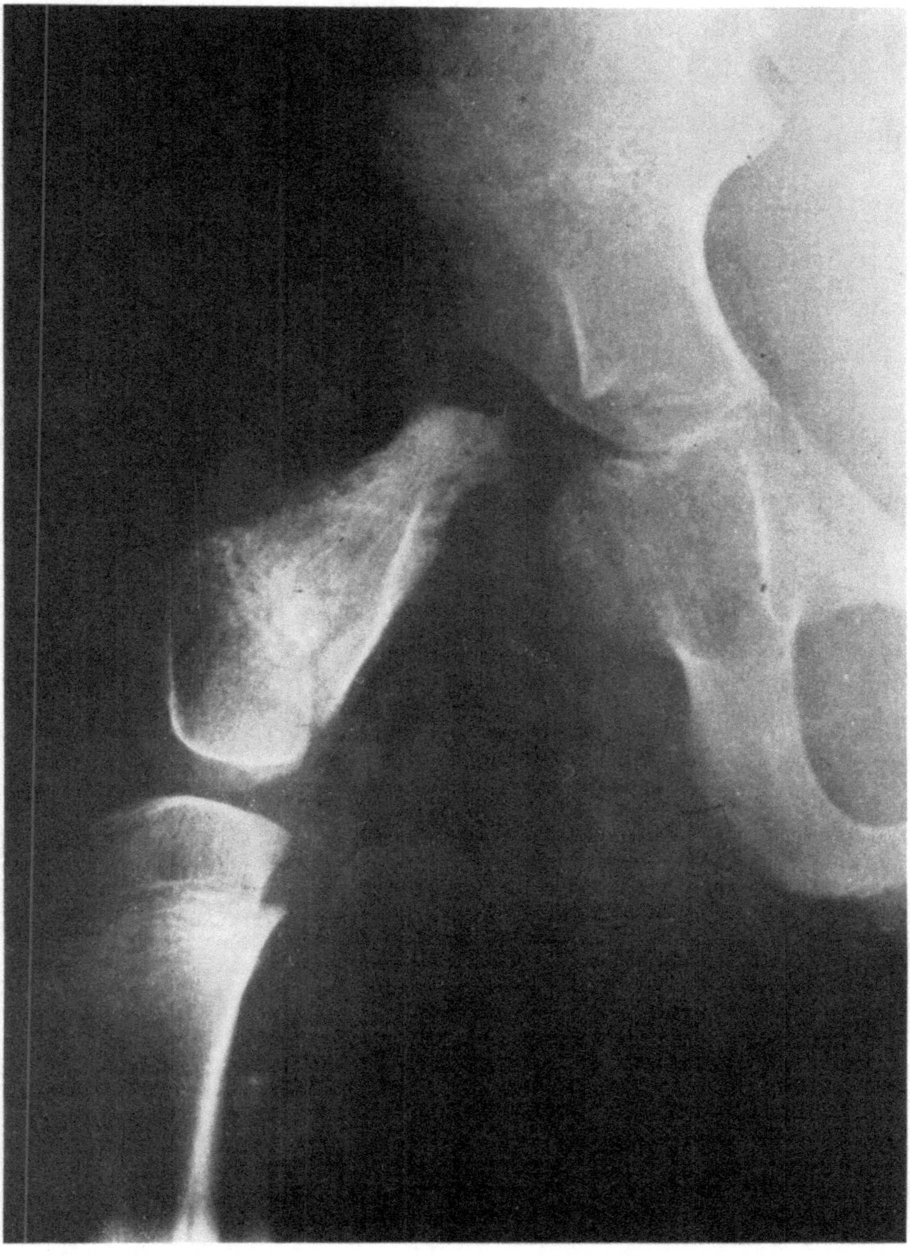

Fig. 6: Proximal focal femoral dysplasia is equivalent to L4 - L5 sclerotome subtraction from around the hip joint.

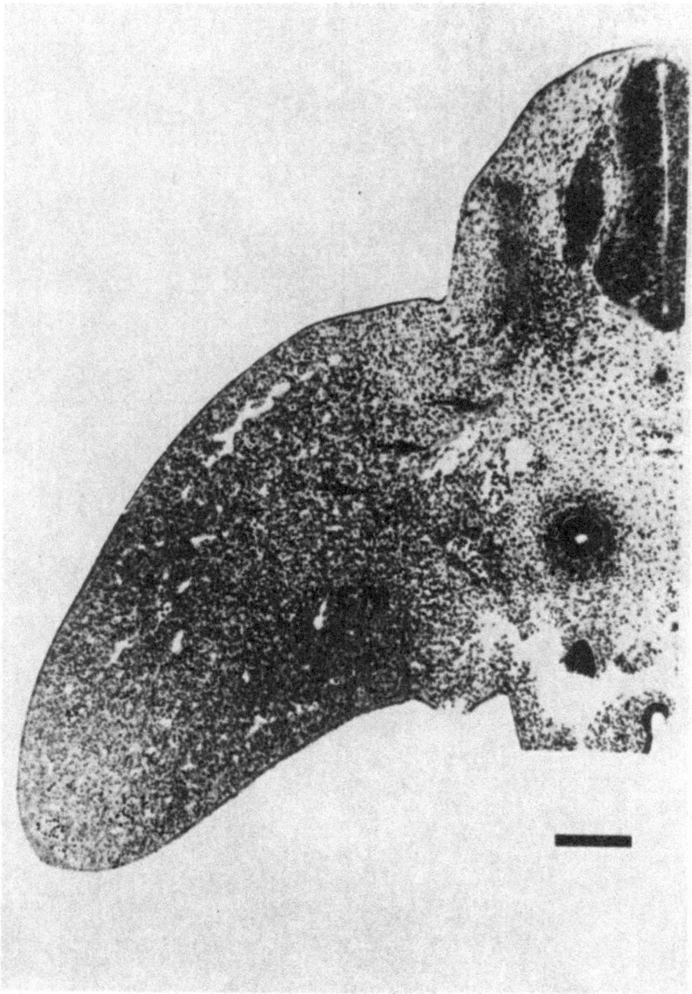

Fig. 7: Nerve trunk within the proximal third of the upper limb bud of rabbit, at 260 - 290 hours gestation. (Reprinted by courtesy of the Lancet).

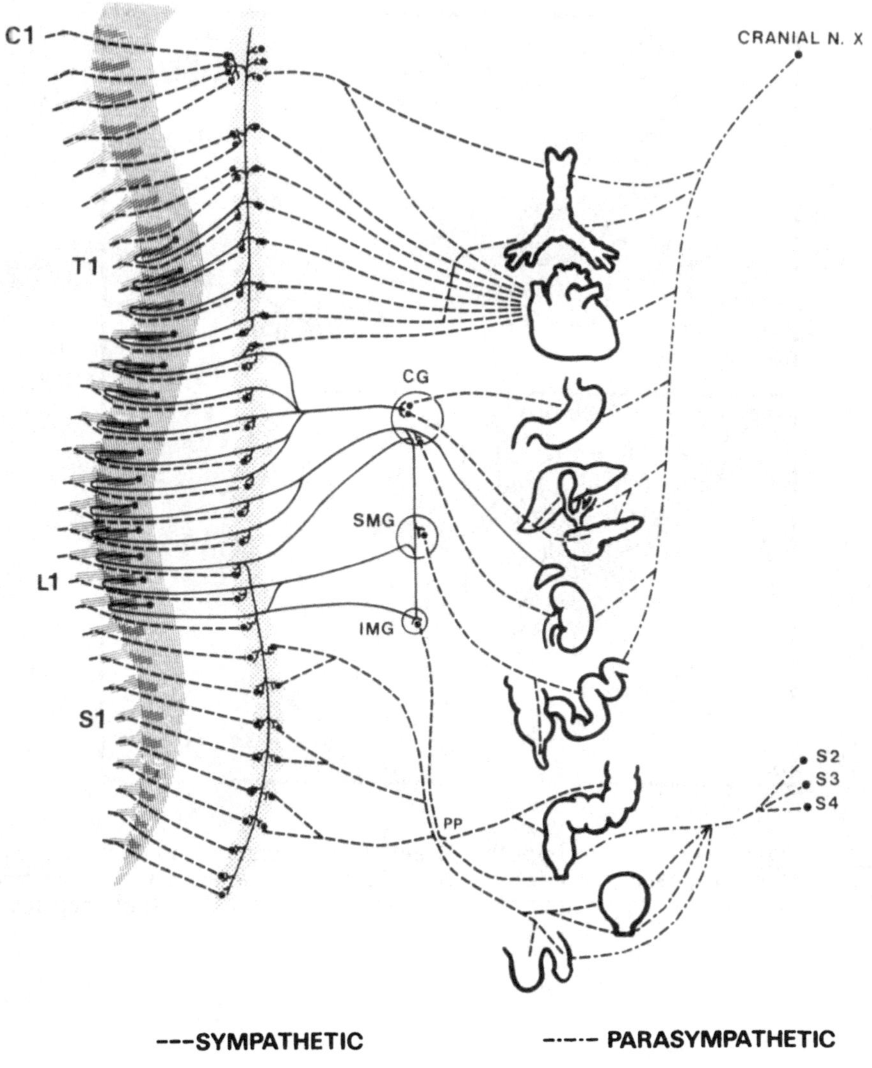

Fig. 8: The segmental arrangement of the autonomic nervous system (after NETTER).

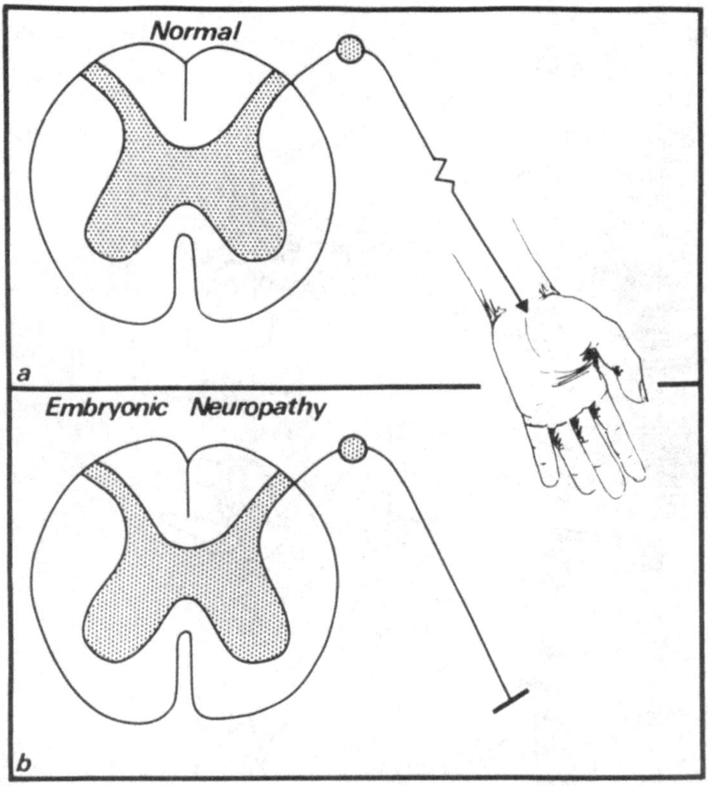

Fig. 9: The neural crest hypothesis and limb defects. Interference with the proposed trophic function (arrow) of a sensory nerve prevents the formation of structures supplied by that segmental nerve.

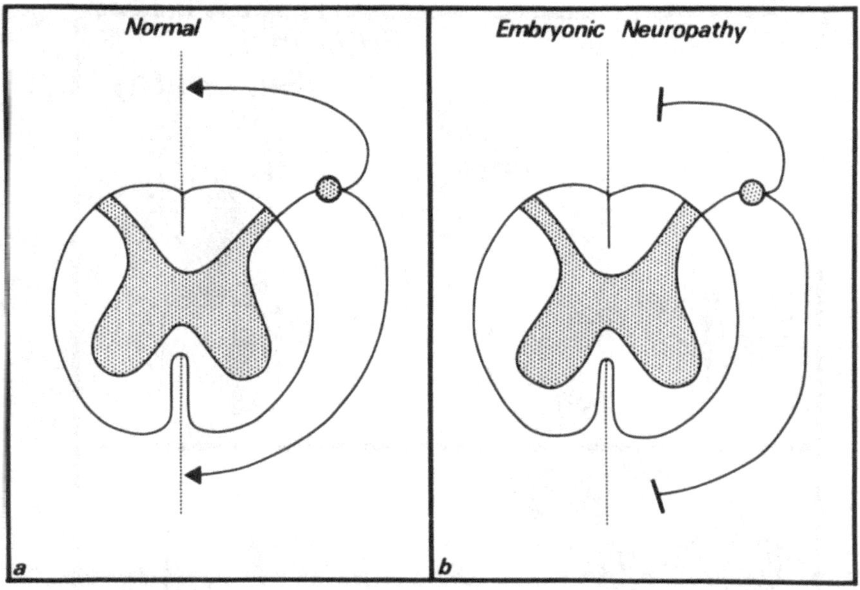

Fig. 10: The neural crest hypothesis and midline defects. Failure of the proposed trophic influence of intercostal and lumbar nerves upon structures which they supply causes cessation of growth, short of the midline destination. Various body wall and other midline deficiencies may be explained as neural crest injury.

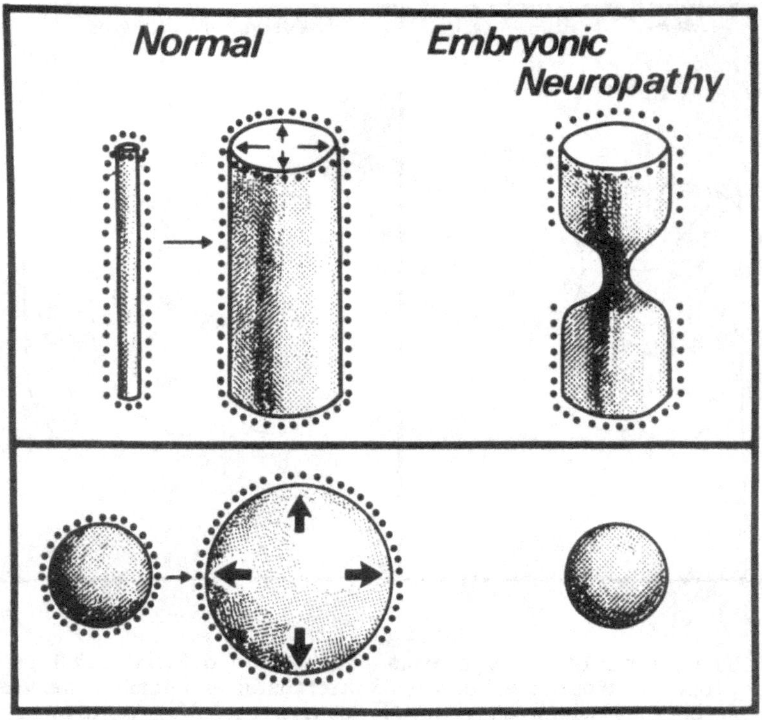

Fig. 11: The neural crest hypothesis and visceral defects. Failure of neural crest migration, or of the postulated trophic function explains atresia, stenosis, aplasia and hypoplasia of various viscera. (Fig. 9 - 11 are reproduced with permission of the Med. J. Aust.).

List of Participants

Dr. H.-J. Barrach
Institut für Toxikologie
und Embryonal-Pharmakologie
Freie Universität Berlin
Garystraße 9
D-1000 Berlin 33

Prof. Dr. Felix Beck
Dept. of Anatomy
University of Leicester
University Road
Leicester LE1 7RH
U.K.

G. Blankenburg
Institut für Toxikologie
und Embryonal-Pharmakologie
Freie Universität Berlin
Garystraße 9
D-1000 Berlin 33

Prof. Dr. G. Bogusch
Institut für Anatomie
Freie Universität Berlin
Königin-Luise-Straße 15
D-1000 Berlin 33

Prof. Dr. B. Christ
Ruhr-Universität Bochum
Institut für Anatomie
Arbeitsgruppe für
Experimentelle Embryologie
Universitätsstraße 150
D-4630 Bochum 1

Prof. Dr. U. Drews
Anatomisches Institut
Österbergstraße 3
D-7400 Tübingen 1

Dr. D.A. Ede
Department of Zoology
University of Glasgow
Development. Biology Building
124 Observatory Road
Glasgow G12 9LU
U.K.

Dr. O.P. Flint
8F27, Pathology
Safety of Medicines
ICI Pharmaceuticals Division
Mereside Alderley Park
Macclesfield, Cheshire SK10 4TG
U.K.

Dr. K. Grundmann
Institut für Toxikologie
und Embryonal-Pharmakologie
Freie Universität Berlin
Garystraße 9
D-1000 Berlin 33

Dr. M. Gumpel-Pinot
Institut d'Embryologie
49 bis, Avenue
de la Belle-Gabrielle
F-94130 Nogent-sur-Marne

Dr. R. Herken
Institut für Toxikologie
und Embryonal-Pharmakologie
Freie Universität Berlin
Garystraße 9
D-1000 Berlin 33

Dr. J.R. Hinchliffe
The University College of Wales
Department of Zoology
Penglais
Aberystwyth SY23 3DA
U.K.

Dr. L.S. Honig
Lab. of Developmental Biology
School of Dentistry
University of S. California
University Park, GER-317
Los Angeles, Cal. 90007
U.S.A.

Dr. A. Hornbruch
Department of Biology
as Applied to Medicine
The Middlesex Hospital
Medical School
Cleveland Street
London W1P 6DB
U.K.

Dr. J.-J. Houben
Laboratoire d'Anatomie et
d'Embryologie humaines de la
Faculté de Médecine
Université Libre de Bruxelles
97, rue aux Laines
B-1000 Brussels
Belgium

Dr. H.J. Jacob
Ruhr-Universität Bochum
Institut für Anatomie
Arbeitsgruppe für Experimentelle Embryologie
Universitätsstraße 150
D-4630 Bochum 1

Dr. E.A. Kaprio
The Children's Hospital
University of Helsinki
Stenbäckinkatu 11
SF-00290 Helsinki 29
Finland

Dr. M. Kieny
Laboratoire de Zoologie
et Biologie animale
Université scientifique et
médicale de Grenoble BP53X
F-38041 Grenoble Cédex
France

Prof. Dr. W. Kocher
Institut für Toxikologie
und Embryonal-Pharmakologie
Freie Universität Berlin
Garystraße 9
D-1000 Berlin 33

Dr. U. Kocher-Becker
Institut für Toxikologie
und Embryonal-Pharmakologie
Freie Universität Berlin
Garystraße 9
D-1000 Berlin 33

Prof. Dr. W. Lenz
Westfälische Wilhelms-Universität
Institut für Humangenetik
Vesaliusweg 12/14
D-4400 Münster

Prof. Dr. V.G. Leone
Istituto di Zoologia
Università di Milano
Via Celoria 10
Milano 20133
Italy

Dr. J. Lewis
Department of Anatomy
King's College
London WC2R 2LS
U.K.

Dr. S. Lilja
Institut für Toxikologie
und Embryonal-Pharmakologie
Freie Universität Berlin
Garystraße 9
D-1000 Berlin 33

Prof. Dr. G.M. Lösch
Medizinische Hochschule Lübeck
Klinik für Plastische Chirurgie
Ratzeburger Allee 160
D-2400 Lübeck 1

Prof. Dr. W. McBride
Foundation 41
The Women's Hospital
Crown Street
Sydney 2010
Australia

Dr. J. McCredie
Department of Surgery
The University of Sydney
Sydney, N.S.W. 2006
Australia

Prof. Dr. J.C. McLachlan
Department of Zoology
University of Oxford
South Parks Road
Oxford OX1 3PS
U.K.

Dr. H. Meinhardt
Max-Planck-Institut
für Virusforschung
Spemannstraße 35
D-7400 Tübingen

Prof. Dr. H.-J. Merker
Institut für Toxikologie
und Embryonal-Pharmakologie
Freie Universität Berlin
Garystraße 9
D-1000 Berlin 33

Prof. Dr. J. Milaire
Laboratoire d'Anatomie et
d'Embryologie humaines de la
Faculté de Médecine
Université Libre de Bruxelles
97, rue aux Laines
B-1000 Brussels
Belgium

Prof. Dr. D. Neubert
Institut für Toxikologie
und Embryonal-Pharmakologie
Freie Universität Berlin
Garystraße 9
D-1000 Berlin 33

Prof. Dr. A. Ornoy
Department of Anatomy
and Embryology
The Hebrew University
Hadassah Medical School
P.O. Box 1172
Jerusalem
Israel

Dr. K.T. Rajan
East Glamorgan
General Hospital
Church Village
Nr. Pontypridd, Mid.Glam.
U.K.

Dr. M. Rooze
Laboratoire d'Anatomie et
d'Embryologie humaines de la
Faculté de Médecine
Université Libre de Bruxelles
97, rue aux Laines
B-1000 Brussels
Belgium

Dr. P. Sengel
Laboratoire de Zoologie
et de Biologie animale
Université scientifique
et médicale de Grenoble, BP53X
F-38041 Grenoble Cédex
France

Dr. R.A. Siddall
ICI Pharmaceuticals Division
Mereside Alderley Park
Macclesfield, Cheshire SK10 4 TG
U.K.

Prof. Dr. R.G. Skalko
East Tennessee State University
College of Medicine
Department of Anatomy
P.O. Box 19960A
Johnson City, Tennessee 37601
U.S.A.

Dr. H. Sterz
Abt. MF - 2T
Medizinische Forschung
Boehringer Mannheim GmbH
Postfach 51
D-6800 Mannheim 31

Dr. D. Summerbell
Medical Research Council
National Institute for
Medical Research
The Ridgeway, Mill Hill
London NW7 1AA
U.K.

Prof. Dr. H. Tuchmann-Duplessis
Laboratoire d'Embryologie
Faculté de Médecine
45, rue des Sts. Pères
F-75270 Paris Cédex 06
France

Prof. Dr. H.-G. Willert
Orthopädische Klinik
der Universität Göttingen
Robert-Koch-Straße 40
D-3400 Göttingen

Dr. B. Zimmermann
Institut für Toxikologie
und Embryonal-Pharmakologie
Freie Universität Berlin
Garystraße 9
D-1000 Berlin 33

Index

FSC
www.fsc.org
MIX
Papier | Fördert
gute Waldnutzung
FSC® C083411

Kolibri 360 GmbH
Ferdinand-Jühlke-Straße 7
99095 Erfurt, Deutschland
produktsicherheit@kolibri360.de